INTERNAL MEDICINE

MEDICAL EXAMINATION MANUAL

INTERNAL MEDICINE

MEDICAL EXAMINATION MANUAL

Manuel M. Villaverde, M.D.

VNR VAN NOSTRAND REINHOLD COMPANY
NEW YORK CINCINNATI ATLANTA DALLAS SAN FRANCISCO
LONDON TORONTO MELBOURNE

Van Nostrand Reinhold Company Regional Offices:
New York Cincinnati Atlanta Dallas San Francisco

Van Nostrand Reinhold Company International Offices:
London Toronto Melbourne

Library of Congress Catalog Card Number: 79-10377
ISBN: 0-442-25094-0

Manufactured in the United States of America

Published by Van Nostrand Reinhold Company
135 West 50th Street, New York. N.Y. 10020

Published simultaneously in Canada by Van Nostrand Reinhold Ltd.

15 14 13 12 11 10 9 8 7 6 5 4 3 2 1

Library of Congress Cataloging in Publication Data

Villaverde, Manuel Maria, 1905-
Internal medicine.

Includes index.
1. Diagnosis–Outlines, syllabi, etc. 2. Semiology –Outlines, syllabi, etc. 3. Internal medicine– Outlines, syllabi, etc. I. Title. II. Series.
[DNLM: 1. Internal medicine–Examination questions.
W18.3 V727i]
RC71.V67 616.07′5 79-10377
ISBN 0-442-25094-0

Contents

INTERNAL MEDICINE

MEDICAL EXAMINATION MANUAL

1. Respiratory Diseases

Systemic Diseases with Nasopharyngeal Symptoms

Common cold symptoms may be the beginning of:
- Influenza (epidemics, serologic confirmation).
- Eruptive diseases (followed by the characteristic rash).
- Nasal diphtheria, and farcy or glanders.

Symptoms of rhinitis may:
- Be the beginning of any of the above.
- Differentiate from sinusitis.

Pharyngolaryngeal symptomatology may indicate the beginning of:
- Influenza (fever, aches, weakness, epidemic outburst).
- Adenoviral infections (young children, winter epidemics).
- Pharyngoconjunctival fever (summer, swimmers).
- Acute respiratory disease (military recruits).
- Eruptive diseases (measles, scarlet fever – followed by the characteristic rash).
- Rheumatic fever (angina plus one or more of the following symptoms: joint pains, cardiac or neurologic involvement, skin reactions).
- Diphtheria (tonsils and pharynx are covered with a grayish membrane that leaves a bleeding surface when detached).
- Agranulocytosis (starts abruptly with angina, local ulcers, septic fever, and regional adenopathy, mostly in patients under treatment with certain drugs).
- Acute leukemia (similar to the former, with dermic symptoms, such as petechiae, or other forms of bleeding).
- Herpangina (picture of a common angina together with herpetic vesicles).
- Zoster angina (occurs only on one side of the pharynx).

Common Cold

The characteristic symptoms of acute rhinitis, common cold, are:
- Nasal discomfort (burning, itching, fullness, and secretion).
- Sneezing, shortly followed by mucoid and then purulent discharge.
- Later on, signs of obstruction, dryness, hoarseness, and coughing.

At physical examination it will be noted:
- That the mucosae of the nose are red and swollen.

What are the suggested traits to differentiate it from influenza?
- The symptomatology is milder in common cold.
- There is not an epidemic of influenza going on.
- Serologic confirmation may be performed, if needed.

What is the suggested treatment for the common cold?
- Only symptomatic treatment is advisable.

Allergic Rhinitis

The symptoms of allergic rhinitis compare with those of common rhinitis as follows:

In allergic rhinitis there are:	In common rhinitis:
paroxysmal attacks of evident sneezing;	sneezing is more or less violent, but it is not paroxysmal;
profuse, watery discharge;	discharge is mucoid or purulent;
cojunctival itching, burning, and lacrimation.	very seldom is there a conjunctival reaction.

Other frequent findings in allegic rhinitis:
- There may be nasal congestion, usually appearing boggy and pale blue.
- Red and swollen conjunctivae are not rare.
- Large amounts of eosinophils are found in secretions.
- Not rarely an allergen is the known cause of the disease.

Antihistamines are given:
- At the beginning of the season, but they fail in 20–40% of cases.

Corticosteroids:
- Are advisable only in severe cases, when antihistaminics of other similar measures do not work adequately.
- Have to be discontinued as soon as possible.

Desensitization to known allergens may work:
- In some cases, not all, when given before the "season."

Atrophic Rhinitis

The outstanding symptom in atrophic rhinitis is:
- The extreme nasal fetor (ozena).

What other symptoms and signs will call attention to this disease?
- Progressive atrophy of the mucosae of the nose.
- Excessive crust formation.

Obstructed nasal breathing.
Dryness and irritation of the nose.
Anosmia or disturbed sense of smell.

Rhinoscopy will show:
Ample space within the nose (there may be atrophic bones).
Excessive crust formation.
Abundant scabs and pus adherent to the mucosae.
A glazed, dry mucosa.

The best treatment should be:
Frequent irrigations with hot saline and bicarbonate (a gentle flow to avoid entrance of the fluid into the ear).

Sinusitis

What are the characters of fever in sinusitis of the acute type?
May vary from mild to severe, usually according to the nature of the disease.
May be accompanied by chills, malaise, and headache.

What are the characteristics of the headache in acute sinusitis?
Worse during the day, and subsides during the evening.
Increases together with the sinusal pain in certain positions of the head that augment pressure over the sinus.
Accompanies facial pain also.

What other pains are felt in acute sinusitis?
Besides the above-mentioned headache, facial and sinusal pain, there are also tenderness within the nose, sore throat, tooth pain, pain when moving the eyes, pain on the roof of the orbit.
The pain in the nose is accompanied by swelling and obstruction.
The sore throat is usually due to the purulent nasal discharge (postnasal drip), and is usually accompanied by coughing.
The teeth hurt (a feeling of long teeth) in maxillary sinusitis.
In acute ethmoiditis the pain is felt behind the eyes and during eye motion.
In frontal sinusitis the pain is felt in the roof of the orbit.

Is pain as severe in chronic sinusitis?
There is no pain in most cases.

What are, then, the symptoms of chronic sinusitis?
A mild postnasal discharge, or profuse purulent discharge.
Nasal obstruction.
Peculiar odor of secretions (like a musty odor).
Nonproductive cough.

Mention also other, less common symptoms of sinusitis:
Vertigo, anosmia, photophobia, generalized pains, and periorbital edema. Other symptoms may indicate a complication.

The essentials of treatment consist of:
Adequate drainage of the affected sinus.
Adequate use of specific antibiotics.
Cautious help from vasoconstrictors.

Epistaxis

Where can the blood be seen in cases of epistaxis?
Obviously, from the anterior nares.
Postnasal drip of blood, either seen or, if unnoticed at the beginning, when the patient presents hematemesis.

When is epistaxis noted more easily?
External trauma to the nose (nose-picking, forceful blowing of the nose, or more obvious injuries).
Nasal lesions, such as polyps, tumors, etc.
Blood dyscrasias, hypertension, or other causes of congestion.
Certain infectious diseases (rheumatic fever).

What procedures are to be followed in cases of epistaxis?
Stop bleeding as soon as possible; keep the patient in a sitting position, and press over the area (bleeding stops in many cases); if needed, pack the nose.
Use the specific measure in each case.

Pharyngitis

How can you evaluate fever and sore throat to diagnose pharyngitis?
Fever varies from mild to a more severe type, at times with chills, usually falling in a very few days.
The sore throat also shows dryness, together with thick, sticky mucus, dysphagia, hoarseness, and cervical lymphoadenopathy in many cases.

What signs can you see accompanying the above symptoms?
The pharynx is red, mildly swollen; it appears dry, but with thick, sticky mucus, and in some cases with a membrane also present (more frequently in streptococcal pharyngitis, Vincent's angina, diphtheria).
Lymphoadenopathy is not rare.
Some stiffness of the neck may be present

When do you think of chronic pharyngitis?
When coughing accompanies dryness with thick mucus.
When there are frequent bouts of increased symptomatology together with some soreness of the throat.

What do you see on examination of the pharynx in chronic pharyngitis?
Erythema, edema, and frequently an associated follicular enlargement.
An easily bleeding mucosa.
A thick, tanacious exudate present at times.
Atrophic signs of a glazed mucosa with crust formation.

Treatment must include:
Symptomatic care, with rest and nonirritating irrigations.
Antibiotics whenever needed.

Removal of chronic crusts with saline; and avoidance of all irritating causes of chronic cases.

Tonsillitis

What is the essential feature in acute tonsillitis?

The presence of very painful, red, swollen tonsils with pus and exudate and more or less enlarged crypts, and notable erythematous reactions of the pillars and the rest of the pharyngeal wall.

What is the general syndrome of acute tonsillitis?

Sudden onset of fever, with chills, sore throat, malaise, headache, and anorexia.

Cervical, painful lymphoadenopathy; possibly stiffness of neck.

What complications may be found with acute tonsillitis?

Terminal chronic tonsillitis.

Otitis, sinusitis, nephritis, osteomyelitis, rheumatic fever, pneumonia.

What do you expect to find in chronic tonsillitis?

Recurrent sore throat, nasal discharge, cervical lymphadenopathy, persistent dull hyperemia of tonsils, mild edema and scarring, abnormal secretions of the crypts, cough, and bad breath.

How local relief of pain can be obtained:

By frequent gargles or irrigations with nonirritating solutions, together with analgesics.

How can you treat the causative infection?

With the specific antibiotic, if known.

What is the best treatment for chronic tonsillitis?

Operative procedure, in most instances.

Peritonsillar Abscess (Quinsy)

When do you consider the occurrence of peritonsillar abscess?

When suddenly one side of a tonsillitis case becomes more severe, dysphagia becomes acute, trismus may be noted, and the breaking of the infection through the tonsillar capsule is evident because it pushes both tonsil and pillar toward the midline.

What other symptoms may be present?

Swelling of the soft palate.

Displacement of the uvula.

Fluctuation that occurs from 3 to 5 days.

How peritonsillar abscess is treated:

Incise and drain the abscess.

Use the adequate antibiotic.

Do not allow closing of the drained abscess.

Perform tonsillectomy after subsidence of symptoms to prevent recurrences.

Ludwig's Angina

How do you diagnose this cellulitic or abscess formation of the floor of the mouth?

There is marked inflammation of the mouth.

The tongue is pushed upwards (to the roof of the mouth).

The movements of the tongue are sharply limited and painful.

There may be an obstruction of the airways.

Not rarely the infection spreads to the neck.

How this serious infection can be treated:

Very large doses of antibiotics are needed.

If there is abscess formation, incise and drain under local anesthesia.

Be prepared for a tracheostomy.

Retropharyngeal Abscess

When you should expect this to occur:

When the patient is very young.

When a suppurative lymph node infection follows a tonsillar, nasal, or sinus infection.

When fever develops, with difficulties in swallowing and breathing.

When the posterior pharyngeal wall protrudes and is tender.

What will you do in these cases?

Use antibiotics and hydration.

If fluctuation occurs, incise and drain (Trendelenburg position).

Be prepared for tracheostomy.

Parapharyngeal Abscess

What are the symptoms and signs of parapharyngeal abscesses?

Fever and other evidence of sepsis.

Bulging of one of the lateral pharyngeal walls.

Trismus.

Dilated veins noted in neck and scalp.

Later development of brawny swelling and redness in the neck, below the angle of the mandible.

General rules for treatment:

Administer antibiotics in large doses.

Provide hydration, and incision for drainage (beware of large vessels!).

Be prepared for tracheostomy.

Tuberculous Ulcer in Oral Cavity

When ulcers are to be thought of tuberculous origin:

Generally they grow larger.

There is considerable induration.

They are undermined and quite painful.

Lymphoadenopathy is usually absent.

They are associated with pulmonary tuberculosis and frequently preceded by small circumscribed submucosal nodules.

Laryngitis

What is the outstanding symptom of acute laryngitis?

Hoarseness, which may lead to aphonia.

What other symptoms usually accompany hoarseness?
- There may be a fever syndrome.
- There may be dysphagia, pain, and cough.
- If edema is marked, there will be stridor and dyspnea.

Laryngoscope examination will disclose:
- There is inflammation and redness of the mucosa.
- There is more or less marked edema, with or without exudate.
- Inflammation may extend into the bronchi.
- There may be limited vocal cord movements.
- There may be a membrane, in which case suspect diphtheria.

What are the usual findings in chronic laryngitis?
- Hoarseness, the chief symptom, which is more rarely causative of aphonia.
- Cough, a sensation of dryness, and expectoration of tenacious mucosities.
- Other symptoms of acute laryngitis, but less marked.
- Chronic inflammation of the cords, thick and edematous mucosa, polyps, and possibly ulcers and secretions.

General rules for the treatment of acute laryngitis:
- Voice rest in a well-humidified room.
- Symptomatic care of cough or pharyngeal irritation.
- Care of the causative factor, including antibiotherapy.

General rules for the treatment of chronic laryngitis:
- Same as above.
- Antiallergic measures, when needed; stop smoking.

Laryngotracheobronchitis (Croup)

When you would suspect this syndrome to occur:
- There are hoarseness, cough resembling the sound of a seal, and inspiratory obstruction.
- There is stridor at inspiration, but no pain on swallowing.
- There is xiphoid and suprasternal retraction.
- A sudden onset with elevated fever and marked prostration and dyspnea will indicate acute supraglottic edematous laryngitis.
- Violent paroxysms of cough may indicate a foreign body.

Essentials of treatment:
- Use steam inhalations and hydration.
- Be on the alert for a life-saving tracheostomy.

Foreign Bodies

What are the natural events in these cases?
- There may be sudden onset while eating (or having something in the mouth).
- Also, there may be sudden onset while unconscious.
- Dentures or bones may be the cause, in the case of adults.
- Bodies lodged in the larynx cause cough, gagging, stridor, and hoarseness, always with the risk of partial or complete air obstruction.
- With bodies lodged in the bronchial tree there is an initial sudden cough, and after a more or less prolonged time there will start again the cough, wheezing, pulmonary infection, and atelectasis.
- With bodies lodged in the esophagus there will be immediate coughing, gagging, and the sensation of something stuck in the throat; at times there will be pain, and difficulties in passing salive.

What to do in each particular case:
- All foreign bodies will be removed.
- Try to expel the foreign body by a sudden pressure over the epigastric area (use both hands, place yourself behind the patient).

Vocal Cord Nodules

Why these nodules usually occur:
- Because of abuse or misuse of the voice, particularly screaming.

What is the main trouble they cause?
- Hoarseness; or a change of voice in a later stage.

What is the logical approach to solve these cases?
- Extirpation, and voice rest.

Tumors of the Larynx

What are the initial differences between benign and malignant tumors of the larynx?
- None; they begin with identical initial symptomatology, only to be differentiated by biopsy.

What are the symptoms that usually denote a tumoral growth in the larynx?
- Hoarseness, which may produce a later change in the quality of the voice of a particular patient. Be suspicious with patients over age 40.
- Cough, which may also be an early symptom.
- Hemoptysis, which may accompany cough.
- Pain, in the form of sore throat or pain in the ear, or a particular sensation in the throat (such as "sticking").
- Dysphagia or respiratory obstruction.

What the laryngeal examination reveals:
- Fullness or swelling, or a frank mass or an ulceration.

Bronchitis

How the clinical picture of acute bronchitis usually starts:
- Cough is the main initial symptom.
- Cough begins dry and nonproductive.
- After 1 or 2 days some secretion appears, viscid first, and more abundant mucoid or mucopurulent later.

What other symptoms of upper respiratory infection (URI) are also noted?
- Febrile syndrome with coryza-like symptoms, sore throat, and general pains, mainly muscle pains.

What are the usual auscultatory signs of acute bronchitis?
- Sibilant or sonorous rales.
- Occasional, at the bases, crackling or moist rales.

In chronic bronchitis what are the symptoms to establish the diagnosis?
- There is productive cough, without other symptoms in many cases.

In older patients there are usually other symptoms of emphysema (dyspnea, prolonged expiratory sounds, barrel-chest thorax, and overaerated lung fields).

With the progress of the disease, obstructive symptoms may also be evident, and other complications may also take place.

Other symptoms may occur, such as cyanosis, dyspnea, asthma, and progressive deterioration.

How bronchitis should be treated:

In both cases, by rest, adequate hydration and ventilation, control of cough and sputum, and the adequate use of antibiotics.

Bronchiectasia

How will you expect a patient to present a case of bronchiectasis?

By presenting a chronic cough accompanied with unusually large amounts of purulent sputum, and maybe hemoptysis, as well.

What are the clinical symptoms and the regular course of the disease?

Onset is insidious, not rarely following other pulmonary infections.

Congenital cases apparently follow the same course.

The increase of cough is peculiar, noted mostly in the morning, late in the afternoon, and on retiring, and depends on expectoration.

The sputum may be abundant (not always so) and distribute in three layers (with pus at the bottom, turbid at the middle, and frothy at the top).

Hemoptysis, dyspnea, recurrent attacks of infections, and clubbing of fingers and toes may accompany the disease.

Atelectasis may be a symptom, particularly with children.

In physical examination, what do you expect to find?

Rales and ronchi, particularly at the lower lobes (if they are absent, the diagnosis is questionable). Check before and after postural drainage.

In more advanced cases, there are retraction of the chest walls and diminished thoracic excursions.

Symptoms of complicating diseases will occur.

General, specific, and surgical measures to be taken in these cases:

Provide clean air, dry and warm.

Avoid all sort of irritants to the respiratory tract.

Control secretions as much as possible.

Control infections with adequate antibiotic therapy.

Consider surgery for those who can bear it easily, or those who present very severe symptomatology.

Asthma

Describe an attack of bronchial asthma:

It begins with tightness on the chest rapidly followed by dyspnea, wheezing that is heard from a distance, and not rarely cough that ends with some sputum production. Dyspnea and wheezing characterize the attack, which lasts 1 hour or less.

The characteristic of these attacks is their recurrence.

Other symptoms of asthma:

There is freedom from symptoms between the attacks.

At the beginning of the attack there is more wheezing and dyspnea than later.

At the end of the attack the cough increases, and there is expectoration of thick, tenacious mucus.

When the symptoms are persistent and there is not a clearing of symptoms in due time, there is a status asthmaticus.

Stethoscopically, the evidence of asthma is characterized by:

There are prolonged expiration sounds.

There are sonorous and sibilant rales, also more marked during expiration.

Respirations are labored, but the rate is normal.

In severe attacks the chest may become distended and the patient cyanotic.

Between attacks respiration is usually normal, but may show expiratory sibilants, particularly in forced expiration.

In treating asthma there will be drugs for the acute attack, and others for chronic treatment:

For the acute attack, epinephrine, aminophylline, nebulized drugs to give in mild attacks, corticosteroids, and others.

For status asthmaticus, aminophylline, corticosteroids, and assisted respiration.

For chronic treatment, desensitize and use some of the drugs also used for the acute attack, such as aminophylline, ephedrine, and others.

Loeffler's Syndrome or Pulmonary Infiltrations with Eosinophilia

Also called the PIE syndrome, it usually presents as follows:

There is such meager symptomatology that it is discovered by accident.

Fever is ocassionally present.

Cough, with or without side pain, may be present.

Pulmonary lesions may disappear or migrate (important for diagnosis).

Physical signs may show:

Hyperresonance, and harsh sounds.

Fine crepitation in localized patches.

When the PIE syndrome mixes with asthma, what are the usual findings?

The bronchopulmonary sounds are more bizarre and less related to definite pulmonary areas.

There is usually an increase in the symptoms of asthma.

There is frequently a weight loss.

Skin tests are different (sensitivity to germs, parasites, or other types of asthmatic reactivity).

Treatment:

Treatment is largely symptomatic.

Corticoids may help

The disease is benign and runs a limited course.

Pneumonia

What are the basic symptoms for the clinical diagnosis of pneumonia?

Sudden onset.

Rapidly rising fever, with shaking chills.

Stabbing pain on the diseased side of the chest, worsened by efforts or movements, and possibly with a heterotopic spread to other areas (shoulder, flank, or abdomen).

Annoying cough.

Production of sputum, which in many cases may show distinctive features for helping the diagnosis of the variety.

Other general symptoms, such as abdominal distention, jaundice, painful tachypnea, tachycardia, a picture similar to appendicitis or cholecystitis, delirium, and convulsions.

How does the sputum differ physically from one variety to another of pneumonia?

First pinkish, then rusty, and finally yellowish purulent in pneumococcal pneumonia.

Reddish, sticky (difficult to expectorate), and mucoid if due to *Klebsiella.*

Copious, purulent or blood-streaked, with salmon tinge, if staphylococcal.

Sticky, bloody, apple-green in *Hemophilus influenzae.*

Scanty and mucopurulent in viral pneumonia.

Auscultation of the lungs helps the diagnosis of pneumonia as follows:

First stage, with fine rales and diminished breath sounds.

Second stage, with evidence of consolidation with bronchial breathing and often friction rub.

Third stage of resolution, reappearance of rales.

Identification of the causative microorganism:

Laboratory and X-ray findings will do the principle work.

In *Klebsiella* pneumonia the disease may be fulminant, cyanosis is noted early, and there is a profound toxicity.

In *Pseudomonas, Proteus,* and *Serratia* the patient will be a debilitated one (chronic lung, heart, alcoholism); delirium and consolidation are of early appearance; there is multiple abscess formation, and maybe also a case of superinfection.

In streptococcal pneumonia the patient soon becomes severely toxic and cyanotic, and pleural effusion and empyema are early complaints.

In staphylococcal pneumonia there may be a previous relatively mild disease that suddenly turns severe.

In *Bacteroides* pneumonia a foul smell may give the diagnosis.

In *Pneumocystis carinii* pneumonia the patient suffers from leukemia or is in immunosuppressive treatment.

In terminal pneumonia the disease is insidious, but the patient is very seriously ill from other causes.

In mycoplasmal pneumonia the disease is mild and the symptomatology scanty.

In aspiration or lipoid pneumonia the disease is linked to the passage of some abnormal material into the lungs.

Please give a brief reminder of the treatment of each kind of pneumonia:

In pneumococcal pneumonia	Penicillin (cephalosporin)
In *Klebsiella* pneumonia	Kanamycin (cephalothin, gentamycin)
In *Hemophilus influenzae*	Ampicillin (chloramphenicol)
In streptococcal pneumonia	Penicillin (erythromycin)
In staphylococcal pneumonia	Oxacillin (nafcillin)
In viral pneumonia	Tetracyclines
In *Pneumocystis carinii*	Trimethoprim plus sulfamethoxazole
In aspiration pneumonia	Ampicillin and corticosteroids
In *Pseudomonas, Proteus, Serratia*	Gentamycin plus carbenicillin
In *Bacteroides* pneumonia	Penicillin (clindamycin)
In terminal pneumonia	The specific or ampicillin
In mycoplasmal pneumonia	Nothing or a tetracycline

Silicosis

Silicosis is usually a diagnosis made on X-ray films; how can you select the cases for study?

Those exposed for a long time to silica dusts.

Frequent upper respiratory infections, including pneumonia.

Dyspnea on exertion, as a frequent complaint.

Cough, initially dry, then becoming productive.

Hemoptysis (may be severe and even fatal).

Other diseases, such as tuberculosis, pulmonary insufficiency, and cor pulmonale.

Treatment to be followed:

Symptomatic, or that of the concomitant disease.

Anthracosis

Coal dust may cause symptoms as follows:

Ordinarily the disease appears to be a benign one.

It may appear as a progressive fibrosis or emphysema.

There may be a silica component in this disease.

The recommended treatment is:

None.

Asbestosis

Asbestos dust is the cause of asbestos bodies, which may provoke:

Early dyspnea, with tachypnea and hyperpnea.

Productive cough, which is dry in the beginning.

Cyanosis on exercise and pulmonary insufficiency.

Embedded particles, which may appear in the extremities as "corns."

Increased susceptibility to pulmonary cancer, but not tuberculosis.

These cases are to be treated:

Symptomatically.

Byssinosis

This sort of sensitization to protein in cotton dust may cause:

Symptoms similar to those occurring in other forms of air pollution.

Periodic symptoms of bronchoconstriction (after nonexposure lasting for more than 1 week).

Later symptoms of chronic bronchitis and emphysema.

Treatment advisable for this condition consists of:

Care of chronic bronchitis and emphysema.

Berylliosis

Fumes or dust containing beryllium cause symptoms as follows:

In acute exposure there are upper respiratory symptoms, with bronchitis first, and pneumonia later.

In chronic forms the symptoms of respiratory insufficiency are out of proportion to physical findings.

The chronic symptoms are dyspnea (of the hyperpneic form) with cyanosis and cough, weight loss, skin lesions, pulmonary insufficiency, and cor pulmonale.

There is a better prognosis for the acute form than for the chronic, which may terminate in progressive deterioration of respiration.

Drugs that may give good results in berylliosis are:

Corticosteroids, particularly if they are given early in the disease.

Coal Miner's Pneumoconiosis

Coal dust retained in the lungs will cause symptoms as follows:

In simple pneumoconiosis, the impairment is not severe.

In simple pneumoconiosis, the association of emphysema makes the situation worse.

In progressive massive fibrosis, dyspnea and cough cause disabling symptoms.

Advisable treatment for progressive massive fibrosis:

The same as for diffuse obstructive pulmonary emphysema.

Farmer's Lung and Bagassosis

The exposure to moldy hay (farmer's lung) and exposure to moldy pulp of sugar cane (bagassosis) provoke similar symptoms, which are:

In the initial phase, fever, dyspnea, and hypoxia.

With repeated exposures, irreversible disabling pulmonary symptoms.

Advisable treatment:

As for acute bronchitis; use corticoids in severe cases.

Silo-Filler's Disease

The inhalation of fumes from silos or from burning nitrocellulose film causes symptoms that appear as an initial phase, and then by a second acute phase, as follows:

Following exposure there are cough, dyspnea and weakness.

After a quiescent phase, though with some dyspnea and weakness, an acute stage occurs with fever, chills, malaise, and increasing cough, and there is a disabling dyspnea with tachypnea and tachycardia.

What is heard on auscultation?

Disffuse rales and ronchi.

What measures are used?

Assisted respiration, oxygen, corticosteroids, and antibiotics.

Pulmonary Tuberculosis

How the primary complex will be differentiated from influenza:

In pulmonary tuberculosis:	In influenza:
fever of varied character will last 2 or 3 weeks, rarely with chills.	fever lasts only 2 or 3 days, most frequently with chills.
the accompanying symptoms consist more of drowsiness, fatigue, and weight loss.	there is more prostration and generalized aches, headache, and weakness.
erythema nodosum frequently appears (tender, red nodules in the anterior aspect of legs).	no erythema nodosum appears.
there is gradual recovery.	

If there is progressive primary tuberculosis, how will it be detected?

After the second or third week there will be no defervescence, and the disease will evolve slowly into progressive pulmonary tuberculosis of the adult type.

In progressive pulmonary tuberculosis of the adult type what are the more important diagnostic traits?

There is a gradual onset, with weakness, anorexia, and weight loss.

Some cases will also show evening fever and malaise for a few weeks.

After the disease is well established, there will be fever, profuse sweating during the night, and increased weakness.
There is cough, which increases as the disease progresses; at the start, only during the morning; thereafter, more severe.
Sputum is scanty at first; in caseous forms, it is green and purulent; in established chronic forms, it is yellowish and mucoid.
Hemoptysis may be the first alarming symptom, from a few drops streaking the sputum to a very important, even fatal, hemorrhage.
Chest pains, dyspnea, and hoarseness generally indicate some of the complicated forms (pleural, pneumothorax, pharyngeal).

By examining the chest you may note:
Possibly, nothing.
Fine localized and persistent rales in upper lobes, better heard after asking the patient to cough.
Rarely, other signs of wheezing, rales, consolidation, deviation, etc.

Basic therapy in the treatment of tuberculosis includes:
Start treatment with three drugs, such as isoniazid, streptomycin, and also rifampin or ethambutol.
To patients previously treated for tuberculosis, give a drug not yet administered to them: aminosalicylic acid, ethambutol or rifampin, and some of the second class like cycloserine, viomycin, etc.

Psittacosis

How will you differentiate psittacosis from a regular pneumonia:
The history of exposure to birds of the parrot family is helpful.
A mucopurulent sputum is usually produced after a period of dry coughing.
Pulmonary migratory lesions may be present.
The signs of pneumonitis may be delayed.
There may be epistaxis, rose spots, and splenomegaly.
For the rest, the clinical picture is almost identical with pneumonia.

Treatment for psittacosis:
A tetracycline; plus oxygen and sedation, if required.

Lung Abscess

Following a previous pneumonia, a possible aspiratiôn of foreign material, or some sort of obstruction, what are the evident symptoms of lung abscess?
One or two weeks later, a septic fever, chills, and sweating will start.
Periodically, there will be expectoration of large amounts of an extremely foul-smelling purulent sputum, of a brown or gray color.
There will be cough, usually nonproductive at the onset.
There will be pain, particularly at coughing.
Rarely, the sputum will not present a foul odor, but will be green or yellow musty sputum.
Hemoptysis will not be rare, or only blood-streaked sputum.
If the abscess becomes chronic, there will be anemia with weight loss and pulmonary osteoarthropathy.
Dyspnea will be noted only in massive infections.

Can the abscess be easily detected at examination?
Signs may be minimal, or totally absent.
Small areas of consolidation due to pneumonitis are the most frequent findings, with dullness and suppressed breath sounds.
Moist rales may also be heard.
When the pneumonic area does not resolve, consider that the abscess is formed.

To solve this situation the best procedure is:
Intensive antibiotherapy.
Surgery.

Pulmonary Cancer

Symptoms that may indicate cancer:
There will be cough, either as a starting symptom, or a symptom already present but which changes in character. This is symptom number 1.
The cough is mostly nonproductive at the start; later a scanty sputum may be produced.
The cough is persistent.
Hemoptysis occurs in some cases.
Chest pain, unilateral, constant, and severe, is very frequent.
Sputum is usually scanty, mucoid, and may be tinged with blood; but when it appears in large amounts, watery or mucoid, it may be considered pathognomonic of bronchiolar carcinoma.
Check for pulmonary cancer when there are:
Hypertrophic ostearthropathy with clubbed fingers and toes
Myasthenia gravis
Peripheral neuritis
Corticocerebellar degeneration
Cushing syndrome
Gynecomastia, in males
Hypercalcemia or hyponatremia
Polycythemia
Pancoast's syndrome (Horner's syndrome plus shoulder-arm pain).
Carcinoid syndrome
There will be localized wheeze or frank evidence of atelectatic obstruction of a bronchus.
Metastases are important: to the cervical and supraclavicular lymph nodes, bones, brain, etc.
Additional symptoms noted in advanced disease are anorexia with weight loss, weakness, pulmonary infections, other respiratory symptoms, pulmonary extension or spread of the disease, etc.

Other helping signs to establish the diagnosis:
- Localized wheezing.
- Evidence of obstructive atelectasis.
- Signs of pleural or mediastinal invasion.

Means of treatment:
- Early surgical removal, the best hope for cure.
- Radiotherapy.
- Chemotherapeutic agents

Sarcoidosis

Sarcoidosis may provoke symptoms other than pulmonary; please establish first the pulmonary and then the nonpulmonary corresponding symptoms:
- Very frequently there are not pulmonary symptoms.
- Cough and dyspnea (due to compression) are among the most common symptoms, but occur mostly late in the disease; notwithstanding, if the onset is acute, they may appear at an earlier stage.
- Most patients belong to the black race.
- General symptoms are minimal or absent, namely, weight loss, night sweats, or fever.
- Skin lesions are nodules or infiltrations noted on face, ears, nose, and extensor surfaces.
- Erythema nodosum may be seen.
- Salivary glands may enlarge, without any pain.
- Ocular symptoms may occur (lacrimal, conjunctiva, iris, etc.)
- Paralysis and other symptoms may also occur, but not too frequently.

Other signs may help in evaluating the disease:
- Hilar adenopathy, which has to be differentiated from Hodgkin's disease and from tuberculosis.
- Extensive lesions with scarce symptomatology.

The treatment:
- There is none, and the prognosis is favorable overall.
- Corticosteroids may help some cases; if no results occur in one month, the medication should be discontinued (slowly).

Granulomatosis

Clinical evidence of Wegener's granulomatosis occurs as follows:
- Symptoms of sinusitis.
- Epistaxis and hemoptysis.
- Also symptoms of pulmonary consolidation.
- Hemorrhagic skin lesions.
- Progressive renal failure, which accounts for the final prognosis.
- Febrile symptoms that point out an acute disease.
- Diagnosis dependent on the biopsy findings.

Explain how treatment can be worked with better efficiency:
- The earlier treatment occurs, the better, to reach a possible control of the disease.
- This may be possible with corticosteroids, alone or with azathioprine.
- Also, heparin may help in early phases to control vascular symptoms.
- Once the disease is well established, there is no treatment available.

Pulmonary Infarction

Findings that may lead to the diagnosis of pulmonary infarction:
- Frequently, not always, the patient suffers from thrombophlebitis.
- Consider it when a clinical picture opens abruptly; though do not forget that there are minor grades of embolization noted by a gradually developing dyspnea.
- The outstanding symptoms are dyspnea and anxiety, which are characteristic.
- Fever rises suddenly, not infrequently being the first and only symptom of this disease.

How the clinical symptoms are completed and the picture develops:
- Silent intervals interrupt the symptomatology.
- Chest pain occurs in a large number of cases.
- The character of chest pain may be either pleuritic or anginal (but not related to any previous angina).
- Cough occurs in one-half of the cases.
- Hemoptysis occurs in one-third of the cases.
- There may be evidence of frank pulmonary edema, but not always.

Other related events that may occur:
- Syncope occurs, not too rarely.
- There may also be evidence of right heart failure.
- Some cases will present less severe dyspnea and pleuritic pain.
- Some cases will present milder cough.
- In these cases, dyspnea, pain, and cough occur some hours after the thromboembolism and characterize the infarction; particularly if there is also hemoptysis.

Pulmonary signs of the disease are:
- Signs of consolidation of the lungs.
- Pleural friction rub.
- Occasional pleural effusion, secondary to infarction.

Cardiovascular signs of pulmonary infarction are:
- Tachycardia.
- Increased second pulmonary sound.
- Loud systolic murmur.
- Protodiastolic gallop.
- Cyanosis and collapse.

Emergency measure to be carried out are:
- Assist respiration, with oxygen.
- Give heparin.
- For severe pain, give morphine or meperidine.
- In the case of shock use vasopressors.
- Place a central venous catheter (for pressure and fluids).

Is there some helpful surgical procedure?
Always be ready to perform an embolectomy, if feasible.

Pulmonary Emphysema

Who are those to be suspected of pulmonary emphysema, because of a previous condition?
Those with a chronic pulmonary infection.
Long-standing cases of asthma.
Those with a chronic fibrotic pulmonary disease (fibrosis, silicosis).
Starting symptoms of emphysema:
Insidious onset.
Dyspnea and cough, the most important symptoms.
Characteristics of dyspnea in cases of emphysema:
It is only exertional at the start.
In some cases dyspnea will occur at rest.
Orthopnea may be seen in some cases.
Dyspnea at rest and orthopnea occur most frequently in late phases.
Bouts of wheezing are not rare.
These symptoms may become extremely severe in cases of intercurrent respiratory infections.
Cough characteristics in cases of emphysema:
The cough is productive.
The cough results are inefficient for clearing out the airway.
The cough is worsened even by mild infections of the respiratory system.
Other symptoms provoked by respiratory difficulties are:
Hypoxia that may cause weakness, anorexia with weight loss, and lethargy.
In more advanced respiratory insufficiency, headache, miosis, papilledema, and tremors.
Auscultation of the thorax will reveal:
There may be diminished movements, inspiratory and expiratory, but with prolonged expiratory sounds.
There is wheezing, mostly of the sibilant type, but some ronchi are also heard.
Symptoms of chronic bronchitis are not rare.
Heart sounds are heard distant.
Symptoms of cor pulmonale are not rare.
The examination of the thorax will also reveal:
There is diffuse hyperresonance of the whole thorax, masking the normal dullness of the heart and the liver.
The chest is maintained in the well-known barrel-shape inspiratory position.
There is an increased anterioposterior diameter of the chest.
As a consequence of the above changes, what other signs may appear?
Diminished or totally absent movements of the diaphragm.
Respiration maintained only by the accessory muscles, including the intercostals.
A resultant short neck.
Total time of emptying the lungs (total vital capacity) above 5 seconds.
The liver found in a lower position.
A ruddy or cyanotic face.
Cyanosis of lips and nails.
Peripheral edema.
Main steps in treatment are:
Relieve bronchial obstruction with bronchodilators and with liquefiers of the secretions.
Use corticosteroids in the severe cases.
When the clinical picture is evident, treat the chronic pulmonary heart disease.
Give the specific antibiotic in case of infections.

Pulmonary Edema

An excess of fluid in the extravascular spaces of the lungs, pulmonary edema, may be diagnosed by the following symptomatology:
The onset may be either rapid or slow.
Cough is the most important symptom of the start.
Cough may be either mild or severe.
A frothy sputum may occur; may be pinkish, abundant in severe attacks.
Oppression may cause chest pain, possibly of an anginal type.
Auscultation of the chest in pulmonary edema will reveal:
There is wheezing, because of bronchiolar spasm.
There are fine rales (not crepitant) of a very humid character.
These rales are heard first at the base of the lungs, very rarely at only one side.
The rales extend upward to the whole lungs, as the disease progresses.
Other signs and symptoms that occur because of the mentioned changes:
There are tachypnea and orthopnea as forms of dyspnea due to chest oppression.
The frothy sputum appears, spilling from the mouth.
There may be sweating, pallor, and cyanosis.
Bouts of mild attacks may appear in patients with mitral stenosis who perform exhaustive exertion.
Severe forms may occur to hypertensive patients.
In very ill patients symptoms of pulmonary edema may appear at a slow pace.
Previous conditions or activities may help for diagnosis:
A previous serious pulmonary or cardiac disease.
Exposure to irritant inhalations.
Schematize treatment:
Provide general care in a sitting position.
Assist respiration (watch for CO_2 retention).
Bronchodilators may help (but avoid sedation).
Some sedation may be given in case of left ventricular failure, to control restlessness and dyspnea, except in respiratory depression.

Diuretics are a very good help.
Consider when phlebotomy or cardiotonics may be of help.

Respiratory Distress Syndrome

This syndrome, also called "shock" or "pump" lung, may be caused by:
Injury leading to shock.
Aspiration pneumonia.
Other forms of pneumonia, particularly viral.
Inhalation of irritant substances, including smoke.
Fat embolism.
Heart-lung perfussion techniques.
What are the outstanding symptoms at the start?
Dyspnea and cyanosis.
The findings noted in respiratory examination are:
Some sort of bronchiovesicular harsh respiration.
Evidence of progressive consolidation of the lungs.
Retraction of the intercostal spaces.
Is there any indication of the disease noted during treatment?
The pressure needed to maintain a relatively normal tidal volume is progressively higher.
Treatment techniques advisable in these cases:
Treat shock as soon as possible with avoidance of fluid overload.
Use intravenous diuretics if they seem needed.
Assist respiration.
Give corticoids in cases of aspiration, septic shock, and fat embolism, or when the patient does not respond adequately to the regular treatment.
Give antibiotics if there is an important sepsis in progress.

Respiratory Failure

Diagnosis of respiratory failure is suspected when any of the following symptoms and signs appear:
There is evidence of hypoxemia as indicated by headache, tachycardia, hypotension, warm extremities, restlessness with confusion, and final unconsciousness.
There is evidence of respiratory acidosis as indicated by headache, tachycardia, confusion, tremors, sweating, miosis and papilledema, and final coma.
(The best procedure for monitoring oxygen and carbon dioxide concentrations is by measuring arterial blood gases.)
The appearance of the above symptoms and signs will be most informative that respiratory failure is occuring in:
Patients with obstructive lung disease, as follows.
Cardiac disorders with severe pulmonary congestion.
Asthma, chronic bronchitis, or emphysema.
Diseases of the type of pneumonia, atelectasis, pneumothorax, or pleural effusion.
Fibrosis of any type.
Cases of restricted respirations due to abdominal distention, obesity, etc.
Cases of restricted respirations due to abnormalities, injuries, or neuromuscular cause (trauma or infection, drugs, etc.).
Schematize the treatment for respiratory failure:
The essentials depend on the nature of the causative disease and the clinical condition of the patient.
Give assisted respiration if needed in the particular case.
Otherwise, give oxygen, relieve bronchiospasm with aminophylline or an aerosol, and try a nebulizer for continuous humidification.
Advise cleansing of the lungs by coughing and deep breathing; also with diuretics, potassium chloride.
When necessary, resort also to corticoids, digitalis, and even intubation.
Main characteristics of chronic respiratory failure:
Cor pulmonale.
Polycythemia.
Possible milder symptoms of the acute condition.
Schematize the treatment for these chronic respiratory failures:
Session of oxygen therapy.
Other forms of aerosol therapy (bronchodilators, mucolytics).
Physical therapy.
Attention to the causative condition.

Atelectasis

Main symptoms of the disease:
There are sudden dyspnea, cyanosis, and fever, in the acute stage.
There are also tachycardia and chest pain.
Wheezing and cough are not rare.
In chronic atelectasis there are very few, if any, symptoms.
Results of physical examination are as follows:
Decrease of chest motion, with narrowing of intercostal spaces.
Shift of the trachea and the cardiac apex towards the involved side.
Diminished sounds on the affected side (vocal fremitus, breath).
Occasionally, bronchial respiration.
Tachycardia.
The patient can help to improve his condition by:
Coughing and hyperventilating the lungs.
If patient's own help does not work, because of lack of cooperation or lack of effect, what are the best steps to follow?
Introduce a transtracheal tube to pass saline to stimulate coughing.
Try bronchodilation with medication given by aerosol.
Try bronchodilation with an intermittent positive pressure apparatus, with which bronchodilators and mucolytic substances will be given.

When the above measure fail, is there some procedure to be followed?

Bronchoscopy may be necessary in some cases.

Pulmonary Vasculitis

What the term "pulmonary vasculitis" includes:

Hypersensivity of vasculitis in systemic diseases.

The immunologic reaction with type III antibody formation responding to various antigens (streptococcus, serums, drugs).

A pulmonary vasculitis reaction is seen in any of the following circumstances:

Interstitial pneumonitis.

Wegener's granulomatosis.

Serum sickness.

Systemic lupus erythematosus.

Polyarteritis nodosa.

What can be done for these patients:

Use corticoids and immunosuppressive agents.

Avoid the offending substance, if known.

Extrinsic Allergic Alveolitis

Patients most easily affected by this disease are:

Those exposed to moldy dusts with fungi.

Those exposed to thermophilic actinomycetes (infected air conditioning systems).

Those with farmer's lung, byssinosis, bagassosis.

How this extrinsic allergic alveolitis caused by type III antigen-antibody reaction is clinically manifested:

There is a regular clinical picture of acute pneumonia.

This pneumonia occurs following relatively closely one of several clinical exposures to the offending agent.

What can be done for these patients:

Use corticoids.

Avoid exposure to the offending substance.

Alveolar Proteinosis

The characteristics of the clinical picture of this disease are as follows:

Progressive onset.

Cough and dyspnea.

Evidence of pulmonary insufficiency.

Intermittent fever.

Easy development of fungal infections.

What can be done for these patients:

Use pulmonary lavage to remove the proteinaceous material by means of saline or heparin.

Interstitial Pneumonia or Fibrosis

After exclusion of other forms of pulmonary fibrosis (infections, toxics, inhalants, and the like), what symptoms will suggest this disease?

Chronic cough.

Progressive dyspnea.

Symptoms of cor pulmonale.

The clinical examination that will confirm the above symptoms will reveal:

Crackling rales.

Clubbing of the fingers (usually an early sign).

Diminution of lung volume and vital capacity.

Treatment of the disease:

Use corticosteroids; but they are not always efficient.

Alveolo-Capillary Block Syndrome

Name the principal diseases in which this syndrome can be present:

Miliary tuberculosis.

Bronchiolar carcinoma.

Mitral stenosis.

Scleroderma.

Sarcoidosis, asbestosis, and beryllosis.

Principal symptoms of the complex are:

Cyanosis.

Dyspnea, with hyperventilation and tachypnea.

In spite of the above, symptoms of hypoxemia.

Principal finding in medical examination:

Decreased lung volume.

Treatment is as follows:

Care for the underlying disease; final results depend on this factor.

Use corticosteroids to prevent fibrosis from becoming established.

Pickwickian Syndrome

Who are the patients that may present this syndrome?

Extremely obese patients.

What are the traits of the syndrome?

A lack of heart or lung disease, until the syndrome is well developed.

Cyanosis, with secondary polycythemia.

Periodic respirations, hypoxia, hypercapnia.

Somnolence, which may be complicated with insomnia.

In advanced cases, right ventricular hypertrophy and heart failure.

Treatment is as follows:

Weight reduction.

Progesterone, which may counteract hypoxia.

Goodpasture's Syndrome

Clinical features of this syndrome consist of:

Pulmonary hemosiderosis and glomerulonephritis.

The principal symptomatology consists of:

Cough.

Recurrent hemoptysis.

Dyspnea.

Progressive glomerulonephritis with renal failure.

Signs of the syndrome are:

Iron deficiency anemia.

The treatment may consist of:
Corticosteroids or immunosuppressive drugs.
Bilateral nephrectomy with transplantation of one kidney, if feasible.

Fibrinous Pleurisy (Dry Pleurisy)

When fibrinous pleurisy may develop:
Secondary to a pulmonary disease, usually preceding the development of pleural effusion.
These primary diseases usually are:
Pneumonia, of most varieties.
Pulmonary infarction.
Cancer, also most of the varieties of pulmonary cancer.
The principal, and almost only, symptom is:
Chest pain.
Explain its characteristics:
There is pleuritic pain, most marked during inspiration.
Pain is referred to the shoulder and neck (central portion of the diaphragm involved).
Pain is referred to the abdomen (peripheral portion of the diaphragm involved).
Pain greatly diminishes or even disappears when no inspiratory movements are performed (withholding inspiration or splinting of ribs).
Auscultatory findings are as follows:
Pathognomonic pleural friction rub.
Treatment procedures are:
Treat the causative disease.
Relieve pain, with analgesics or strapping.
In very severe cases procaine infiltration of intercostal nerves may be needed.

Pleural Effusion

Is idiopathic pleural effusion prone to occur?
There may be a possibility, but in the greater number of instances it will prove to be of a tuberculous origin.
What are, then, the most frequent causes of pleural effusion?
Tuberculosis.
Malignant tumors.
Pneumonia.
Pulmonary infarction.
Previous fibrinous pleurisy (dry pleurisy).
The outstanding symptoms of pleural effusion are:
Chest pain.
Decreased chest movements.
Dyspnea.
Is the chest pain in pleural effusion similar to that in dry pleurisy?
There may be no symptoms at all.
Chest pain is present when fibrinous pleurisy starts the picture.
The characteristics of this pain are the same as in fibrinous, dry pleurisy, whether or not it precedes the disease (see above entry).
Are there other symptoms also present in pleural effusion?
Dyspnea is ordinarily mild in mild effusions, and severe in more important ones, depending also in the speed of the accumulation.
There may be fever and sweats.
Cough and expectoration may also occur.
Evidence of cardiac failure may also occur.
Also, evidence of the causative disease will be present.
Auscultatory evidences of pleural effusion:
Diminished or abolished sounds in the site of the effusion, notably on the bases of the lungs, depending on the amount of fluid.
Egophony over the fluid level, like a bleating voice.
More rarely, bronchial breath sounds or bronchophony also present over the fluid area (generally in rapidly forming large effusions).
Other evidences noted in physical examination:
Decreased motion of the chest.
Dullness on percussion (flat percussion).
Diminished or absent perception of tactile fremitus.
Usually, hyperresonance above the fluid level.
Changes that are prone to occur in this disease:
The mediastinum will shift away the lesion in large effusions.
The shift will be toward the fluid if there is atelectasis.
Signs similar to those of consolidation may occur in large rapidly forming effusions (dullness, bronchophony, and bronchial respirations).
If the initial pain is due to dry pleuritis, it may diminish when the pleuras are separated by some amount of effusion.
Large amounts of fluid accumulating rapidly may cause heart impairment; but at a slower pace even large amounts can be better tolerated.
Succusion splash may be heard when there is also pneumothorax.
General lines of treatment are:
Specific treatment of the causative disease.
Aspiration of fluid.

Pneumothorax

How can the entrance of air into the pleural cavity occur?
Spontaneously, during a previous disease or of unknown cause.
By traumatic injuries that perforate the chest.
By a tear from a fractured rib or other foreign object.
By therapeutically induced pneumothorax, as formerly was a routine in the treatment of tuberculosis.
Tell the usual clinical picture of pneumothorax:
The initial symptom is most frequently a sudden chest pain.
Pain is sharp and mostly interferes with respiration, thus decreasing chest motion.
The pain is referred, at times, to the shoulder, or to the arm, and also to the abdomen.

There is some sort of dyspnea.

Shock and cyanosis will occur in tension pneumothorax (elevated intrapleural pressure).

Other symptoms of circulatory collapse may also occur.

Most signs of distress will subside after the intrapleural and intrapulmonary pressures equalize.

The initial sudden chest pain in pneumothorax is always an intense symptom?

Most frequently there is some pain, but it may be overlooked because it is minimal.

Explain how other changes may occur:

There may be a dry cough.

The start of pain may occur at any time during daily life, and not necessarily be related to overexertion.

Pain is worsened by exercise and deep respirations.

Pain is usually of a sharp character.

Pain should not be mistaken for an acute abdomen, or an infarction.

The collapse of the lung may close the openings causing the entrance of air, those leading the way to improvement.

But also, there may be openings of a "valve type" that allow the entrance of air and prevent its escape, thus worsening the prognosis.

Usual results of clinical examination of these patients reveals:

Decreased breath and voice sounds.

Augmented corresponding sounds on the normal lung.

Hyperresonance over the fluid level.

"Tapping" sound frequently heard on the left side.

Shift of mediastinum and trachea, as above (see above entry).

Trends of treatment are:

Advise bed rest, and avoidance of pain and cough.

Aspirate air, if needed, even with an implanted catheter.

In tension pneumothorax, which is an emergency, aspirate air as soon and effectively as possible; the catheter is better left in place with a water pump.

Hydropneumothorax

What characterizes the presence of a hydropneumothorax?

The presence of a transudate that shows a specific gravity below 1.015 and/or protein content of 3 grams in 100 ml.

The clinical symptoms of hydropneumothorax will be:

In general, the same as pleural effusion, but the gradual development will present a mild clinical picture.

What is the most common cause of hydropneumothorax?

Congestive heart failure.

Other less common causes are:

Hepatic cirrhosis, particularly that with ascites.

Obstruction to blood circulation of the superior vena cava or azygos.

How to treat this occurence:

Remove the fluid by thoracentesis.

Treat the causative disease.

Note: In most instances there is only a hydric effusion in these cases, and we should call it "hydrothorax." In other instances, there is a mixture of air and fluid, and it is a "hydropneumothorax" proper. Consequently, answers will be evaluated somewhat for each instance.

Hemothorax

Explain by what means blood may enter into the pleural space:

Traumatic injuries.

Pulmonary infarction.

Tuberculosis.

Cancer.

Will symptoms and signs vary widely from those of pleural effusion?

Essentially are the same, q.v., above.

Essentials of treatment are:

Remove all blood from the space, as soon as possible.

Use an intercostal tube, with water-seal drainage.

Thoracotomy will be indicated as a last resort.

Pneumomediastinum

In pneumomediastinum, how can the air enter into the mediastinal space?

By a perforation of the respiratory tract.

By a perforation of the intrathoracic esophagus.

By ruptured alveoli into perivascular interstitial tissues.

From the neck, due to an open would or a secondary neck emphysema due to a chest wound.

From pneumothorax, particularly of the tension type.

The characteristics of the symptoms due to pneumomediastinum itself:

In most cases, the symptoms are very mild.

Dyspnea may be present, but also is of little intensity.

If the air is transmitted to the subcutaneous tissues close to the mediastinum, there will be puffing of the neck and face.

According to the route that air follows to escape from the mediastinum, what are the characteristic facts to consider?

Due to retroperitoneal "dissection" there will be anal pain in cases accompanying tension pneumothorax; also sudden sharp retrosternal pain radiating to shoulders and arms.

Other signs of pneumomediastinum are:

Rarely, elevated pressure in the mediastinum will cause compression of the heart and great vessels, evidenced by severe dyspnea, shock, and even death; symptoms and changes are similar to those of pericardial tamponade.

Subcutaneous crepitus on palpation is usually noted in the neck and upper portions of the chest.

Usually in left-sided lesions crackling syncronous with heartbeats will be heard.

What are the essentials of the treatment?

To treat the causative disease.

Mediastinitis

The clinical course of mediastinitis can run:
- Acute mediastinitis.
- Chronic mediastinitis.

Acute mediastinitis may be due to:
- Retropharyngeal abscess.
- Other closely related infections in the area.
- Perforation of the esophagus, by either cancer or instrumentation.
- Perforation of the trachea by a foreign body or instrumentation.

Chronic mediastinitis may be due to:
- Histoplasmosis.
- Tuberculosis.
- Sarcoidosis.

Clinical features of acute mediastinitis are:
- Acute onset following within 24 hours the action of the causative problem.
- Pain noted in chest and neck.
- Dysphagia and dyspnea.
- Other evidence similar to pneumomediastinum.
- Fever, chills, and other evidence of toxicity.

Clinical features of chronic mediastinitis:
- Are minimal, or those due to a local mass.
- In the case of a mass, there may be evidence of pressure on the superior vena cava, the inferior vena cava, or the azygos, with developing edema.

Findings in medical examination of these patients are:
- Subcutaneous crepitus on palpation (neck, chest).
- Evidence of compression of heart and great vessels (dyspnea, shock, other symptoms similar to cardiac tamponade).

Regular features of treatment:
- In acute mediastinitis, give antibiotics and perform surgery for drainage whenever indicated.
- In chronic mediastinitis, use corticosteroids and treat the cause.

Tumors of the Mediastinum

Mediastinal tumors may reach important clinical proportions, no matter what the histologic character, because of:
- The proximity of heart, great vessels, nerves, air passages, and esophagus, which may be damaged.

Is there pain in tumors of the mediastinum?
- There is no pain until the mass reaches a large size.
- When there is pain, it is usually substernal.
- The pain spreads to the shoulder or arms, neck, and even the back, at times reminding of cardiac pain.

Respiratory symptoms in mediastinal tumors:
- There may be cough, usually of bronchial character.
- Respirations may be noisy, with retraction of suprasternal spaces.
- Respirations are dyspneic.
- Hoarseness will appear if the left recurrent laryngeal nerve is involved.
- There may be more or less severe dysphagia.
- There may be evidence of superior vena cava or Horner's syndrome.

What are the symptoms of *Horner's syndrome?*
- Sinking of the eyeball.
- Ptosis of the eyelid.
- Miosis.
- Narrowing of the palpebral fissure.
- Anhydrosis.
- All the above symptoms present at the same side of the lesion.

What are the symptoms of the *superior vena cava syndrome?*
- Dilation of the veins of the neck.
- Developing of collateral veins on the walls of the thorax.
- The face appearing round, full, or chubby.

At clinical examination, what are the findings noted?
- Tracheal shift, when the tumor displaces the organ.
- Palpable lymph nodes, in some cases.
- Radicular pain or compression of the spinal cord in some cases of neurofibroma.

A *teratoma* in the anterior mediastinum may give origin to symptoms:
- So mild that it may be clinically silent.
- May open into a bronchus provoking cough with expulsion of tissues belonging to the teratoma, such as hair, teeth, etc.

Symptoms corresponding to *Hodgkin's disease* or other lymphomatosis are:
- The systemic symptoms, usually well marked.
- Fever.
- Pruritus.
- Anemia.
- Cachexia.
- Lymphadenopathies palpable in other areas.

Symptoms of *enlarged thymus:*
- Frequent in infants, mainly with respiratory symptoms if too large.
- Rare in adults, where it is frequently malignant except in cases of myasthenia gravis.

Changes that *neurofibromas* localized in the posterior mediastinum may cause:
- There may be radicular pain.
- There may be compression of the spinal cord.
- Lack of generalized symptomatology is not rare.

The treatment of these mediastinal tumors depends on:
- The causative factor.

2. Cardiovascular Diseases

Frequency of Congenital Anomalies

What is the generally found frequency of congenital cardiovascular anomalies?

Atrial septal defect	20%
Patent ductus arteriosus	13
Pulmonary stenosis	12
Tetralogy of Fallot	11
Coarctation of the aorta	9
Ventricular septal defect	9
Aortic stenosis	3
Pulmonic stenosis	3
Eisenmenger's syndrome	3
Tricuspid atresia	1.5

What other anomalies are less frequently found?

Transposition of great vessels.
Single atrium.
Single ventricle.
Other anomalous pulmonary vein drainage.

Pulmonary Stenosis (Congenital)

Clinical features of pulmonary stenosis in its pure form, that is, without reversed interatrial shunt, are as follows:

Asymptomatic in mild cases, requiring special studies for diagnosis.
Exertional dyspnea.
Chest pain.
Possibly, fainting.
In very severe cases, evidence of right ventricular failure, with increased dyspnea, easy fatigability, and edema.

Clinical findings on medical examination of former patients are:

There is a systolic murmur in left second and third interspaces close to the sternal border.
The systolic murmur is loud and harsh.
There is a palpable right ventricular heave.
A thrill may be noted on palpation.
If the stenosis is infundibular, the murmur is heard a little lower (third and fourth intercostal spaces).
In severe cases the auscultatory sounds are diminished.

Procedures to follow:

Surgery.

If the stenosis presents reversed shunt, what are the symptoms? (See also page 17.)

There will be arterial unsaturation, with cyanosis.
Exertional dyspnea.
Polycythemia.
Clubbing of digits.

Procedure to follow:

Also, surgery.

Coarctation of the Aorta

If in coarctation of the aorta the blood pressure is elevated at the cardiac side of the stricture and lowered on the distal side, what will the symptoms be?

Pulsations are marked and strong at the neck and suprasternal notch.
Femoral pulsations are weak or absent.
Femoral pulsations are slightly delayed relative to the radial pulse.

Other clinical findings:

Hypertension is noted in the arms, but with normal or somewhat lower blood pressure in the legs.
After exercise, that difference is exaggerated.
Collateral arteries may appear in the intercostal spaces or in the scapular area.
Systolic ejection murmurs are heard at the base.
The systolic ejection murmur may be heard better at the back of the thorax.

Procedures to follow for treatment:

Surgery is the best advice.

Aortic Stenosis (Congenital)

When and how symptoms will develop in aortic stenosis:

Disease almost asymptomatic for long periods of time.
Exertional dyspnea.
Fatigue and syncope.
Anginal pains.
Rarely, cardiac failure.

Clinical findings will be:

Ejection systolic murmur, usually of a loud character, over the aortic area.
Thrill noted over the aortic area.
The thrill possibly radiating to the neck.
Narrow pulse pressure.

Treatment for congenital aortic stenosis:
Discuss the convenience of direct valve surgery, use of artificial valves, or grafts.

Atrial Septal Defect

In the case of small or moderate defects, what is the symptomatology?
Disease is mostly asymptomatic.
In the case of larger defects, what is the common symptomatology?
Exertional dyspnea.
Other evidence of cardiac failure.
At examination, what is found in atrial septal defect?
Systolic ejection murmur at second and third intercostal spaces.
Second sound results split.
Apical mid-diastolic murmur.
Palpable and easily visible right ventricular pulsations.
The logical treatment approach is:
Surgical.

Patent Ductus Arteriosus

How the clinical course of the patent ductus arteriosus develops:
There are no symptoms, initially.
The course develops with left ventricular failure symptoms.
At physical examination of the patient, what are the most important signs noted?
Continuous "machinery" murmur is heard high at the left border.
The murmur may become systolic (raised pulmonary pressure).
Second sound may split (left ventricular hypertrophy).
A forcefull apex beat is generally noted.
Thrills may be present.
The diastolic pressure is low, together with an elevated pulse pressure.
Procedures to follow for treatment:
Try prostaglandins inhibitors (chloroquine or indomethacin).
If the above do not work, discuss the convenience of surgery.
Do not delay surgery.

Ventricular Septal Defect

Characteristic symptomatology of ventricular septal defects:
None in smaller defects.
Progressive symptoms of pulmonary vascular disease in larger defects.
Clinical features found in examination of these patients:
There are loud heart sounds.
Second heart sound may split.
Apical diastolic murmur may appear.
Loud systolic murmur, together with thrill, noted in the left third and fourth intercostal spaces, which may be the only finding in smaller defects.
Approach to treatment:
Discuss with an expert the timing for surgery.

Tetralogy of Fallot

Are all the cases with tetralogy of Fallot of the same clinical severity?
There is a mild, acyanotic variety.
There is a severe variety, symptomatology of which starts soon after birth.
What are the usual manifestations of the severe form of tetralogy of Fallot?
Start at about 3 or 6 months of age.
Delayed growth.
Poor tolerance to exercise (squat).
Notable cyanosis of the skin.
Polycythemia.
Clubbing of fingers.
Other symptoms of cardiac failure.
Treatment to be followed:
Discuss with expert the more convenient surgical procedure.

Transposition of Great Vessels

Common symptoms of transposition of great vessels:
Cyanosis, increasingly severe.
Lack of growth.
Very severe dyspnea.
All these symptoms starting soon after birth.
Common signs of transposition of the great vessels:
Greatly enlarged heart.
Steps of treatment:
Emergent surgery, initially.
At a later age, definitive surgery.

Pulmonary Stenosis with Reversed Interatrial Shunt

Clinical findings are usually as follows:
Cyanosis.
Exertional dyspnea.
Easy fatigability.
Polycythemia.
Clubbing of digits.
The common signs noted at examination are the following:
Long, systolic murmur in the pulmonic area.
Thrill.
At times, evidence noted of pulsation of right pulmonary artery.
Treatment of this condition will be:
Surgery.

Eisenmenger's Syndrome

Pulmonary hypertension in congenital heart disease is noted by:

Exertional dyspnea, either moderate or severe.

Evidence of ventricular septal defect, mainly with cyanosis, polycythemia, and clubbing of digits.

Cyanosis of the lower legs and toes occuring with reversed ductus.

The accompanying signs of this syndrome are:

Systolic murmur on the left border of the heart.

In some cases a pulmonic systolic ejection click.

Pulsations palpable from the right ventricle and the pulmonary artery.

What can be done to treat these cases:

Treat symptoms; there is no any kind of surgery available.

Tricuspid Atresia (Congenital)

How does tricuspid atresia occur congenitally?

An isolated tricuspid atresia.

Tricuspid atresia associated with stenosis of the pulmonary artery and atrial defect.

Tricuspid atresia with ventricular septal defect.

Tricuspid atresia with ductus arteriosus.

What are the principal signs of this lesion?

Systolic murmur.

Thrill on the left border of the heart.

A marked apical impulse.

Cyanosis, polycythemia, and clubbing of digits.

Treatment:

Discuss the outcome of anastomosis of the subclavian to the pulmonary artery.

Mitral Stenosis (Acquired)

The most frequent symptoms associated with mitral stenosis are:

Frequent hemoptysis.

Dry cough.

Dyspnea, which may be worse on recumbency, and may reach orthopnea.

Easy fatigability.

Long-standing cases may present cardiac failure or pulmonary edema.

Atrial fibrillation develops in a good number of patients.

Some of the above patients will develop thrombi (brain or other sites).

Other patients may develop right ventricular failure.

Three out of four patients are women under 45 years of age.

Auscultatory signs of mitral stenosis may be:

A presystolic crescendo and presystolic murmur heard at the apex of the heart.

A snaping first mitral sound of high intensity.

What other clinical signs may appear?

There may be malar flush.

Thrill may be noted at the apex (pre- or mid-diastolic).

Precordial bulge is noted in many cases.

There is evidence of pulmonary congestion in many cases.

Treatment to be advised:

Evaluation of surgical procedures.

Mitral Insufficiency (Acquired)

Enumerate the clinical evidences of mitral insufficiency:

Cyanosis in a good number of cases.

Exertional dyspnea, which may lead to orthopnea and paroxysmal dyspnea.

In many cases atrial fibrillation developed, more than those with mitral stenosis.

Emboli to other areas of the body occurring less frequently than in cases with mitral stenosis.

Auscultatory characteristics of mitral insufficiency:

Very typic systolic murmur at the apex, which propagates to the axilla.

Delayed opening snap present in some cases.

Clinical signs usually present in mitral insufficiency:

Enlarged cardiac area; notably more marked than in cases of stenosis.

Percussion area enlarged to the left.

Steps to follow in the treatment of mitral insufficiency:

In the first asymptomatic stage (diagnosed by auscultation and other procedures), which may last for a few years, just observe.

As soon as it begins, treat congestive heart failure.

If needed, consider surgical prosthetic replacement.

Aortic Stenosis (Acquired)

The regular symptomatology of aortic stenosis is:

Exertional dyspnea, at times leading to syncope.

Easy fatigability.

Pounding of the heart.

Anginal pains.

Finally, congestive heart failure.

Four out of five patients men.

Auscultation of patients with aortic stenosis:

Loud systolic murmur on the second intercostal space at the right.

Diminished or absent second aortic sound.

Thrill.

Other findings from clinical examination of patients with aortic stenosis:

Characteristic slow-rising pulse.

Possibility of a coexisting defect of the mitral valve.

Possibility of a later combination of aortic stenosis and insufficiency.

Management of patients with aortic stenosis:

Care of cardiac insufficiency and anginal pains.

Surgical correction, to be performed as soon as needed.

Aortic Insufficiency (Acquired)

Are symptoms always manifested in aortic insufficiency?
No, many patients are asymptomatic for many years.

When the symptoms become evident, what are the most common ones?
- Exertional dyspnea, even with mild efforts.
- Progressively developing paroxysmal nocturnal dyspnea.
- Congestive heart failure, possibly with acute pulmonary edema.
- Easy fatigability, even with orthopnea.
- Anginal pains, or just chest pains.
- Possible sudden death.

Auscultatory findings in aortic insufficiency:
- Diastolic murmur, better heard over third and fourth intercostal spaces, but at the left side of the sternum.
- Murmurs appearing also, in some patients, at the base or at the apex of the heart, always systolic.

Other examination findings in aortic insufficiency:
- Diastolic blood pressure elevated, but frequently late in the disease.
- Enlargement of the heart area (left and down).

Management of cases with aortic insufficiency:
- Care of cardiac failure.
- Surgical replacement of the valve.

Tricuspid Stenosis (Acquired)

What can suggest that a patient has tricuspid stenosis:
- A previous mitral stenosis with rapid development of right heart failure.
- Hepatic congestion.
- Hepatic cirrhosis, of cardiac origin.
- Ascites of a relatively severe character.
- Dependent edema.
- Possibility of development of atrial fibrillation.
- Easy fatigability.

Auscultatory evidence of tricuspid stenosis:
- A rumbling murmur presystolic-diastolic along the lower left sternal border, with some resemblance to the murmur of mitral stenosis.

Other evidence of medical examination in tricuspid stenosis:
- Presystolic pulsation of the liver (only in sinus rhythm).

Management of tricuspid stenosis:
- Discuss the convenience of surgery.
- If tricuspid stenosis is of the congenital type, special surgical procedures will be carried out.

Tricuspid Insufficiency (Acquired)

When tricuspid insufficiency is to be suspected:
- When there is a previous right ventricular failure.
- When the veins of the neck are distended.
- When there is hepatomegaly.
- When there are pleural effusion and ascites.

What auscultation reveals in tricuspid insufficiency:
- Systolic murmur on the left sternal border, different from mitral murmur.

Management of tricuspid insufficiency:
- Usually recedes when the accompanying diseased mitral valve is replaced.

Rheumatic Heart Disease

What are the most frequent valvular diseases due to rheumatic heart disease?
- Pure mitral lesions are number one.
- A combination of mitral and aortic lesions is number two.
- Aortic lesions are number three.
- Triscuspid lesions are usually associated with mitral or aortic lesions.

The regular course of rheumatic heart disease is as follows:
- A murmur is usually the first symptom to appear.
- There are the symptoms of each individual valvular disease.
- Symptoms of heart failure occur as a final stage.

Management of rheumatic heart disease:
- While patient is in the asymptomatic stage, prevent acute recurrences.
- In all other instances, discuss the individual treatment of each disease.

Endocarditis

Depending on the intensity of the infections, what are the clinical forms of endocarditis, regarding its course?
- Acute bacterial endocarditis (ABE)
- Subacute bacterial endocarditis (SBE)

In acute bacterial endocarditis, what is the common course?
- The course if fulminating, and the patient seems to be toxic.
- Fever is the usual onset, but may be absent in some cases, particularly with the aged.
- Chills are common, but not always present.
- There are night sweats.
- There are multiple pains (joint or muscle pains, principally)
- There is redness or swelling of the joints.
- There are embolic symptoms, in the brain, the lungs, the kidneys, the spleen, or the mesenteric vessels.

Clues that are useful in establishing the diagnosis of acute endocarditis are:
- The patient has had an acute infection.
- Patient has recently been treated surgically or subject to some sort of instrumentation.
- Patient is addicted to narcotics, particularly those injected with needles.
- There are other minor symptoms, such as anorexia, weight loss, malaise, and fatigability, nosebleeds, petechiae, etc.

Changes of preexisting cardiac murmurs are noted.
There is early occurrence of heart failure.

In subacute bacterial endocarditis, the clinical course is described as:

Essentially the same as in acute endocarditis, but less acute and less rapid in course.
Usually accompanied by a history of a previous heart disease.
A continuous fever, not rarely with chills, but also less marked in some cases, particularly among the elderly.
Multiple pains (joint and muscle, principally).
Easy fatigability.
Anemia and weight loss.

Other clues that may help the diagnosis of subacute bacterial endocarditis:

Tachycardia.
Petechiae in the skin, in the ocular fundi, beneath the nails, or in the mucous membranes.
Splenomegaly and clubbing of digits.

Auscultatory findings in these patients with endocarditis:

There are heart murmurs.
The heart murmurs may change in character.

What other clinical circumstances may suggest the occurrence of endocarditis?

A sudden embolic syndrome.
Petechiae that appear without a cause.
Previous heart murmurs that change in character.
Unexplained elevation of temperature.
Rapid occurrence of heart failure without logical explanation.
Any of the above occurring during antibiotic treatment (which may be insufficient or inappropriate for the problem involved).

Management of endocarditis:

Provide a sufficient and effective antibiotic therapy.
Also treat all additional symptoms.

Angina Pectoris

The limited amount of oxygen delivered to the heart by some sort of insufficiently functioning coronary arteries will be announced as follows:

There may be a distressing sensation felt in the middle of the chest, as pain, squeezing, a pressure-like feeling, burning, choking, or whatever other quality is suggested by the fantasy of the patient.
The sensation sets retrosternally or somewhat to the left.
The sensation may radiate to the left shoulder, to the left upper arm, or even below in this same arm (elbow, wrist, or fingers 4 and 5).
Other forms of radiation may exist, but are not common.
Not rarely, the initial pain is felt in the lower jaw, in the neck (base or back), between the scapulae, or in the upper part of the back.

Onset and subsidence of pain follow this course:

Pain appears rapidly after exertion.
The amount of effort is the same for each particular patient.
Patient prefers to stay upright until the pain subsides.
After a characteristic short time the anginal pain subsides.
If the patient stops his effort immediately, the attack may last less than 3 minutes.
In other circumstances, the attack may last even 20 minutes, rarely more.
The use of nitroglycerin will shorten the attack duration.

Findings usually noted during medical examination at the time of the attack:

Gallop rhythm during the attack.
Elevated blood pressure (both diastolic and systolic).
Palpitations, sweating, or digestive disturbances.
Dyspnea, dizziness, or faintness.
Possibly cardiac arrhythmias.

Do not mistake angina pectoris for:

Hiatal hernia.
Cholecystitis.
Psychophysiologic cardiovascular reactions.
Anterior chest wall syndrome.
Different forms of neuritis.
Peptic ulcer.
Cardiospasm.
Spontaneous pneumothorax.
Other less frequent complaints.

Management of angina pectoris:

During the attack, use nitroglycerin or any similar antianginal drug.
For prevention of further crises, use nitroglycerin, other nitrates, xanthines, propanolol, etc.
Consider bypass for suitable cases.

Myocardial Infarction

Premonitory symptoms of myocardial infarction could be:

A change of the usual pattern of anginal attacks.
A typical angina pectoris of sudden onset.
Other discomfort related to the chest, such as indigestion, or the like.

Regular symptoms of the attack of myocardial infarction:

There is a chest discomfort similar to angina pectoris, not usually related to effort.
The chest discomfort is similar to angina, but usually more severe and accompanied by anxiety and apprehensiveness.
The pain does not subside with rest, nor is it alleviated by nitroglycerin.
The initial attack is rapid, but not instantaneous; it progresses to a maximum in a matter of minutes and usually lasts for several hours, if not relieved.
The pain may reach unbearable proportions, thus requiring the use of narcotic analgestics for relief.
The patient appears restless, and does not like to stay quiet.

Other symptoms accompanying the attack of myocardial infarction:

Arrhythmias.
Hypotension.
Cardiac failure.
Syncope or shock.
Cold sweating, weakness, lightheadedness.
Cough, dyspnea, orthopnea, nausea, etc.

What happens when painless myocardial infarction occurs?

In a few cases the pain is almost absent or very minor in character.
In most of these instances there are other problems, such as acute pulmonary edema, a rapid acute heart failure, cerebral thrombosis, or the regular symptoms of syncope or shock.

Physical signs obtained in medical examination may be:

Tachycardia.
Gallop rhythm.
Other forms of arrhythmia or bradycardia.
Rales heard on auscultation of the lungs.
Hypotension (even in the case of a previous hypertension).
Fever.

Differentiate myocardial infarction accurately from:

Acute pulmonary embolism.
Acute pancreatitis.
Acute cholecystitis.
Spontaneous pneumothorax.
Dissecting aortic aneurysm.
Acute pericarditis.

During the course of myocardial infarction watch for:

Congestive heart failure.
Development of syncope or shock.
Pulmonary embolism.
Arrhythmias of any kind.
Perforation of the ventricular septum.
Cerebrovascular accidents.
Ventricular aneurysm or the rare heart rupture.

Management of myocardial infarction:

Rest, analgesia, oxygen, and anticoagulants.
Prevention or care of complications.
Surgical procedures whenever needed.

Tachycardia

What is the rhythm that characterizes sinus tachycardia?

A rhythm of 100 beats or more, which may reach 160 or rarely 180 every minute.

Is the same speed rhythm characteristic of other forms of tachycardia?

In paroxysmal tachycardia the usual rhythm varies between 170 and 220 every minute, but may reach 240, or perhaps somewhat more.
Similar rates are present in junctional tachycardia or in paroxysmal ventricular tachycardia.

When sinus tachycardia will occur:

After exercise.
After emotional disturbances.
Usually after eating.
After the use of certain drugs.
Usually accompanying fever.
As a response to hemorrhage.
In cases of hyperthyroidism.
In cases of heart failure.

What are the characteristics of *paroxysmal atrial tachycardia*?

It is characterized by the abrupt onset and termination of the attack.
The rhythm is totally regular, and does not change because of exercise or other causes.
There are no other symptoms, excepting in long-lasting attacks when the patients will complain of dyspnea or tightness of the chest.
The regular length of the attack is a few hours; some may last days.

Management of paroxysmal atrial tachycardia:

Try to end the attack by simple maneuvers (carotid sinus pressure, Valsalve's maneuver, holding the breath, bilateral eye pressure, vomiting, etc.).
If the above fail, use drugs, such as propanolol, procainamide, or digitalis; edrophonium is also recommended. Consider cardioversion.
Avoid further attacks by using quinidine, procainamide, or propanolol.

How *junctional tachycardia* may be diagnosed:

It may be due to a severe myocardial disease, be present in cor pulmonale, digitalis toxicity; but sometimes it is only a benign condition.
The diagnosis has to be made by the joint efforts of clinical examination and electrocardiography; but in some instances cardiac catheterization is needed.

Management of junctional or auriculoventricular nodal tachycardia:

Just like above.

Paroxysmal ventricular tachycardia will be diagnosed as follows:

It usually occurs following myocardial infarction or digitalis intoxication.
When it is due to myocardial infarction, pain, hypotension, and syncope or shock are usually noted.
The rhythm is regular, but with less regularity than in atrial tachycardia.
In auscultation, there is a variation from beat to beat of the first heart sound.

Management of paroxysmal ventricular tachycardia:

Use countershock, except in milder cases.
Administer lidocaine in first instance; as alternates, use quinidine, procainamide, diphenylhydantoin.
Treat shock.
Transvenous cardiac pacing may be a temporary help.

Bradycardia

What is the rhythm that characterizes sinus bradycardia?
- It is less than 60 beats a minute.
- Differentiate it from slow rhythms due to heart block.

When bradycardia may occur:
- In cases of increased vagal tone.
- In cases of heart disease (mainly coronary occlusion).
- In cases of meningitis or other forms of increased intracranial pressure.
- In some cases of gastrointestinal disturbances.
- Following an initial tachycardia in cases of profuse hemorrhages.
- In many patients with jaundice.
- In all forms of stimulation of the carotid sinus.

Symptoms will occur in what circumstances with bradycardia?
- If there is any form of coronary insufficiency.
- In very severe cases it will cause syncope or convulsions.
- In the elderly there may be weakness or confusion, or even syncope.

What is considered the *sick sinus syndrome*?
- An alternation of tachycardia and bradycardia.
- Other symptoms resulting from inadequate blood perfusion of vital organs or symptoms due to the rapid cardiac rate.

Management of the above conditions:
- No treatment is usually needed for bradycardia; but in some cases atropine may give good results.
- In the sick sinus syndrome a pacemaker should be considered.

Pulsus Bigeminus

What characterizes the pulsus bigeminus?
- The pulse seems to occur in pairs; two beats come close together and appear somewhat separated from the following two pulsations.

Symptoms and management of pulsus bigeminus:
- Most frequent it indicates digital toxicity.
- In most senses it resembles premature contractions, q.v. Sedatives, quinidine, or procainamide may be used.

Atrial Premature Beats

Our knowledge of atrial premature beats is that:
- They are pulse beats that start closer to the preceding beat and are followed by a slightly longer pause.
- They do not ordinarily tell anything important about the heart.

Fibrillation

Fibrillation may be atrial or ventricular, and should be differentiated as follows:
- The pulse is rapid and irregular in both cases, but there are slightly more marked spaces between some of the beats in the auricular than in ventricular fibrillation, where the irregular beats are closer together.
- In auricular fibrillation there is usually a sensation of tightness of the chest, a possibility of palpitations, pallor, nausea, and even syncope. Syncope may occur, but is rare.
- In ventricular fibrillation the heart sounds become inaudible and the blood pressure falls considerably. Shock may occur, and death may follow the cardiac standstill that frequently occurs.

What common causes may precede atrial fibrillation?
- Excessive alcohol intake.
- Hyperthyroidism.
- Arteriosclerotic heart disease.
- Rheumatic heart disease.
- Infections, poisoning, or trauma.
- And there are cases that occur without known cause.

Ventricular fibrillation may follow:
- Coronary insufficiency.
- Over dosage with digitalis, quinidine, emetine, papaverine, or other drugs.
- And may occur during anesthesia or surgical procedures done to the heart.

Management of fibrillation:
- In atrial fibrillation start with digitalis; and if there is not a good result, proceed to cardioversion.
- In the chronic stage of atrial fibrillation use digitalis, quinidine, or propanolol, or proceed to cardioversion.
- In ventricular fibrillation give emergent countershock.
- In ventricular fibrillation, if there is no possibility of countershock, give external cardiac massage and intravenous lidocaine, procainamide, or diphenylhydantoin.

Flutter

Again, flutter may be atrial or ventricular, and should be differentiated as follows:
- In cases of atrial flutter the pulse is rapid, but pulsations are almost equal (usually one pulsation for each two atrial contractions).
- In cases of rapid ventricular contractions during atrial flutter, not all the beats are felt (this is called the pulse deficit).
- In atrial flutter the first heart sound may vary from beat to beat.
- Ventricular flutter is rapidly fatal.

The common causes that precede flutter are:
- Usually the same as for atrial fibrillation.
- In the case of ventricular flutter, it is usually a severe myocardial disease, and is precipitated by the use of digitalis, quinidine, or even epinephrine.

Management of flutter:
- Countershock is the management of choice.
- In atrial flutter, digitalis should be tried.

Pulsus Alternans

How can the alternating large and small pulsations of the disease be noted?

- If the difference is sufficient, they will be noted in the radial arteries.
- If the pressure cuff is gradually inflated, it will provoke the disappearance of the smaller pulsations.
- In the pulmonary circulation alternans may also occur, but they are not detectable clinically (only by catheterization).
- A gallop rhythm is frequent.

Management of pulsus alternans:

- There is no therapy. Treat any underlying problem present.

Ventricular Premature Beats

Ventricular premature beats are manifested as follows:

- The interval between the extra systole and the next normal beat is slightly larger than in the case of atrial premature beats.
- There may be sudden death when they occur in a case of coronary insufficiency.
- The premature ventricular beats may disappear with exercise.
- Palpitations may occasionally be felt.

Management of ventricular premature beats:

- Only if needed, potassium chloride will be given in digitalis toxicity (the digitalis has to be discontinued).
- It is important to note that they may occur in the case of heart disease when an insufficient amount of digitalis is given (to check it, withdraw digitalis and treat heart failure effectively by other means).

Sino-Atrial Block

Sino-atrial block is evidenced by:

- Regularly or irregularly absent beats, thus causing some sort of bradycardia.
- Clinically, by absence of cardiac sounds during the pause.
- In the presence of pauses that are too long, by faintness or syncope.

Management of sino-atrial block:

- Either do nothing or try atropine; or in some more severe cases, consider a pacemaker.

Bundle Branch Block

Bundle branch block may be assumed in what circumstances?

- Some of the normal beats fail to be produced.
- If the pause between beats is too long, there may be dizziness, convulsions, or syncope.
- The beats that fail can be noted on auscultation.
- Palpitations or other chest sensations may be noted.
- The final diagnosis depends on electrocardiography and other clinical procedures.

Adams-Stokes syndrome is a variant of bundle block characterized by:

- Attacks of temporary loss of consciousness.
- Convulsions.
- Very slow bradycardia.
- The loss of consciousness (syncope) occurs suddenly, and the convulsions appear after a short interval if consciousness is not regained.

Management of heart block:

- Try to eliminate all causative factors.
- Discuss the convenience of a pacemaker.
- Use drugs in other cases (isoproterenol, epinephrine, corticosteroids).

Wolff-Parkinson-White Syndrome

How can this accelarated conduction syndrome be diagnosed?

- There are no clinical symptoms.
- The only clue is the electrocardiographic record of a short P-R interval.
- The consequences are: paroxysmal tachycardia, atrial fibrillation, and atrial flutter.

Management of these patients:

- Use quinidine to prevent other forms of arrhythmias.

Hypertension

Hypertension is characterized by the following:

- Casual finding by a routine examination of blood pressure.
- Psychological symptoms caused by anxiety about known hypertension: headaches, fatigue, dizziness, palpitations, tinnitus, insomnia, etc.
- Readings of blood pressure over 90 to 110, 111 to 130, 131 to 150 or over 150 for the diastolic figure; these according to severity.

In long-lasting hypertension, what are the ocular changes?

- There may be hemorrhages, exudate, papilledema, or other forms of arterial compression.
- Arterial narrowing of mild consideration is the first symptom.
- There is a second stage of more marked narrowing and nicking between arteries and veins.
- A more marked third stage occurs with hemorrhages and exudates.
- Papilledema will mark the more severe stage.

In long-lasting hypertension, what are the cardiac symptoms?

- Cardiac hypertrophy.
- Cardiac asthma.
- Paroxysmal nocturnal dyspnea.
- Anginal pectoris or myocardial infarction.
- Congestive heart failure.

In long-lasting hypertension, what are other vascular symptoms?

- Epistaxis is not rare.
- Other forms of hemorrhage may also occur.
- Peripheral artery disease causing intermittent claudication may occur.

There may be low back pain (narrowing of terminal aorta).
Impotence may occur in men (narrowing of the terminal aorta).
Involvement of cerebral arteries will cause hypertensive encephalopathy.
In hypertensive encephalopathy there are severe headaches, vomiting, convulsions, mental changes, and a terminal accident of thrombosis or hemorrhage.

In long-lasting hypertension, the renal symptoms are:
Polyuria and nocturia.
Proteinuria, cylindruria, and hematuria.
Poor concentration and nitrogen retention.

Hypertension due to pheochromocytoma will present:
Attacks of anxiety, with profuse perspiration, pallor, and trembling.
Palpitations.
Nausea and vomiting.
Weakness or paralysis, in some cases.
Marked rises of blood pressure during the attacks.

What characterizes malignant hypertension?
Rapid course, with marked rise of blood pressure, which is progressive.
Rapidly progressive renal damage.
Retinopathy with papilledema.
Not rare incidence of hypertensive encephalopathy.

What characterizes the hypertensive encephalopathy?
Acute attacks of headache.
Mental changes and transient neurological signs.
Nausea, vomiting.
Blurred vision, convulsions, coma.
Rapidly and steadily rising blood pressure.

What causes of hypertension frequently occur?
Essential hypertension.
Renal hypertension (vascular, parenchymal).
Pheochromocytoma.
Cushing's syndrome.
Some patients with acromegaly.
Some patients with hyperthyroidism.
Coarctation of the aorta.
Pre-eclampsia and eclampsia.
Some contraceptive agents.
Polyarteritis nodosa (late stages of the disease).
Scleroderma.
Disseminated lupus erythematosus.
Neurogenic bladder.
Increased intracranial pressure.

Management of hypertension:
Some variations occur according to the level of hypertension.
For 90/110 levels: give chlorothiazide or hydrochlorothiazide; or methyldopa, reserpine, etc.
For 111/130 levels: same as above, plus methyldopa; or hydrazine.
For 131/150 levels: same as above, but instead of methyldopa give guanethidine.
For levels above 150: same as above, but methyldopa and guanethidine given simultaneously.
In the case of complications consider congestive heart failure, azotemia, cerebrovascular insufficiency, or coronary insufficiency as the most important ones.

Cardiac Failure

Since the heart has a right and a left group of chambers, are the symptoms of heart failure identical in each case, or not?
Left ventricular failure is noted mainly by dyspnea, cough, rales, gallop rhythm, cardiac enlargement, and pulmonary congestion.
Right ventricular failure is noted by hepatomegaly and edema.
There is a dual failure with a combination of symptoms.

Cardiac failure most commonly occurs in:
Coronary artery insufficiency and other forms of myocardial diseases.
Hypertension.
Hypertrophic diseases of the heart.
Diseases of cardiac valves.
Congenital heart diseases.
Hyperthyroidism, and hypothyroidism.
Anemia.
Arteriovenous fistula.
Pregnancy.
Endocarditis, and pericarditis.
Some cases of beri-beri.
Pulmonary diseases.
Arrhythmias.
Systemic lupus erythematosus, polyarteritis, scleroderma, amyloidosis.
Chagas' disease.
Hemochromatosis, Paget's disease.

In left ventricular failure the clinical features are:
Exertional dyspnea, leading to orthopnea, nocturnal paroxysmal dyspnea.
Cough, which may be one of the initial symptoms.
Wheezing, which may occur during dyspneic attacks (cardiac asthma).
Mild dependent edema, occasionally.
Easy fatigability and weakness.
Nocturia.
Pulmonic rales, gallop rhythm, pulsus alternans, all rare.
In severe cases the patient becomes disabled, dyspnea occurs at rest, patient becomes cyanotic, cerebral symptoms may appear, and there will finally be cachexia and total deterioration.

In right ventricular failure the symptoms are:
Dependent edema noted by ankle swelling, but at the beginning it subsides during night rest; thereafter, it becomes continuous.
Hepatomegaly, with pain at palpation.
Ascites and pleural effusion, resulting more or less promptly in the disease.

Congestion of abdominal viscerae (anorexia, indigestion, constipation).
Also, bloating or exertional right abdominal pains.
Oligura during the day, and polyuria at night.
Easy fatigability.
Not rarely, respiratory manifestations.
In severe cases, mental changes.

In advanced congestive heart failure the patient will present:

Total inability to do any work.
Disabling respiratory distress, even at rest.
Cyanosis not only of nail beds, but evident in other areas of the body.
Total asthenia, because of an extremely easy fatigability.
Loss of concentration, and confusion (more noted in the elderly).
Loss of memory, more or less marked.
Final total deterioration of the patient.

Signs to be found in medical examination of cases with heart failure:

Tachycardia or other arrhythmias may be present.
Heart is enlarged in most instances.
Murmurs may be heard; a gallop rhythm is a frequent manifestation.
Respiratory wheezing is heard in those with cardiac asthma.
Rales, which do not clear on coughing, are heard in some patients.
Pulsus alternans and gallop rhythm are noted in many cases.
An accentuated second pulmonic sound is noted.
There is evidence of symptoms and signs of a causative disease.

Management of heart failure:

The main features are rest, diuretics, and cardiotonics.
Also, care of the diet (low salt intake), oxygen therapy, and mechanical drainage of retained fluids may be employed.

Cor Pulmonale

Cor pulmonale presents the following main symptoms initially:

Cough, permanent and productive.
Wheezing respirations.
Exertional dyspnea.
Marked asthenia.

As cor pulmonale advances, it will present:

Evidence of right ventricular failure.
The initial symptoms, more marked.
Dependent edema, particularly in the ankles.
Digestive discomfort, including pain in the hepatic area.
Cyanosis.
Clubbing of digits.
Full pulses and warm extremities.

Medical examination of patients with cor pulmonale will reveal:

Evidence of pulmonary emphysema.
Gallop rhythm.
Prominent veins in the neck, and marked pulsation in the epigastric or lower sternal areas.
Tender hepatomegaly.
Ankle edema.

Beware of the following incidences that may occur in cor pulmonale:

Respiratory infections, which worsen the condition.
CO_2 narcosis (somnolence, disorientation, coma, convulsions).

Management of cor pulmonale:

Give antibiotics when convenient.
Use assisted respiration, with intermittent positive pressure.
Treat heart failure.

Cardiac Arrest

In the inadequacy or absence of cardiac contractions that characterize cardiac arrest, what symptoms may be found?

A previous ventricular fibrillation, usually present.
A complete cardiac standstill.
Sudden unconsciousness.
Absence of perceptible pulsations or auscultable heart sounds.
Apnea.

The emergent treatment requires:

Starting no more than 5 minutes after occurrence, to avoid brain damage.
Putting into practice the resuscitation procedure.
Further treatment of the condition.

Shock

The state of shock usually follows these causes:

Very severe infections.
Myocardial infarction, and valvular diseases.
Severe hemorrhages.
Important traumas (including surgery).
Dehydration, including burns.
Poisoning and drug reactions.
Pancreatitis, peritonitis, and severe liver diseases.
Bradycardia and hypotension.
Pulmonary embolism.

Shock, when due to deficient venous return, presents the following symptoms:

The skin is pale, cool, and moist.
Veins appear collapsed, as noted in the flat neck veins.
There is tachycardia.
There is a very weak or almost absent peripheral pulse.
There may be unconsciousness; but the patient may still be conscious, though agitated or apathetic.

Shock, when cardiogenic in origin, presents the following symptoms:

Notable asthenia.

Dyspnea.

Sweating, and a nauseous state.

Some form of chest discomfort, or pain.

Ventricular fibrillation or cardiac standstill, causing collapse.

Symptoms of myocardial infarction, in some cases.

Paleness, coldness, dyspnea, irregular pulse, and low blood pressure, in some patients.

Pulmonary edema, with engorged neck veins.

On auscultation, a diastolic gallop, and also rales in the lungs.

Hepatojugular reflux.

Shock, if due to peripheral vascular deficiency, will present:

A somnolent patient.

Warm skin.

Pulse bounding and collapsing.

Hypotension.

Management of shock:

Depends on its severity and its cause.

Lowering of the head may suffice, in some instances.

Try to counteract the cause of shock, and its effects upon the body.

Rest, elevation of the feet, sedation, epinephrine, and venous infusions may be utilized.

Give corticosteroid and vasoconstrictors (these not for too prolonged a time).

Some forms of shock need a causative treatment (myocardial infarction).

Pericarditis

In *acute pericarditis* what are the principal symptoms?

Fever, which may be moderate or really elevated, with or without chills.

Chest pain, precordial or substernal.

Usual sudden onset of pain.

Pain steady or increased with respirations (pleuritic type).

Pain radiating to the epigastrium, left shoulder, or neck, or the back.

Pain increased by swallowing, and lying supine.

Tachycardia.

Pericardial friction rub at auscultation.

Effusion in the pericardium will cause:

Fever, depending on the causative factor.

Dysphagia, a very important symptom.

Variable chest pain, from absent to acute.

Pain, substernal or precordial.

Cough and dyspnea, forcing the patient to sit and lean forward for relief.

Enlarged cardiac area.

Friction rub may persist in spite of the effusion.

When the effusion is large enough to constitute *"cardiac tamponade"*, the symptoms will be:

All the above symptoms.

Distended neck veins increasing during inspiration.

Paradoxic pulse (decreases in size during inspiration).

Narrowed pulse pressure.

Hepatomegaly.

Ascites and leg edema.

In acute cases, also shock.

Chronic constrictive pericarditis symptoms will be:

Dyspnea and progressive asthenia.

Leg edema, and also edema of the scrotum in male patients.

Abdominal distention, with ascites.

Neck veins markedly distended.

Hepatomegaly.

Frequently found atrial fibrillation, and absent systolic pulsations (with marked diastolic retraction).

Enlarged heart.

Tachycardia and very soft heart sounds.

Blood pressure with high diastolic and low pulse pressure.

Paradoxic pulse.

Management of acute pericarditis will be:

Treat the underlying disease.

Relieve pain with analgesics.

If it is rheumatic in origin, give salicylates and corticosteroids.

Management of pericarditis with effusion will be:

Drain the fluid by paracentesis.

Treat the causative factor according to its nature.

Management of cardiac tamponade will be:

Drain the fluid by paracentesis.

Use surgery if symptoms recur or are not well controlled.

Management of chronic constrictive pericarditis will be:

Give low-sodium diet and diuretics if there is cardiac failure.

The surgical approach seems to be the procedure of choice.

Myocarditis

Most cases of myocarditis are due to a previous infection, and the symptoms will be:

The symptoms due to the causative factor.

The above symptoms possibly obscuring the whole myocardial disease.

Chest pain.

Dyspnea.

Easy fatigability, dizziness.

Nausea and vomiting.

Syncope, shock, or sudden death.

In the case of primary myocardial disease, the symptoms will be:

Similar to the above, but acute, subacute, or chronic.

Peripheral emboli and heart failure when the primary myocardial disease is caused by other forms of heart disease.

In all the above cases, also fever, and the following symptoms.

Tachycardia, with faint heart sounds, changing murmurs, and arrhythmias.

Cardiac enlargement and congestive heart failure.

Gallop rhythm and pulsus alternans possibly noted.

Distended neck veins.

Emboli to the brain or other organs.

Summarize the causes of myocarditis (infectious and others):

Diphtheria	Heart failure, heart block, shock
Influenza and other viral causes	Heart failure, mild symptomatology
Meningococcal	Enlarged heart
Cardiac amyloidosis	Rare heart failure
Sarcoidosis	Arrhythmias, heart block, cor pulmonale, and heart failure
Hyperthyroidism	Tachycardia and arrhythmias; and heart failure in older patients
Hypothyroidism	Enlarged heart, pericardial effusion, coronary insufficiency
Acromegaly	Heart enlargement
Hurler's syndrome	Oligophrenia, developmental defects, valvular disease, angina, heart failure
Systemic lupus erythematosus	Murmurs, myocarditis, pericarditis
Dermatomyositis	Enlarged heart
Rheumatoid arthritis	Myocardial lesions, aortic insufficiency
Polyarteritis	Enlarged heart, coronary insufficiency
Alcoholism	Heart failure

How these diseases should be treated:

Generally speaking, the treatment is poor.

Corticosteroids or symptomatic treatment may help some cases.

Surgery or the use of pacemakers may also be of help.

Tumors of the Heart

Myxoma of the left atrium is the most common tumor of the heart; what are its symptoms?

Fever, with tachycardia.

Symptoms of tricuspid or of mitral stenosis.

Symptoms of emboli.

Symptoms of hemolytic anemia.

Feeling worse in the upright position.

Intermittent symptoms of dyspnea, vertigo, and syncope.

Changing murmurs.

In some cases, clubbed digits.

Symptoms of *rhabdomyosarcoma* are:

Oligophrenia.

Adenoma sebaceum.

Tuberous sclerosis.

Other *metastatic tumors* may present the following symptoms:

Cardiac arrhythmias.

Pericardial effusion.

Heart failure.

What can be done for treatment of these patients?

Symptomatic treatment.

Aneurysmatic Diseases

In *aneurysms of the thoracic aorta* the main symptomatology is as follows:

Initially, there is paucity or absence of symptoms.

Pain will be present in the chest (substernal), the back, or the neck.

There will be dyspnea, cough, and stridor if there is tracheal pressure.

Dysphagia occurs in cases of pressure on the esophagus.

Hoarseness is a symptom when the left recurrent laryngeal nerve is involved.

Edema in neck and arms may occur, because of pressure on the superior vena cava.

There may be distended neck veins (pressure on the superior vena cava).

Erosion of vertebras or Horner's syndrome is suggestive.

Aortic insufficiency may occur.

Finally, there may be rupture of the aorta.

The management of these aneurysms is:

Surgical.

Dissecting aneurysms of the aorta will cause the following symptoms:

There is chest pain (anterior or middorsal), spreading to the abdomen and the hips.

The pain is sudden and severe.

The constant, persistent pain is only somewhat decreased in the prerupture hypertensive stage.

When the dissecting aneurysm of the aorta causes partial or complete occlusion of the branches from its arch, what symptoms may occur?

Hemiplegia.

Paralysis of the lower extremities.

Convulsions, or even shock (at least in later stages).

What other circulatory symptoms and signs may occur?

Pulse may disappear or become unequal in the wrist, the carotid, or any other peripheral site.

Blood pressure is markedly lower in the legs than in the arms.

Arterial murmurs may be heard.

If the dissection occurs near the heart, a diastolic murmur may reveal the resultant aortic insufficiency.

Hypertension is a common initial factor.

Fever rarely is absent.
Most patients are male.

What is the most difficult factor in diagnosing the dissecting aneurysm of the aorta?

It must not be taken for myocardial infarction.
The clinical study may be insufficient, and more elaborate laboratory and radiological procedures may be needed.

Management steps to be taken in these cases:

Prepare the patient for surgery.

In aortic *aneurysm of syphilitic origin,* what symptoms will originate?

On the site of the aneurysm there will be heard a tambour-like second aortic murmur and also a systolic murmur.
A diastolic murmur may reveal secondary aortic insufficiency.
Other symptoms may be anginal pain or heart failure.

Aneurysms set on the *abdominal aorta* will be revealed by the following symptomatology:

There will be a pulsating abdominal mass in the abdomen (mid- or upper), with no other symptoms, or perhaps hypertension.
When symptoms appear, pain will be the important one.
Pain will appear in the abdomen or in the back, of a boring character and intense severity.
The pain will be constant or intermittent.
Finally, rupture will be announced by increased severity of the pain, which occurs suddenly.
Shock will occur soon or be delayed.
Subcutaneous ecchymoses may be present.

Management of abdominal aorta aneurysms:

Surgery for most cases; and emergent in the case of rupture.

Symptomatology of *intracranial aneurysms:*

There is usually very little or no symptomatology.
There may be exertional headache.
Rarely, a cranial bruit will be heard at the site of the aneurysm.
There may be symptoms due to impairment of ophthalmic, oculomotor, or trigeminal cranial nerves.
Rupture of the aneurysm is noted by a sudden severe headache, nuchal rigidity, and a brief loss of consciousness or convulsions.

Management of intracranial aneurysms:

Use antifibrinolytic agents.
Discuss convenience of surgery.

Arteriosclerosis

Discuss the terminology related to arteriosclerosis:

Arteriosclerosis	There is a loss of elasticity marked by thickening and hardening of the arteries.
Atherosclerosis	There is a lesion of large and of medium-sized arteries, with fat deposition in the intima.
Mönckeberg's arteriosclerosis	There are extensive deposits of calcium in the medial coat.
Arteriolosclerosis	There is hyalinization of the small arteries.
Arteriosclerosis obliterans	Proliferation of the intima causes the characteristic obliteration.

Sclerotic arteries are usually silent until the appearance of:

Stenosis, with further occlusion.
Aneurysm.
Thrombosis.
Emboli.
Coronary insufficiency or hypertension in men over 50 years of age.

Atherosclerosis of the *cerebral vessels* is known by:

Behavioral changes of the patient.
Forgetfulness, mainly of recent events.
Confusional states.
Transient weakness or numbness of arm or leg (contralateral).
Transient loss of vision, partial or total (ipsilateral).

In the case of *carotid insufficiency* to irrigate the brain, the symptoms will be:

Mostly the same as above, plus the following.
Aphasia.
Weakness of the face muscles.
Possibility of complete hemiplegia.
Possibility of coma.

In the case of insufficient irrigation from the *vertebral and basilar arteries,* the symptoms will be:

Vertigo, particularly when the patient stands up.
Unsteady gait.
Blurred vision, or diplopia.

The *subclavian steal syndrome* is noted by:

Symptoms of claudication and of central nervous system impairment on exercise of the left arm.

What is the final outcome of most of these situations?

Repeated "little strokes."
Final stroke.

In case of *coronary insufficiency* there will be any of the following:

Angina pectoris.
Myocardial infarction.
Cardiac arrhythmias.
Cardiac failure, following repeated ischemic attacks.

In cases of *insufficiency of the aorto-iliac arteries,* the symptoms are as follows:

There is evidence of claudication of the lower extremities.
Pain is progressively more intense, until it will not allow the patient to walk over a block, sometimes even less.

Feet are usually cold.
Impotence is frequent among men.
Pulses are absent or weak in the lower limbs.
Murmurs may be heard over the arteries (aorta or iliacs).
Oscillations are notably diminished, even absent, in the lower arteries.

Insufficient flow through the *renal arteries* will cause:
Renovascular hypertension.
Possibility of hearing a murmur on abdominal auscultation.
Frequent sudden onset of hypertension, particularly with young patients.
Final diagnosis dependent on special findings (renin, X-ray studies).

Insufficiency of the *femoral and popliteal arteries* will cause:
Claudication of the corresponding leg, but it may be bilateral.
If bilateral, more marked claudication in one of the legs, usually.
Pain usually limited to the calf and foot.
Acral coldness.
Popliteal and pedal pulses very weak or totally absent.
Oscillations very weak, or totally absent, in the leg.

Insufficiency of the lower leg and foot blood supply will cause:
Same symptoms of intermittent claudication, or even rest pain.
Muscle cramps lasting only a few minutes, usually leaving more durable soreness at the site.
Very weak or totally absent pulses in some or all of the involved arteries.
Oscillations diminished or absent; most distal arteries can be tested by modern methods.
Change of color of the feet (bluish-red). Also, cyanosis may be present.
The foot becomes pale when elevated.
Local coldness.
Skin changes may occur (smoothness, loss of hair, nail changes, etc.).

Advisable treatment to be followed in each particular case:

General measures in arteriosclerosis	Anti-hyperlipidemia diet; avoidance of smoking; exercise; if needed, drugs for hyperlipidemia; anticoagulants if occlusion threatens.
Cerebral insufficiency	General treatment until there is a stroke: rest, relief of agitation, anticoagulant therapy; surgery when possible and needed.
Carotid insufficiency	As above; surgery (endarterectomy, bypass).
Verterbral and basilar arteries insufficiency	Same as for carotid insufficiency, above.
Subclavian steal syndrome	As for the two entries above.
Coronary insufficiency	See entries for angina pectoris and myocardial infarction.
Aorto-iliac arteries insufficiency	Prosthesis by arterial graft, thromboendarterectomy; possibly with sympathectomy.
Renal arteries insufficiency	Discuss convenience of saphenous vein bypass, or the removal of the stenosis. Nephrectomy only for pure urologic problems.
Femoral and popliteal insufficiency	As for aorto-iliac insufficiency, q.v.
Insufficiency of lower leg and foot arteries	For claudication, exercise the leg under tolerance; take care of diseased feet (ulcers, infections, gangrene), even to the point of amputation. Consider sympathectomy for selected cases.

Thromboangiitis Obliterans (Buerger's Disease)

Who are the usual patients with this disease?
Young smokers.

Claudication in Buerger's disease presents some characteristics as follows:
The pain may be noted in the foot; also there may be pain in the palm of the hands.
Pain is mostly persistent, and felt even at rest.
Pain is usually more intense than in atherosclerosis.

Indicative of an accompanying neuropathy are:
Hypoalgesia and numbness.
Burning and prickling.

Vascular findings may be present, such as:
Small, red, tender chords indicative of superficial thrombophlebitis, preferently in saphenous tributaries, usually segmental and migratory.

The foot will show the following changes:
One, more than one digit, or the entire distal portion of the foot pale, cold, with little change with change of position.
Frequent feeble or absent pulses.
Trophic changes, also frequently noted (check nails with care).

Other changes to be noted:
Not rarely, involvement of both feet (unequal changes).
Not rarely, involvement of hands and lower arms.
Not rarely, the Raynaud's phenomenon present in digits or toes.

Main differential findings when compared with atherosclerosis:

Pain is more intense.

There are differences in claudication pain and discomfort.

More marked changes are noted in one extremity.

The course is more acute and dramatic than in atherosclerosis.

Raynaud's disease affects preferentially young women, and does not affect pulsation.

Treatment measures to be followed:

Stop smoking.

Give regular care to foot lesions.

Discuss extent of surgery for each particular case.

Aortic Arch Syndrome (Martorell's Syndrome, Takayasu's Disease)

These two conditions are also called "pulseless disease" because of:

Narrowing or total occlusion of one or more of the arteries from the aortic arch or the thoracic aorta.

What are the differences between Martorell's syndrome and Takayasu's disease?

There are more localized symptoms in Martorell's syndrome.

In Martorell's syndrome there are atheromatous changes of the arteries; in Takayasu's disease the cause is unknown, and the atheromatous changes are secondary.

What are the common symptoms of pulseless disease or reversed coarctation?

Blood pressure is elevated in the legs, and low or unobtained in the arms.

Pulse is weak or absent in arteries of the arms, head, and neck.

There is evidence of collateral blood flow in the chest, neck, and shoulders.

There are transient central nervous system disturbances, eventually ending in permanent damage.

The transient symptoms may be dizzy spells or visual disturbances.

The permanent damage may be hemiplegia.

Other symptoms may be syncopal or epileptiform attacks, claudication of the arms, facial atrophy, aphasia, etc.

The visual disturbances may be transient blindness, cataracts, atrophy of the iris and retina.

Management of these cases:

Surgery (endarterectomy with autogenous or Dacron graft, replacement of the aortic arch).

Anticoagulation, if surgery is not feasible.

Temporal Arteritis

What is the usual age to suffer from temporal arteritis?

Old age.

What are the usual manifestations that precede the arterial manifestations?

Symptoms of polymyalgia rheumatica.

The outstanding symptoms of temporal arteritis or giant cell arteritis:

There is headache, frontal or occipital, generally of a throbbing type.

There are tenderness and pain over the temporal arteries.

The arteries are usually pulseless and appear to be nodular cords, firm and tender.

Other symptoms of giant cell arteritis are:

Visual disturbances (sudden or gradual blindness, involvement of the central retinal artery, ischemic optic neuritis).

Localized erythema at the site of the lesion.

Arterial complication leading to myocardial or cerebral infarct.

Dissecting aneurysm of the aorta.

Management of temporal arteritis:

Stop smoking, and relieve pain.

Start corticosteroid therapy as soon as possible.

Raynaud's Phenomenon and Raynaud's Disease

What is the difference between Raynaud's phenomenon and Raynaud's disease?

Raynaud's phenomenon is a secondary manifestation to occlusive diseases of the arteries, thoracic outlet syndromes, collagen diseases, traumas, drug intoxication, etc.

Raynaud's disease occurs when there is not a known cause.

What is the characteristic symptomatology?

Usually, following cooling or emotional upsets, the tips of one or more fingers (more rarely the toes) blanch and become cyanotic, or cyanosis follows blanching (more rarely the changes may reach proximal sites).

The attacks are intermittent.

Usually, the thumbs are not involved.

Symptoms that may be found with the attack are: numbness, hypoalgesia, pain, and possibly stiffness.

The recovery phase is accompanied by throbbing pain, swelling, and more intense rubor.

In long-standing cases there may be skin changes (atrophy and gangrene, sclerodactyly, ulcers), mainly affecting the distal area of the finger.

The attacks may last from a few minutes to a few hours; and as the problem continues, they become more prolonged and more frequent.

The symptoms of the causative factor should be found in Raynaud's phenomenon.

Management of these problems:

In Raynaud's phenomenon find the causative factor and treat it.

Protect the fingers from cold, and stop smoking (vasoconstrictor).

Use reserpine, nicotinyl alcohol, papaverine, or other vasodilators.

Discuss sympathectomy, but at an early stage of the symptoms.

Causalgia

What is the characteristic symptom of causalgia?

As the name, causalgia, implies, it is a burning pain.

The pain is excruciating.

Also it is characteristic that it follows an irritation or an injury to a peripheral nerve, most usual, affecting an extremity.

There is not a firm relationship between the intensity of the damage to the nerve and the symptoms of causalgia.

Symptoms that are also usually present in causalgia:

Vasomotor changes (heat, redness, or cyanosis; dry, swollen, ridged nails; long hair; etc.).

Protective immobilization of the affected extremity, usually held in a splinted position, thus provoking disuse atrophy of the muscles, osteoporosis of the bones, and in the long run the extremity becoming cool, clammy, developing trigger points for pain, stiffness of joints, glossy and atrophic skin, and other evidence of disuse of the extremity.

Management of causalgia:

Try conservative treatment first, with protective measures and tranquilizers.

Discuss surgery with a specialist (sympathetic block, sympathectomy, electronic biostimulator).

Erythromelalgia

Other names for this disease; also meaning pain and/or redness of a limb:

Erythermalgia.

Acromelalgia.

Describe the outstanding changes in this disease:

There are paroxysmal attacks, usually bilateral, of feet (more rarely of hands).

The attacks last from a few minutes to a few hours.

The attacks present: a burning pain, with redness, heat, and pain.

The involved areas are the soles (or palms), but when the disease progresses, include the whole extremity.

The attack follows vasodilation (heat, exercise, etc.).

Other accompanying changes are:

Increased skin temperature.

Increased sweat in the affected area.

Increased pulsations.

Disability, in some of the long-lasting cases.

Differentiate from similar symptomatic diseases:

Vasodilating attacks are transient in erythromelalgia and permanent or continuous in acrocyanosis.

In occlusive arterial diseases there are usually skin changes.

In neuritis there are also skin changes, plus nerve disorders.

Management of erythromelalgia:

Protect from heating, which provokes the attack.

Acetylsalicylic acid gives good relief.

Discuss surgery in severe cases (section or crushing of nerve).

Acrocyanosis

Acrocyanosis presents an outstanding symptom:

Acral cyanosis, that is, cyanosis of the distal parts of the extremities, mainly the hands, more rarely the feet; more rarely arms or legs.

The cyanosis is symmetrical.

Other symptoms are:

Acrocyanosis worsens during cold weather.

Acrocyanosis does not completely recede during the warmest months.

Acrocyanosis improves with advancing age.

The affected area is of a bluish discoloration (cyanosis) due to poorly oxygenated blood, cold, humid, and somewhat edematous.

Management of acrocyanosis:

No treatment is needed, in almost all cases.

Some help could be offered by advising patient to avoid coldness, to use a vasodilator (nicotinyl alcohol), and in extreme circumstances to have a sympathectomy performed.

Venous Insufficiency

What is the symptom that will suggest venous insufficiency?

Ankle edema, since venous insufficiency occurs in the legs, mostly.

Regularly accompanying symptoms, which usually occur at a later stage:

At times, discomfort is noted after standing for long periods.

Varicosities may develop.

There may be pain (mostly if ulceration is present).

There may be itching, due to eczema, with intense oozing.

Skin changes will occur in most instances: atrophy, thin and shiny; cyanotic with a brownish pigmentation; subcutaneous fibrosity and ulceration from stasis.

Avoid confusion with the following:

Edema from heart failure (this has a history of heart disease, while venous insufficiency has a history of thrombophlebitis).

Edema from renal disease (more diffuse).

Pure varicosities (there is no history of thrombophlebitis).

Lymphedema, which does not disappear after elevation of the leg.

Management of this form of venous insufficiency:
- Advise rest with elevation of the legs, intermittent elevation of the legs during the day, use of elastic supports.
- Treat all features involved, such as ulceration, dermatitis, varicosities, and the like.

Superior Vena Cava Obstruction

Attitudinal behavior of the patients that may lead to diagnosis:
- They try to stay seated most of the time.
- They avoid lying down as much as possible.
- They avoid bending forward.
- They avoid all sorts of physical exertion.

Superior vena cava obstruction is indicated by what symptoms?
- Edema of the eyelids.
- Dilatation of the cutaneous veins of the upper body.
- General swelling of head and arms, developing at a later stage.
- If congestion is severe, engorged veins and cyanosis.
- Also, in severe cases, possibly some central nervous symptoms.

Search for, as the cause of the obstruction:
- A tumoral mass in the mediastinum (cancer or lymphomas).
- Extensive cancer of the lung.
- Aneurysm of the aortic arch, or constrictive pericarditis.
- Thrombophlebitis (mostly propagated from neighboring veins).
- Chronic fibrotic mediastinitis (mostly tuberculous).

Management of superior vena cava obstruction:
- Treat the cause, whenever present.
- Discuss convenience of surgery.

Varicosities (Veins)

The objective evidence of varicosities is:
- Mainly noted in the legs; there will be enlarged and tortuous veins, generally with localized dilated sacs bulging from the affected ones at the length of their course.

Symptomatology of varicose veins:
- Varicosities of the legs are better noted on standing.
- Obese people may present hidden varicosities (special procedures for detection).
- Symptoms are as in venous insufficiency, q.v., in the above entry.

The Trendelenburg's test—how to proceed, and what to find:
- With the patient on the bed, elevate the leg; varicosities will empty immediately.
- Place a tourniquet around the thigh; ask the patient to stand, and if there is a slow filling of the long saphenous vein, the valves close to the saphenousfemoral junction are incompetent; but if the filling is rapid, the communication of superficial and profound veins is incompetent.
- After releasing the tourniquet, in the first instance, a rapid filling of the veins from above confirms the incompetence; in the second instance, an increase in filling will confirm the incompetence, but if not, the valves in the saphenousfemoral junction are competent.

Secondary varicosities are usually due to:
- Chronic venous insufficiency.
- Arteriovenous fistula, often with bruit and thrill.
- Retroperitoneal vein obstruction.
- Malformations.

Management of varicosities:
- Use of elastic stockings.
- Surgical approach, including sclerotherapy.

Phlebitis and Thrombophlebitis

Discuss words related to this topic:

Phlebitis	Inflammation of the vein wall.
Thrombophlebitis	Same as above, but with the added formation of a thrombus.
Phlebothrombosis	Formation of a thrombus, but with minimal or absent inflammation.
Phlebolithiasis	The formation of phleboliths or vein stones.
Phlebosis	Irritation of a nonseptic character of a vein; nonseptic inflammation.
Phlebostasis	Ratardation of the blood flow of a vein.

Frequency of evident symptomatology of thrombophlebitis:
- Only about half of the cases will present evident symptomatology; the other half may be diagnosed because of pulmonary embolism.

The symptoms in thrombophlebitis, when present, will show:
- There is local pain of the leg, where practically all these cases occur.
- The character of the pains varies from a dull ache to severe intensity.
- The pain increases on walking, but some patients will feel worse pain while standing and are more comfortable while walking.
- Pain notably improves on rest.
- Dorsiflexion of the foot causes pain (Homan's sign).
- There is swelling of the calf, with tenderness and induration or spasm of the muscles.
- The affected leg appears warm.
- There is other evidence of skin changes, as in venous insufficiency, q.v., above.
- Fever and tachycardia may be present.

Do not mistake thrombophlebitis for:
- Cellulitis.
- Diseases of the heart, liver, or kidney, with bilateral edema.
- Lymphangitis.
- Arterial occlusion.
- Strain or contusions to the calf muscles.

In cases of thrombophlebitis be on the alert for:
- Embolism (in the lungs).

Measures that will be followed to prevent thromboembolism:
- Special care before and after surgery.

Management of thrombophlebitis:
- Positional care, and elastic stockings.
- Anticoagulation.
- Fibrinolytic drugs for thrombolysis.
- Discussion of convenient surgery.

Lymphangitis

Lymphangitis usually follows a previous attack of:
- Cellulitis.
- An infection caused by a hemolytic streptococcus.

What are the common symptoms of lymphangitis?
- Red streaks spreading from the area of cellulitis.
- Symptoms of infection, generally developing rapidly (fever mostly with chills, tachycardia, sweating, anorexia, etc.).

Management of lymphangitis:
- Local measures and the specific antibiotic.

Lymphadenitis

The characteristic symptoms of lymphadenitis:
- Regional lymph nodes are enlarged.
- Lymphadenopathy is usually painful.
- Lymphangitis precedes the attack of lymphadenitis.

Management of lymphadenitis:
- Essentially the same as for lymphangitis, q.v., in the above entry.

Lymphedema

The impairment of lymph flow that occurs in lymphedema is noted by:
- Soft and pitting edema enlarging one of the extremities.
- At a later stage the edema becomes nonpitting and firm.
- In the long run, the extremity becomes enormous (elephantiasis).
- Frequently, multiple infections develop in this area.
- There is no pain, except for the recurrent infections.
- The regular forms of infection are cellulitis and lymphangitis.

Preceding lymphedema, there may be:
- A congenital abnormality.
- A hereditary form, also known as Milroy's disease.
- Abnormal lymph vessels in pubertal females (lymphedema praecox).
- Filariasis.
- Interference with lymph flow (surgical, radiological, recurrent lymphangitis).

Do not mistake it for:
- Lipodystrophy.
- Stasis dermatitis.
- Lymphangiomas or hemangiomas.

Management of lymphedema:
- Low-sodium diet, diuretics, graded compression.
- Surgery.

3. Gastrointestinal Diseases

Reflux Esophagitis

The outstanding symptom of reflux esophagitis is:

Pyrosis, the burning sensation felt from the epigastrium to the pharynx, also called heartburn, which is accompanied by sour eructations.

How is this sensation of pyrosis or heartburn characterized?

It is usually severe, more intense in the recumbent position, relieved by sitting or standing, and generally starts after eating.

It is accompanied by actual pain, felt at the lower tip of the sternum or upper epigastrium.

This pain radiates to the back (interscapular area), neck, arms, or jaw.

Sour eructation results from the reflux of gastric contents, which may reach the pharynx and cause sialorrhea.

Other symptoms of reflux pharyngitis are:

Not only dysphagia, but also odynophagia is noted when there is a spasmodic component involved, or there are ulcers, etc.

Hematemesis or melena may also be present in a few cases.

Regurgitation may be present at night, with cough and dyspnea if aspiration occurs.

What is the cause of reflux esophagitis?

Hiatal hernia, which because of the reflux from the stomach contents becomes symptomatic.

Do not confuse reflux esophagitis with:

Peptic ulcer.

Coronary insufficiency.

Management of reflux esophagitis:

Reduce intra-abdominal pressure, if it exists.

Patient should avoid going to bed immediately after eating.

He should sleep at night with the head elevated.

Recommend antacids.

Consider surgery in selected cases.

Esophageal Diverticulosis

Zenker's diverticulum in the pharyngoesophageal area is noted by:

Nocturnal coughing and halitosis.

Dysphagia with regurgitation.

Gargling sounds.

When this diverticulum is filled with food it provokes:

A swelling noted at one side of the neck.

Esophageal compression (ordinarily from behind), which makes swallowing very difficult in some instances.

As a final consequence, weight loss.

If the diverticula are mideosphageal in location, the symptoms will be:

Absent in most instances.

In some cases, dysphagia.

On rare occasions, esophagobronchial fistulas or mediastinal abscesses.

If the diverticula are immediately above the diaphragm, located in the lower portion of the esophagus, what will the symptoms be?

There will be mild or no symptoms.

In later stages they will produce dysphagia and possibly pain.

Achalasia and pulmonary complications may occur.

Clarify the diagnosis, ruling out:

Esophageal ulcer (epiphrenic diverticula).

Tumors, particularly malignant ones.

Other esophageal diseases.

Management of esophageal diverticula:

Surgery.

Esophageal Stricture

What are the two main symptoms of esophageal stricture?

Dysphagia, particularly related to solid foods, not to liquids.

True odynophagia or just a sensation of a "hang-up" of food.

When these symptoms appear:

Relatively soon after the initial cause (caustics), or years later.

What are the frequent causes of esophageal strictures?

Reflux esophagitis.

Infections of bacterial or viral etiology.

Ingestion of caustic substances.

How to manage esophageal strictures:
Dilation.
If dilation fails, surgery.

Achalasia of the Esophagus

Failure to relax the smooth muscle fibers at the lower portion of the esophagus together with an impaired coordination of peristalsis is noted by:
Dysphagia, not usually accompanied by chest pain.
Regurgitation, which may be the cause of symptoms of aspiration.
Marked dilatation of the upper segment of the esophagus, which ordinarily takes a sigmoid form.
Symptoms of esophagitis caused by stasis of food in the esophagus.
Patient spontaneously helping the passage of food by drinking plenty of water and performing the Valsalve's manuever.
Frequent symptoms of malnutrition.
Why esophagoscopy has to be performed on these patients:
To check the degree of esophagitis and rule out cancer.
Management of achalasia of the esophagus:
Surgical procedures (dilation, esophagocardiomyotomy).

Esophageal Abnormalities

What are the most common abnormalities noted?
Lower esophageal ring.
Esophageal cysts.
Esophageal webs, alone or with iron anemia (Plummer-Vinson syndrome).
What are the clinical symptoms and management of the *esophageal ring*?
There is dysphagia, if the ring sufficiently reduces the lumen.
The ring must be dilated.
What are the clinical symptoms and management of *esophageal cysts*?
Some cases are asymptomatic.
Some cases may cause dysphagia, dyspnea, cyanosis, cough, or pain.
Most need surgical excision because they may secrete acid.
What are the clinical symptoms and management of *esophageal webs*?
There is dysphagia, at times with laryngospasm.
Esophagoscopy may disrupt the web.
Plummer-Vinson syndrome is diagnosed by the following symptoms:
Frequent evidence of atrophic esophagitis and pharyngitis.
Esophageal webs.
Glossitis.
Spooning of the nails.
Splenomegaly.
Other symptoms of iron anemia.
The great majority of patients are menopausal women.
Plummer-Vinson syndrome should be treated by:
Iron therapy.

Tumors of the Esophagus

Tumors of the esophagus present the following clinical symptomatology:
Progressive dysphagia.
Progressive chest pain, unrelated to eating.
Weight loss.
The final diagnosis depends on special examinations.
Management of these tumors will be:
Surgical or by irradiation.

Acute Gastritis

The most frequent causes of acute gastritis are:
Bacterial or viral infections.
Toxins or other irritants.
Allergy.
The regular symptoms of this common disease are:
Complication of enteritis, thus presenting a clinical picture of gastroenteritis.
Anorexia, the outstanding symptom.
Nausea and vomiting.
Colicky diarrhea.
Epigastric fullness and tenderness on pressure.
Fever, chills, headache, if the cause is a toxin or an infection.
Hemorrhage (melena), with irritant substances.
Dehydration and prostration, in some cases (vomiting, diarrhea).
Management of this occurrence:
Correct electrolyte disturbances, if necessary.
Advise gastric rest, sedatives, and a cautious return to normal feeding.
For corrosive gastritis (corrosive symptoms noted in the mouth) an emergent treatment will be supportive, and the correspondent antidote will be given.

Chronic Gastritis

The symptoms of chronic gastritis are:
Very few or none, in most cases.
Anorexia, nausea, vomiting, and specific food tolerance.
Epigastric sensation of fullness, and mild tenderness on pressure.
Pyrosis, and other symptoms as in peptic ulcer.
Management of chronic gastritis should be:
Similar to that of peptic ulcer, q.v., below.
Those cases associated with pernicious anemia or iron deficient anemia will respond well to treatment of the anemic condition.

Acute Gastroenteritis

This disease, usually due to factors similar to those of acute gastritis, presents a similar but more acute symptomatology, such as:

- Sudden onset, with malaise and prostration.
- Anorexia, nausea, vomiting, and diarrhea.
- Abdominal crampy pains, frequently with rectal tenesmus.
- Abdominal tenderness on pressure, more marked in the lower parts, with muscle guarding when the disease results are severe.
- Abdominal distention, with audible borborygmi.
- Diarrhea possibly containing mucus and blood.
- Possibly fever, particularly in cases of infectious origin.
- Fluid loss may lead to dehydration (check for hypokalemia).

Diseases that may present a similar clinical picture are:

- Surgical cases presenting the so-called acute abdomen.

General treatment of acute gastroenteritis:

- Correct electrolytic balance, and proceed as in acute gastritis, q.v., above.
- In case of food infection, give an antibiotic.

Anachlorhydria

There are no symptoms corresponding to anachlorhydria; how will it be suspected?

- Because of the symptoms of the causative disease.

More frequent diseases causing hypo- or anachlorhydria are:

- Pernicious anemia.
- Sprue, and pellagra.
- Parasitic infections.
- Tuberculosis, chronic alcoholism, chronic nephritis.
- Hyperthyroidism.
- Other chronic debilitating diseases.

Hyperchlorhydria

Hyperchlorhydria is best diagnosed by laboratory means, but there are some symptoms that may suggest the problem:

- Pyrosis, which appears late after eating and is alleviated by ingestion of food and, of course, by the use of alkaline agents.
- Occasional tenderness on the epigastric area.
- Good or even increased appetite.
- Constipation, not too rarely.

Causes that should be treated to avoid hyperchlorhydria:

- The ingestion of irritant food.
- Food to which the patient is sensitive; should be avoided.
- Specific medications and toxic substances; should be avoided.

Dyspepsia

Impaired digestion expresses its discomfort by presenting:

- Nausea.
- More or less profuse meteorism, including aerophagia.
- Accompanying weakness, vertigo, and sweating.
- Pyrosis, and belching.
- Possibility of headache and other neurotic symptoms.

There are several diseases accompanied by dyspepsia; the most important are:

- Chronic gastritis, and most gastric diseases.
- Reflux esophagitis.
- Cardiac failure and chronic renal diseases.
- Tuberculosis, jaundice, migraine, coronary insufficiency.
- Enteropathies and liver diseases.

Management of dyspepsia:

- Eat moderate amounts of food, and slowly.
- Treat the basic cause of dyspepsia.
- Treat symptomatically: nausea (chlorpromazine), meteorism (bethanechol), constipation (bulk laxatives).

Gastric Ulcer

Symptoms of hyperchlorhydria may or may not accompany peptic ulcer; other symptom may occur:

- Epigastric or left subcostal area presents the known "hunger pains" or merely some burning, aching, etc.
- These symptoms appear earlier than in pure hyperchlorhydria.
- Similarly, the symptoms are relieved by alkaline agents, food, or vomiting.
- Nausea and vomiting are not rare.
- Constipation and weight loss are also possible symptoms.
- Exacerbations and remissions occur.

Care will be taken to rule out:

- Gastric cancer.

Care will be taken to watch for hemorrhage, penetration, perforation, or obstruction:

- Hemorrhage produces sudden weakness, dizziness, thirst, wet skin, and other evidence of shock, possibly with low blood pressure.
- Penetration is noted by pain radiating to the back, little help after the ingestion of alkalies or food, and frequently a previous history of peptic ulcer.
- Perforation causes an acute abdomen, with pain that may recede and then increase again; muscle guarding appears later.
- Obstruction is noted by copious vomiting, particularly after meals.

Management of peptic ulcer:

- Diet, antacids, and sedatives may be used.
- For hemorrhage give blood, treat shock, give symptomatic medication, and discuss with surgeon the convenience of surgery.
- Penetration and perforation may need surgery.
- Obstruction may be treated medically (gastric decompression and ulcer therapy) or surgically.

Duodenal Ulcer

The symptoms of duodenal ulcer are practically the same as for gastric ulcer, but there may be some differences, such as:

Distress worsening as the day progresses and reaching its peak at midnight.

Vomiting of acid juice with little or no food retained.

Final diagnosis made by X-ray or endoscopy.

Zollinger-Ellison Syndrome

When a gastrin-secreting tumor is located in the pancreas, the spleen, regional lymph nodes, or the gastrointestinal submucosa, the symptoms that characterize the Zollinger-Ellison syndrome are:

Those of a very severe typical peptic ulcer.

Symptoms that respond very badly to regular medical care.

Frequent diarrhea.

Also, frequent episodes of hemorrhage, perforation, or obstruction.

Management of this situation will be:

Surgical.

Jejunal Ulcer

Following an operation for peptic ulcer, the symptoms of a newly formed jejunal ulcer will be:

The typical ulcer pain is located at a lower position, is felt in a larger area, and radiates to the back.

The pain occurs earlier than in other types of ulcers, and the relief from food or medication is shorter.

They occur more frequently, as hematemesis, nausea, vomiting, and weight loss.

Muscle guarding and an inflammatory mass are usually noted on palpation.

Management of this situation is:

Surgical.

Acute Gastric Dilation

The accumulation of large quantities of gas in the stomach because of loss of its tonus may be due to:

Previous surgical procedures (if nasogastric suction is not used).

Severe myocardial infarction.

Injuries of considerable intensity, including prolonged labor.

Upper mesenteric thrombosis.

Other severe conditions.

What are the usual symptoms that follow?

First, fullness; then, pain.

Persistent regurgitation or vomiting of bile-stained fluid.

Distention and tympanism of the upper abdomen.

Hematemesis in later stages.

Dyspnea.

Thirst and symptoms of dehydration (including alkalosis, tetany).

Shock.

This condition will be suspected when a bed patient with a considerable abdominal distention vomits large amounts of fluid.

What is the difference with high intestinal obstructions?

Borborygmi will be heard in obstruction.

Management of acute gastric dilation:

Constant mild suction from the stomach, and restoration of electrolyte balance.

Hiatal Hernia

What are the characteristics of hiatal hernia?

The same as for reflux esophagitis, q.v., at the beginning of this chapter.

Gastric Tumors

What are the main symptoms of benign gastric tumors?

Most are symptomless.

If large, they may produce fullness or obstruction.

They may cause gastrointestinal hemorrhage.

An epigastric mass may be touched.

What are the main symptoms of malignant tumors?

All are symptomless in the early stages of the disease.

There may be any type of upper gastrointestinal symtom, accompanied by weight loss.

A dislike for meat ordinarily develops.

Hematemesis may occur.

Diarrhea may occur, not rarely with melena.

There may be symptoms of peptic ulcer, even with some relief with antacids.

There may be symptoms of esophageal or pyloric obstruction (the first, progressive dysphagia and regurgitation; the second, stomach fullness and vomiting of recently ingested food).

How the final differentiation will be made:

By X-ray studies and endoscopic biopsy, including direct cytology.

Management of gastric tumors:

For benign tumors, use surgery only when needed.

For malignant tumors, the only hope is an early resection.

Gastrointestinal Hemorrhage

Symptoms that may lead to the diagnosis of gastrointestinal hemorrhage:

Sudden faintness or dizziness.

Sudden weakness.

Sudden chills and moistening of the skin.

Thirst.

Desire to defecate, and passage of bloody stools.

Other symptoms of shock, including low blood pressure, and tachycardia.

What are the common diseases that cause gastrointestinal hemorrhage?

Peptic ulcer.

Gastric tumors, usually malignant.

Chronic or acute gastritis or gastroenteritis.

Enteric and colonic diseases.

Other general diseases, including hypertension, liver diseases, and any cause of acute abdomen.

Disorders due to drugs (aspirin, alcohol).

Management of gastrointestinal hemorrhages:

General care and observation.

Blood replacement.

Symptomatic medication.

Consider emergent operation.

Gastric or Enteric Perforation

Symptoms that will force one to consider perforation:

There is a sudden onset of acute sharp pain.

There is a more insidious onset, particularly for enteric perforation (typhoid, etc.).

The patient usually stays very quiet.

The pain may spread to the right shoulder or the lower quadrant (stomach).

The pain may recede for a while.

There is marked muscle guarding.

Symptoms of shock will develop; also symptoms of peritonitis.

Management of perforations:

Surgical.

Regional Enteritis (Crohn's Disease)

Characteristic traits of regional enteritis will be:

Exacerbations and remissions.

This regional enteritis, ileitis, or enterocolitis presents the following symptoms:

An insidious onset, in most cases.

General symptomatology of fever (low or with chills), malaise, weight loss, and the aspect of a chronically ill patient.

Anorexia, flatulence, and intermittent crises of diarrhea.

Pain in the right lower quadrant of the abdomen.

The character of the pain steady or colicky, mild or severe.

Symptoms increasing with milk or irritating foods.

Tenderness and perhaps a mass in the right lower quadrant, revealed by palpation.

The general course mild or severe.

Frequently, fistulas.

From what diseases must it be differentiated?

Appendicitis.

Intestinal tuberculosis.

Ulcerative colitis.

Other infections of the colon.

Regional enteritis will be treated as follows:

General care.

Sulfonamides, ampicillin, or tetracyclines.

Corticosteroids (toxic and diffuse types of the disease).

Surgery.

Appendicitis

This frequent cause of acute abdomen will show the following symptoms:

There is initial epigastric or periumbilical pain, with vomiting, and fever.

In a few hours the pain will shift to the right lower quadrant of the abdomen, and be aggravated by walking, coughing, or palpation.

One precise painful point is elicited by palpation.

The pain is felt in the MacBurney area, or at any other of the commonly reactive zones according to the direction of the appendix.

Rebound pain is also noted.

Muscle guarding is present.

Peristalsis diminishes or becomes absent.

Anorexia, nausea, and constipation are almost always present.

In old age, symptomatology may be deceiving.

Complications that should be watched for:

Perforation.

Peritonitis that follows perforation.

Other forms of abscess (in the appendix, subphrenic, pylephlebitis).

Other diseases that present similar symptomatology are:

Meckel's diverticulitis.

Acute gastroenteritis.

Regional enteritis.

Salpingitis.

Mesenteric adenitis.

The procedure of choice for treating appendicitis is:

Surgery.

Pseudomembranous Enterocolitis

The most frequent conditions preceding pseudomembranous enterocolitis are:

Vascular collapse or shock (myocardial infarction).

Important traumas, including surgery.

Severe diseases treated with broad-spectrum antibiotics.

Symptoms that will call attention to pseudomembranous enterocolitis are:

Sudden onset, with high fever and prostration.

Profuse and watery diarrhea, with serumlike aspect and necrotic odor.

Diarrhea possibly becomming bloody.

Abdominal distention.

Symptoms of dehydration rapidly following diarrhea of 10 or more liters a day.

Hypotension, tachycardia, and shock.

Oliguria.
The rectal mucosa possibly also involved.

Treatment to be advised:
- Correct shock and dehydration.
- Discontinue antibiotics.
- Give vancomycin orally or intravenously (for the staphylococcic type of the disease), either alone or with a penicillinase-resistant penicillin.
- For other cases use cephalotin, intravenously.

Meckel's Diverticulitis

When this form of diverticulitis occurs, what are the main symptoms?
- In acute diverticulitis, they are identical with appendicitis.
- Symptoms may be of perforation, intussusception, or ulceration.

The advisable treatment will be:
- Surgical.

Whipple's Disease

This rare malabsorption disorder is noted by:
- Insidious onset.
- Abdominal pain and fever.
- Diarrhea, with steatorrhea and bleeding.
- Enlarged lymph noted.
- Signs of polyarthritis.
- Skin changes (edema, hyperpigmentation)

An advisable form of treatment will be:
- A tetracycline or oral penicillin, for about 6 months.

Intestinal Tuberculosis

Symptoms of this form of tuberculosis will be:
- Almost always secondary to pulmonary tuberculosis.
- In some patients, minimal symptomatology, or none.
- Fever.
- Gastrointestinal symptoms (anorexia, nausea, food intolerance, discomfort after eating, meteorism, abdominal pain, and diarrhea).

Treatment should be:
- As for tuberculosis.

See page 42 for additional information.

Mesenteric Vascular Insufficiency

Symptoms of acute mesenteric occlusion are:
- Abdominal pain of severe intensity and sudden onset (rarely, the onset will be gradual), steady or colicky.
- Nausea with vomiting, rarely with blood.
- Diarrhea, usually with blood; abdominal distention.
- Prostration, anxiety, and other symptoms of shock.
- Borborygmi, which may be heard but will disappear lately.
- Late symptoms of peritonitis, with tenderness and rigidity.

The usual diseases that provoke this accident are:
- Endocarditis, congestive heart failure, or shock.
- Diseases that may cause embolism.
- Recent surgery in the abdomen.
- Acute abdominal diseases.
- Diseases of the liver or the spleen.

Advised therapy for these patients:
- Restore fluid and electrolyte balance.
- Give antibiotics or any agent to prevent infection.
- Discuss surgery.

Acute Mesenteric Lymphadenitis

This disease, most frequently affecting children, will present:
- Sudden onset of pain in the appendicular or periumbilical area.
- The pain steady and the area tender to palpation.
- Relatively elevated fever in most instances.
- Anorexia, nausea, and vomiting.
- Diarrhea, in some cases.
- Peritoneal irritation may be very mild or totally absent.

Rule out carefully the following diseases:
- Appendicitis or Meckel's diverticulitis.
- Right lower lobe pulmonary infections.
- Renal colic, or infections.

Is there any treatment for this disease?
- No treatment is needed.

Intestinal Obstruction

Organic obstruction, due to physical causes, follows:
- Hernia (external or internal), and volvulus.
- Surgically provoked adhesions, and foreign bodies.
- Neoplasms, and granulomatous diseases.
- Intussusception.
- Gallstones.

Pseudo-obstruction, not due to any mechanical cause, can be due to:
- Congestive heart failure.
- Pneumonia.
- Pancreatitis.
- Spinal injury.
- Renal failure or electrolyte imbalance.

If pseudo-obstruction follows a chronic course, it may be due to:
- Endocrine disorders (myxedema, hyper- or hypoparathyroidism).
- Sprue, amyloidosis.
- Scleroderma, myotonia distrophica, Hirschsprung's disease.
- Chagas' disease.
- Disorders of the autonomic nervous system.

Adynamic or paralytic ileus is associated with:
- Abdominal surgery.
- Peritoneal irritation of any cause (infectious, hemorrhagic, etc.).
- Vertebral fractures and spinal cord injuries.

Pneumonia and other severe infections.
Diabetic coma.
Renal colic and uremia.

Symptoms of organic obstruction:
There are pain and distention.
Pain is colicky in character and set at the periumbilical area.
Pain becomes more constant and more diffuse with increasing distention.
Distention is diffuse, but may be localized to a loop.
Distention is greater as time passes.
Distention is greater as it localizes at a lower segment.
There are audible borborygmi together with visible peristalsis.
Local signs of hernia, intussusception, tumors, or the like may be present.

Symptoms of pseudo-obstruction are:
Abdominal pain, of the crampy type.
Abdominal distention.
Vomiting, diarrhea, and weight loss.
Exacerbations and remissions, which are characteristic.

Symptoms of paralytic ileus are:
Continuous pain and very severe constipation (practically, no stools are passed).
Very severe abdominal distention, with no audible bowel sounds.
Vomiting, which will turn fecal in character; dehydration will follow.
Evidence of the causative factor.

Treatment advisable for these cases:
Surgery.
Treatment of the causative factor.

Intestinal Tumors

Symptoms of benign tumors:
Most of them are asymptomatic.
Some may present obstruction (lipomas).
Some may bleed (angiomas, leiomyomas).
Multiple polyposis with mucocutaneous pigmentation constitutes the *Peutz-Jeghers syndrome.*
Colonic polyposis with soft tissue tumors and osteomas constitutes the *Gardner's syndrome* (watch for malignant changes).

Symptoms of malignant tumors are:
Obstruction.
Hemorrhage.
A mass that may be palpated.

Symptoms of the *carcinoid syndrome* are:
Vasomotor symptoms, particularly attacks of flushing.
Recurrent attacks of diarrhea with abdominal pain.
Symptoms of disease of the right valvule of the heart.

Management of these conditions should be:
Surgical in most instances.
If the carcinoid syndrome is not operated in time, corticoids.

Mucous Colitis or Irritable Colon

Symptomatic manifestations of irritable colon:
Patients are usually anxious.
Symptoms vary form case to case.
There is abdominal distention.
There are abdominal cramps at the left side, or the right iliac fossa.
The pain is sharp in character and may resemble appendicitis.
Discomfort is usually relieved after defecation or passing flatus.
There is constipation, with small or ill-shaped stools.
Diarrheic stools occasionally compensate constipation.
Stools usually contain large amounts of mucus.
Hemorrhoids are usually present.
There is matinal gastrointestinal discomfort.
On palpation, a contracted colon is usually felt.
Patients do not look ill.

Management of mucous colitis or spastic colon will be:
Reassurance of the patient.
Bland diet.
Symptomatic treatment of colonic symptoms.
Treatment of the anxious patient.

Chronic Ulcerative Colitis

The outstanding symptomatology of ulcerative colitis is:
Low abdominal cramps and bloody diarrhea.

What are the other symptoms of the disease?
The above symptoms may be mild or very severe in character.
The diarrhea is bloody and also mucous.
The number of discharges may vary from a few up to 40 a day.
Only blood and mucus are passed on some occasions.
Constipation may occur instead; but there will be blood and mucus.
Anal incontinence may occur.
Anal tenesmus may reach disturbing proportions.
The abdominal pain, crampy in character, rarely is severe.
Febricula or moderate fever will be present.
Anorexia, with weight loss, is usually present.
Asthenia and a general malaise are mostly present.
Abdominal distention may be noted and, if it accompanies fulminant cases, represents an ominous sign.
There is abdominal tenderness, not too severe.
There is intolerance to milk products.

Complications to watch for are:
Hemorrhage.
Rectovaginal fistulas.
Cancer (intestinal, biliary tract).
Other extracolonic complications.

Ulcerative colitis is differentiated from:
Dysentery.
Regional enteritis.

Diverticulitis.
Lymphogranuloma venereum, neoplasms, functional diarrhea.

Management of ulcerative colitis:
Bed rest and general care.
Corticosteroid therapy.
Sulfisoxazole or sulfasalazine.
Surgery.

Granulomatous Colitis

Granulomatous colitis, clinically almost identical with ulcerative colitis, may be differentiated by the following features, besides the most accurate distinction given by pathologic findings:
Bleeding is more rare in this condition.
Fistulas and perforation are more frequent in granulomatous colitis.
Only a very few cases will present symptoms of toxicity.
Perirectal disease may be present even before the development of other symptoms.
There is frequent symptomatology of spondylitis, periarthritis, or erythema nodosum.

Management of granulomatous colitis:
Same as for ulcerative colitis, q.v., above.

Ischemic Proctocolitis

This consequence of infarction of the colon or the rectum presents the following symptomatology:
Sudden onset of lower abdominal pain.
Defecation of pure blood or clots.
Fever and vomiting.
Gangrene in severe cases.

Management of ischemic proctocolits:
Blood replacement.
Antibiotics.
Surgery.
No treatment for milder cases.

Hirschsprung's Disease (Congenital Megacolon)

Stools in congenital magacolon will show the following characteristics:
They will be passed every 4 weeks or more.
Stools are of very large volume.
Stools present a very offensive smell.
There is poor response to cathartics (somewhat better to enemas).

The abdomen will present the following aspect:
Distention to extremely large bulk.
Thinning of the walls, with separation of the anterior muscles.
Visible peristalsis (sluggish movements), and audible borborygmi.
Palpable masses (fecal, bowel loops) through the abdominal walls.

Other symptoms accompanying this disease:
Projecting ribs.
Dyspnea due to pressure of the abdominal contents.
Abdominal hernias.
Edema of the lower extremities.
Poor nutrition and retarded growth.

Management of megacolon:
Avoid high-residue diets; give softeners and lubricants, enemas, and drugs of the acetylcholine or physostigmine type.
Perform surgery in more severe cases.

Toxic Megacolon

The symptoms will be presented by any of the following diseases, which may be watched for its developing:
Ulcerative colitis.
Crohn's disease.
Gastrointestinal diseases of the type of amebiasis, cholera, typhoid fever, and dysentery.

Symptoms of toxic dilatation of the colon are:
Fever, and symptoms of toxicity.
Tachycardia.
Abdominal distention due to colonic dilatation.

Treatment of dilatation of the colon:
Tube for colonic decompression.
Restoration of electrolyte balance, particularly checking for potassium.
Corticosteroids and antibiotics.
Careful observation to determine the convenience or not of surgical procedures.

Diverticulosis

How are these frequent colonic diverticula diagnosed?
There is no symptomatology, in most instances.
They are diagnosed when they are coincidental with other diseases, or because of some other form of special examination.

Management of diverticulosis:
There is none if there are no symptoms.
Treat coincidental disease, if any.
Recommend that patient drink plenty of liquids.

Diverticulitis

When the diverticula are infected, what are the symptoms to be noted?
Acute pain, usually located in the left side of the abdomen.
Symptoms similar to those of appendicitis ("left-sided appendicitis").
Abdominal distention, with some tenderness and muscle guarding on the affected site; frank induration, and palpation of a mass in the left lower quadrant when there is abscess formation.

Nausea and vomiting.
Constipation, obstipation, diarrhea, or alterning diarrhea and constipation.
Fever, with or without chills, and malaise.
Check for developing complications, such as peritonitis, abscess formation, hemorrhage, fistulization, and even irritation of the bladder.

Evolution of the usual cases of diverticulitis:
Localized, with full resolution in a few days.
Intestinal obstruction due to edema or spasm.
Abscess formation, with or without fistulization.
Recurrent attacks of diverticulitis.

Management of diverticulitis:
Chronic or subacute diverticulitis only requires a low-residue diet, local heat, antispasmodics, and stool softeners.
Acute diverticulitis requires bed rest, protection of the bowel, intravenous fluids and electrolytes, analgesics, antispasmodics, and the rational treatment of complications, particularly peritonitis.

Intestinal Polyposis

Intestinal polyposis, setting mostly on the colon and rectum, may give the following symptomatology:
Most of them are asymptomatic and diagnosed only by special examinations.
Some may present acute or chronic blood loss.
Some may present intestinal obstruction.
If they are known to exist, maintain a continuous watch for malignant degeneration.
The Peutz-Jeghers syndrome is characterized by bleeding and skin and mucosal hyperpigmentation; more rarely by hyperpigmentation of the digits of the hands and feet.
Very rarely there are generalized symptoms, like febricula, moderate weight loss, clubbed fingers, and perhaps diarrhea.

Management of intestinal polyposis:
Consider surgery.

Peritonitis

Almost all patients with peritonitis will present a previous history of an abdominal disease, but there may be others, as well; explain:
Perforation or necrosis of the gastrointestinal tract.
Hematogenous or lymphatic dissemination of an infectious disease.
Propagation of an infection of the female genital tract.
Injuries and wounds to the abdomen.
Surgery.
Acute pancreatitis (enzymatic action).

Diagnostic symptoms of peritonitis may be the following:
Abdominal pain.
Other symptoms of fever and toxemia.

Abdominal pain may be characteristic in what sense:
It is a diffuse, severe and constant pain increased by all movements.
The patient remains quiet.
Respirations are shallow.
The maximum of pain is felt over the site of the underlying disease (epigastric, hepatic, appendicular, etc.).
Marked rebound pain on pressure.
Notable muscle spasm.

Other symptoms present in peritonitis are:
Nausea, vomitting, and at times diarrhea.
High fever, usually with chills; finally, symptoms of toxemia.
Tachycardia.
Abdominal distention; and possibility of paralytic ileus.
Shoulder pain, and hiccups.
Symptoms of dehydration and acidosis; final toxic shock.
Keep in mind that elderly patients may have no pain.

Differentiate peritonitis from the following diseases:
Renal colic.
Lower lobe pneumonia.
Gall bladder acute diseases.
Acute intestinal obstruction or hemorrhage.

Management of peritonitis will be:
Continuous gastric suction, intravenous infusions, analgesics, and antibiotics (start with gentamycin or kanamycin).
Surgery at the earlier possible moment.

Tuberculosis of the Gastrointestinal Tract

Tuberculosis of the gastrointestinal tract may be of the ulcerative or the hypertrophic type; what are the principal symptoms of each form?
Symptoms of ulcerative enterocolitis may be crampy pains, abdominal discomfort, and diarrhea.
Symptoms of ulcerative tuberculosis may also resemble appendicitis.
Symptoms of hypertrophic tuberculosis will give symptoms of obstruction together with a palpable mass.

Treatment of gastrointestinal tuberculosis:
The regular antituberculous treatment.

See page 39 for additional information.

Obstruction of the Colon

Explain how to arrive clinically at the diagnosis of colonic obstruction:
Constipation or steady obstipation is the outstanding symptom.
Pain develops gradually.
In case of intensely severe pain, strangulation is to be suspected.
There are abdominal distention and tympanitis.
Borborygmi and bowel sounds are audible.
Palpation of a mass will suggest cancer, strangulation, or intussusception.

In case of perforation there will be peritonitic symptoms.
Nausea and vomiting only appear late in this accident.
Management of colonic obstruction:
Surgical.

Constipation

To what causes is the insufficient voiding of the colon due?
Faulty habits, like sedentarism, incorrect hygiene.
All forms of colitis, particularly those of the chronic type.
Intestinal cancer, and other tumors.
Intestinal tuberculosis or syphilis.
Physical gastrointestinal defects (Hirschsprung's disease, loops, strictures, etc.).
Gynecological and prostatic problems.
Some general diseases, such as hypothyroidism, neurosis, and the like.
Symptomatology of constipation:
There is infrequent or difficult evacuation of the feces, which usually are of a hard consistency.
Diarrhea may alternate with a basic constipation.
The number of depositions is an individual factor, from two a day to one every two or three days.
Management of constipation:
Correct the causative condition.
Use laxatives with caution, and only temporarily.

Impaction

Fecal impaction, usually very hard feces, when collected in the rectum will give the following symptomatology:
There is a clinical picture of constipation, or obstipation.
There are possibly episodes of watery diarrhea.
There may be some blood or mucus noted in the stools.
There is a distended abdomen, with a palpable fecal mass.
Feces may be noted in the rectum by digital examination.
Dislodgement of fecal masses is usually performed:
Digitally.
Sigmoidoscopically.
By colonic irrigations.
At times, by gradual dislodgement (daily oil enemas, digital dislodgement, and saline enemas, for a few days).

Meteorism

Also called flatulence, tympania, tympanism, typanites, or tympany, meteorism refers to the collection of gas in the abdominal cavity, which gives the following symptomatology:
Abdominal dilatation.
Dilatation noted at the central part of the abdomen when the patient is on the bed, and at the upper abdomen when patient is standing up.
On percussion a drumlike sound (tympanism), which is, in fact, a symptom preceding dilation.
Diseases that may cause meteorism are:
Dyspepsia, particularly due to fermentations.
Peritonitis, perhaps the most important cause.
Intestinal obstruction, perhaps second in importance.
Gastric dilatation, and megacolon.
Infectious diseases (typhoid, pneumonia, etc.).
Acidosis.
Other diseases, such as nervous system diseases, vascular diseases, etc.
Management of meteorism:
Treat the basic cause.
Avoid food that may cause fermentation.
In emergent cases use intubation to remove gas.

Diarrhea

What are the symptoms of diarrhea?
Accelerated intestinal transit revealed by identifiable foods.
Increased number of daily depositions.
Soft or liquid character of stools.
What are the most frequent causes of diarrhea?
Acute gastritis, and gastroenteritis.
Not too rarely, the Zollinger-Ellison syndrome.
Gastric tumors.
Intermittent crises in regional enteritis.
Pseudomembranous enterocolitis.
Whipple's disease.
Intestinal tuberculosis.
Mesenteric vascular insufficiency.
Some cases of acute mesenteric lymphadenitis.
Cases of pseudo-obstruction.
Recurrent attacks in the carcinoid syndrome.
Irritable colon, in which occasional attacks may compensate the habitual constipation.
Chronic ulcerative colitis, and granulomatous colitis.
Diverticulitis, where diarrhea may alternate with constipation.
Dysentery and cholera.
Pancreatitis (or there may be constipation).
Salmonellosis and rickettsioses.
Brucellosis, trichinosis, and some of the eruptive fevers.
Psychogenic disorders, and neurological diseases.
Sprue, hyperthyroidism, kwashiorkor, pancreatic insufficiency.
Other diseases, such as allergic syndromes, toxic diseases, etc.
Management of diarrhea:
Treatment of the causative disease.
Correction of changes induced by diarrhea (dehydration, electrolyte imbalance).
Diet and antidiarrheic agents.

Fecal Incontinence

The failure of voluntary control of defecation may be due to:
Injury to the sphincter (homosexuals, surgery, accidental).

Local disease (cancer, rectal prolapsus, etc.).
Cases of severe diarrhea, particularly in ulcerative colitis.
Diseases that may impair neurologic regulation of defecation, such as brain tumor, stroke, diabetes, etc. All cases of mental obnubilation.
Senility.
Congenital anomalies.

Management of fecal incontinency:
Surgery may correct some physical defects.
Whenever possible, treat the causative factor.

Cancer of the Terminal Gastrointestinal Tract

General symptoms of this form of cancer:
Bleeding, the most important symptom (occult or blood in the stools).
Altered customary bowel habit (changes of normal defecation, diarrhea or constipation).

Symptoms of cancer setting on the right colon:
General discomfort progressing to crampy pains.
Occult blood in the stools.
Frequent cases of diarrhea.
Anemia and weight loss.
Palpable mass in the right side of the abdomen.

Symptoms of cancer located in the distal colon:
Possible obstructive symptoms.
Diarrheic bouts; and a small amount of red blood in the stools.
Progressive constipation.
Weight loss.
Palpation of a mass in the left side.

Symptoms of cancer located in the anus:
A painful ulceration is noted.
Bleeding is frequent.

How the final diagnosis can be established:
By special resources (X-ray, sigmoidoscopy, biopsy).

Management or colonic cancer:
Resection, if diagnosed in time.

Sprue

In *tropical sprue* what is the principal symptomatology?
There are foul-smelling, greasy, bulky, frothy, and pale stools.
In the beginning the stools are watery and extremely abundant; thereafter, they turn into the regular type.

In *celiac disease* the principal symptomatology is:
Foul-smelling, soft, pale stools, which are similarly rich in fats.
Symptoms appearing after the ingestion of cereals.

What are the common symptoms, due to *malabsorption*, present in both forms?
Weight loss and deficient developing.
Anemia (of the pernicious type).
Other symptoms of vitamin deficiency (cheilosis, tetany, osteomalacia, hyperkeratosis, peripheral edema, bleeding episodes, hyperpigmented skin, and others).
The progressive course more steady in tropical sprue; may show some quiescent periods in celiac disease.
Also, impaired absorption of glucose, and fats.

A careful distinction should be made to differentiate from:
Tropical sprue from celiac disease, the latter responding very well to a gluten-free diet.
Several malabsorption syndromes, between which jejunal biopsy may give the differential diagnosis.
Diseases due to abnormalities, regional enteritis, Whipple's disease, pancreatic insufficiency, etc.

Management or tropical sprue:
Diet, folic acid (thereafter adding vitamin B_{12}, and a tetracycline.
Supplementation of vitamins.

Management of celiac disease:
A gluten-gliadin-free diet.
Supplementation of vitamins.
Corticosteroids to those who do not respond adequately.

Hemorrhoids

The symptomatology of hemorrhoids (or piles) simply shows:
The external hemorrhoids, which are small rounded masses of a purplish color encircling the anus. These are covered by skin.
The internal hemorrhoids, which are not seen from the outside, but are also small, irregular in shape, and covered by mucosal tissue. These are mostly known because of bleeding.

Other symptoms of hemorrhoids:
There is no pain, except when they are thrombosed; then they also bleed.
When they are thrombosed, there are also tenesmus and pain at defecation.
The external hemorrhoids, after a time, appear as tabs or tags.
The external hemorrhoids may be itchy.
The internal hemorrhoids may prolapse to the outside, which occurrence may be accompanied by thrombosis or strangulation.
The internal hemorrhoids may cause leakage of mucus and itching.

Treatment of hemorrhoids:
Local care, or surgical therapy whenever advisable.

Rectal Prolapse

The protrusion or prolapse of the rectal mucosa through the anus may present:
Incomplete, partial, or mucosal prolapse, with no displacement of the sphincter or anal wall.
A complete prolapse with displacement of the sphincter.
A complete prolapse with no displacement of the sphincter but with herniation of the bowl.

An internal complete prolapse, with intussusception of the upper into the lower part of the rectum; but in this case there is no external prolapse.

Management of rectal prolapse:

Surgical.

Anal Fissure

Regular symptoms of anal fissure:

Acute pain noted during defecation and persisting for a time thereafter.

Streaks of bright red blood tinging the stools.

Voluntary constipation, to avoid pain.

At a later stage, appearance of a hypertrophied papilla, with spasm of the anal sphincter developing (very painful, even to digit examination).

In acute anal fissure, what are the symptoms?

Pain, perhaps less marked, which may disappear if bowels are maintained soft and regular.

Management of anal fissure:

Regulation of defecation habits.

If good results are not obtained, surgery.

Rectal Stricture

Common causes of rectal stricture are:

Congenital.

Traumatic.

Lymphogranuloma venereum or granuloma inguinale.

This fibrotic narrowing of the rectal canal causes what symptoms?

Possible alteration of defecation habits.

Change of form of the stools.

Management of strictures:

Check and correct the cause.

Perform progressive dilatation.

Anal Abscess and Fistula

What is the relation between anal abscess and fistula?

The anal abscess is considered the initial stage of the fistula.

Symptoms of *anal abscess:*

There is a painful red swelling in the border of the anus.

This makes it difficult to walk, to sit, or to defecate.

Internal abscesses (ischiorectal, perirectal) are usually accompanied by fever and present a different symptomatology.

Treatment of the anal abscess:

Incise and drain.

Symptoms of *anal fistula:*

Purulent discharge from the opening of the fistula.

Skin irritation, with local itching and pain.

Discomfort aggravated at defecation.

Recurring abscess formation not too rare.

Management of the anal fistula:

Check the fistula with a probe.

Surgery is the only cure (excise).

Cryptitis and Papillitis

What are the suggestive symptoms of cryptitis and papillitis?

There are pain and burning felt during defecation.

This discomfort is of brief duration, while defecating.

Management of cryptitis and papillitis:

Try mineral oil and suppositories, with local application of phenol.

If this fails, excise crypts and papillae.

Condylomas

The symptoms of anal condylomas are:

A wartlike excrescence growing in the vicinity of the anus.

Usually accompanied by humidity or the discharge of pus.

What is the most important distinction to make?

To differentiate the condition from syphilitic condylomas (dark field or serology).

Management of condylomas:

Treat with podophyllum or electrocoagulation.

Proctitis

The most common causes of inflammation of the rectal mucosa are:

Ulcerative colitis.

Regional iletis.

Lymphogranuloma venereum.

Injury, including foreign bodies.

Several infectious diseases.

Symptomatology of proctitis:

Continuous urge to defecate.

Painful diarrhea, with blood, pus, and mucus.

Continuous rectal discomfort.

Tenesmus felt after defecation.

Other symptoms that may accompany the causative disease (check for local symptoms).

Management of proctitis:

Treatment of the causative factor, when known.

Topical corticosteroids in all instances.

Anal Pruritus

Itching of the anus is felt in what conditions?

Poor hygiene.

Irritation by soaps, clothing, etc.

Local anal diseases.

Intestinal parasites (pinworm).

Other fungal or bacterial infections.

Allergic diseases.

Diabetes, jaundice, uremia, Hodgkin's disease, etc.

The characteristics of anal itching are:

- The urge to scratch is irresistible, although to do so worsens the sensation.
- It worsens at night and by heating.
- There will be skin changes, particularly in most advanced cases (erythema, humidity, excoriations, lichenification, fissuring, etc.).

Management of anal pruritus:

- Treatment of the cause.
- Talc or corticosteroids (this in silicone barrier cream).

4. Diseases of the Liver

Jaundice

When jaundice begins, and when jaundice is seen:

- It begins with a blood concentration of bilirubin over 1.5 mg in each 100 ml.
- It starts to produce symptoms that can be seen when it reaches a bilirubin concentration of 3 mg for each 100 ml.
- Patients with mild jaundice only present the yellowish discoloration visible in the conjunctivae.
- In more advanced cases there is a total yellow discoloration of the skin and the mucosae.
- All types between mild and intense may be noted.

Symptoms that usually accompany jaundice:

- Itching.
- Bradycardia.
- Anorexia, nausea, meteorism, constipation.
- Possibility of bleeding.
- Possible more or less marked nervous depression.
- Hepatomegaly (more marked in retention jaundice) without splenomegaly.
- Coluric, dark urine.
- Acoluric, light-colored stools, only in retention jaundice.
- Other symptoms and sign according to the type of jaundice, such as weakness, malaise, abdominal or back pain, splenomegaly, vascular spiders, asterixis, palmar erythema, ascites, gynecomastia, hairless body, fever, fetor hepaticus, etc.

The principle types of jaundice accepted are:

- Prehepatic, usually hemolytic in character.
- Hepatic, due to a disease affecting hepatic tissue, either congenital or acquired.
- Prosthepatic, due to an extrahepatic retention by obstruction.

Summarized symptoms of prehepatic jaundice:

- Hemolysis, in the first place.
- Weakness.
- Pains with the hemolytic crises.
- Splenomegaly (except in sickle cell anemia).
- No coluric changes of stools and urine.

Summarized symptoms of hepatic acquired jaundice:

- Most of the symptoms usually accompanying jaundice, as listed above.
- Low grade fever.
- Tender hepatomegaly.
- Ascites.
- Hairless body.
- Skin symptoms, besides discoloration, of vascular spiders and palmar erythema.
- Malaise and asterixis.
- Fetor hepaticus.

Summarized symptoms of posthepatic jaundice:

- There are most of the symptoms usually accompanying jaundice, as seen above.
- The jaundice may vary in intensity.
- Discoloration of the stools is of variable intensity.
- There are pain and discomfort on the hepatic area.
- Cancer is suggested by weight loss, blood in stools, and the positivity of Curvoisier's sign or law; that is, there is dilatation of the gall bladder.
- Chills and fever, without gall bladder enlargement, usually indicate stones together with cholangitis.

What other procedures are needed for completion of the diagnosis?

- Laboratory chemistry.
- Percutaneous liver biopsy.
- X-ray studies.
- Liver scanning.

Hepatitis

The general symptoms of hepatitis before the appearance of jaundice:

- There is a flu-like initial symptomatology.
- A less rapid onset may start the disease.
- There are asthenia and generalized pains.
- There is very severe anorexia (an important sign, in disproportion to the apparent disease).
- Upper respiratory and digestive symptoms may occur.
- There is moderate fever.
- Fever improves when jaundice appears.
- Hepatomegaly is noted in about half of the cases.
- There is splenomegaly in a few cases.

The general symptoms during jaundice are:

- Not all the patients develop clinical jaundice (only chemical).
- This phase may occur after 5-10 days of the onset.

Jaundice may appear from the very beginning of the disease.
The present symptoms may worsen when jaundice starts.
Clinical improvement follows.

Diagnosis of the preicteric phase will exclude:
Influenza and upper respiratory diseases.
Initial phase of exanthematous diseases, and other viral diseases.

Diagnosis of the icteric phase will exclude:
Infectious mononucleosis.
Leptospirosis.
Cirrhosis.
Liver amebiasis.
Toxic hepatitis.

The clinical picture of heaptitis A, or infectious hepatitis, usually shows:
A shorter incubation period, one month more or less following contagion.
A relatively sudden onset of symptoms.
The starting symptomatology usually presenting a flu-like syndrome or mimicking a gastroenteritis.
A relatively short clinical course, with subsidence of symptoms.

The clinical picture of hepatitis B, or serum hepatitis, shows:
A long incubation period after transfusion was made.
The onset relatively insidious.
Initial symptomatology that may include fever, skin rash, and joint pains.
A tendency to some sort of chronicity of the clinical picture.

What can be the atypical course of the disease?
Prolonged hepatitis, which may occur in the two types.
Relapsing hepatitis, milder in symptomatology, but which may be repeated.
Cholestatic hepatitis may last almost 1 year, with marked jaundice and itching.
Submassive necrosis runs a very severe course, in almost all the cases with prolonged hepatic coma.
Fulminant hepatitis kills within a few days (fewer than 10 in most instances) in hepatic coma.

Management of viral hepatitis:
Provide good general hygienic care.
Treat symptomatically, avoiding morphine and other toxic drugs or substances.
Use corticosteroids in only the very severe cases.

Hepatic Abscess

The clinical symptoms of hepatic abscess are:
Fever, usually the first to appear.
Pain, also an important sign.
Location of pain: right hypochondrium or epigastrium.
Also, tenderness in the right upper abdomen.
Jaundice, in most cases.
For amebic abscess or amebic hepatitis, see below.

Hepatic abscess is usually preceded by one of the following diseases:
Ascending cholangitis.
Appendicitis.

Treatment of hepatic abscess:
Use antibiotics effective against the gastrointestinal flora, like gentamycin or kanamycin.
If no results are obtained, drain surgically.

Chronic Hepatitis

What are the clinical types of chronic hepatitis?
A benign chronic persistent hepatitis.
A form of active hepatitis usually progressing to cirrhosis, of which there are two types: lupoid hepatitis and the hepatitis with HB_3AG antigen positive.

Symptoms of chronic persistent hepatitis:
No symptoms present, in many cases.
Vague, nonspecific symptoms in other cases (weakness, anorexia).
The diagnosis made only by persistent laboratory findings.

Symptoms of chronic active hepatitis:
Insidious onset, frequently of the clinical type of hepatitis.
Jaundice frequently not present, in spite of elevated bilirubin.
Skin changes, including spider nevi, acne, hirsutism (in females), and cutaneous striae.
Characteristic involvement of several systems, such as skeletal system (arthritis), kidneys, lungs, gastrointestinal system, and blood (anemia).

How the two types of chronic active hepatitis are differentiated:
The lupoid type affects females, and the HB_3Ag type affects males, predominantly.
The presence of the HB_3Ag antigen differentiates the two forms.
Other laboratory evidence is needed for the diagnosis of chronic hepatitis.

Diseases that usually resemble chronic hepatitis are:
Viral hepatitis.
Subacute hepatic necrosis.
Postnecrotic cirrhosis.

Treatment of chronic hepatitis:
Usually no treatment is needed for the benign type.
Use corticosteroids and immunosuppressive agents.

Hepatic Amebiasis

Before hepatic amebiasis develops, what are the common symptoms of amebiasis?
None, only mild gastrointestinal discomfort, or the painful passage of stools with blood and mucus.

Symptoms of amebic hepatitis are as follows:
Discomfort or frank pain in the hepatic area.
The pain spreading toward the right shoulder.

The pain aggravated by motion.
Fever, with chills and sweating.
Nausea, vomiting, and weight loss.
Clinical jaundice of a very mild degree.

Symptoms of amebic abscess are as follows:
Perisistence of symptoms of hepatitis after about one week of treatment.
Tender hepatomegaly, in most cases, but not all.
Final diagnosis made by X-rays or scanning.
Complications may occur as appendicitis or perforation; hematogenous spread of the disease, also.

Treatment of amebic hepatitis:
Metronidazole, diiodohydroxyquin, emetine, and chloroquine are very effective medications. If one fails, use any of the others.

Treatment of hepatic abscess:
Use emetine plus choloroquine, or metronidazole followed by diiodohydroxyquin.
Aspiration is preferable to open drainage, if this procedure is needed.

Alcoholic Hepatitis

Symptoms of alcoholic hepatitis:
There are only symptoms common to other diseases of the hepatobiliary system.
The symptoms may be jaundice, abdominal tenderness with more marked pain in the right upper area, fever, nausea, vomiting, and the usual laboratory findings. "Spiders" and other changes are frequent.
Hepatomegaly with jaundice in a habitual drinker will suggest the disease.
Splenomegaly, ascites, and encephalopathy may also help.
The final diagnosis is given by liver biopsy.

Treatment of alcoholic hepatitis:
General care and hygiene, as for cirrhosis.
Vitamins, particularly folic acid.

Fatty Liver

Conditions preceding fatty liver:
Excessive fat intake (obesity).
Alcoholism, and other toxics, such as yellow phosphorus, chloroform, carbon tetrachloride, tetracyclines, etc.
Disorders of metabolism, such as diabetes, kwashiorkor, Cushing's syndrome, deficient diets (particularly poor for choline and methionine contents).
Chronic infections of the type of tuberculosis.

Resulting symptomatology following fatty deposition in the liver:
Symptoms are identical with those of cirrhosis, amyloidosis, chronic passive congestion of the liver, etc.
A persistently enlarged and tender liver may be suggestive.
Liver biopsy is the only diagnostic procedure of value.

Treatment of fatty liver:
Eliminate the causative factor.
In alcoholism or malnutrition, give a rich protein diet, with vitamins and folic acid.

Cirrhosis

Forms of cirrhosis that are more commonly found in medical practice:
Nodular cirrhosis, of which two forms are prevalent: portal cirrhosis (also called Laennec's cirrhosis) and postnecrotic cirrhosis.
Biliary cirrhosis, of which two forms are prevalent: primary biliary cirrhosis and obstructive biliary cirrhosis.

What are the initial symptoms of *nodular cirrhosis?*
None, or very vague symptomatology.
The onset of symptoms more frequently insidious.
Weight loss, weakness, and asthenia.

Failing liver function symptomatology may be as follows:
Anorexia, nausea, vomiting.
Abdominal discomfort, or pain; hepatomegaly; ascites.
Bleeding tendency (epistaxis, purpura, others).
Diarrhea, or constipation in a few cases.

Other symptoms of nodular cirrhosis:
Amenorrhea in women and impotence in men.
Gynecomastia in men, even testicular atrophy.
Peripheral neuropathy, anemia, parotid hypertrophy, pancreatitis, glossitis, in some patients (alcoholism, malnutrition).

In advanced nodular cirrhosis the symptoms are:
Increased anorexia.
Hematemesis from esophageal varicosities.
Ascites, pleural effusion, or massive edema, which are very important.
Jaundice.
Splenomegaly.
Abdominal collateral veins, and hemorrhoids.

The skin symptomatology will show:
Spider nevus.
Palmar erythema.
Clubbing of fingers and Dupuytren's palmar contraction.

The treatment for nodular cirrhosis should be:
Provide general care and symptomatic measures for diuresis, anemia, hemorrhages, etc.
Treat complication (encephalopathy or coma, etc.), and consider the convenience of surgery, particularly for portal hypertension.

Symptoms of *primary biliary cirrhosis:*
Symptoms are very similar to those of nodular cirrhosis, particularly when the disease is fully developed.
In the first stage there is a gradual onset of jaundice, xanthomatosis, itching, steatorrhea, and an important enlargement of the liver, discomfort over the hepatic area, and other symptoms of jaundice.

In the second stage, after 5 or 10 years of the disease, there will be ascites, peripheral edema, bleeding symptoms, and final coma.
Liver biopsy and percutaneous transhepatic cholangiography are usually needed for a final diagnosis.

Treatment of primary biliary cirrhosis:
There is no treatment available. Treat symptomatically.

Symptoms of *obstructive biliary cirrhosis:*
There is a history of chronic or intermittent jaundice.
The skin takes on a bronze hue.
Fever with chill may occur.
This is nontender hepatomegaly.
There are terminal symptoms of cirrhosis, like ascites, peripheral edema, and generalized bleedings, particularly of the esophageal varicosities.
There are other symptoms of the causative factor of obstruction.

Management of obstructive biliary cirrhosis:
Treat the causative factor of the obstruction.
Provide symptomatic treatment.

Hepatic Coma

This possible ammonia poisoning of the brain starts in the patient with some sort of liver disease (cirrhosis, hepatitis, etc.) with the following symptomatology:
Irritability or confusion, and restlessness.
Asterixis (intermittent lapse of an assumed posture).
Confusion progressing to stupor, finally with true coma supervening.

Management of hepatic coma:
Treat aggressively any of the causative diseases.
Curtail as much as possible protein intake, sedation, and hypokalemia.
During the acute episode, discontinue proteins and give parenteral feeding.
Give neomycin or lactulose to reduce ammonia in the blood.
Treat shock.
Consider the use of corticoids.

Chronic Passive Congestion

This disease, mostly due to cardiac failure, is manifested by:
Symptoms of the previous disease, namely, cardiac failure.
Large, firm, smooth liver, usually tender.
Sensation of discomfort in the hepatic area.
Splenomegaly or jaundice occasionally developing.

Management of passive congestion:
Treat the causative factor, i.e., cardiac failure.

Portal Vein Thrombosis

Diseases usually preceding portal vein thrombosis:
Local infection.
Cirrhosis.
Tumors.

Symptoms presented during vein thrombosis:
Symptoms of the active causative disease.
Sudden midabdominal pain.
Nausea, vomiting, and hematemesis.
Ascites, which may develop in a number of cases, not all.
In severe cases, paralytic ileus, collapse, and death.
All symptoms may be mild or even absent in cases that develop slowly.

Management of portal vein thrombosis:
Surgery: portacaval anastomosis.

Hepatic Vein Thrombosis

Diseases usually preceding hepatic vein thrombosis:
Hepatic cirrhosis or tumor.
Thrombophlebitis migrans.
Pylephlebitis, or the use of contraceptives.
Polycythemia vera.

Symptoms prevalent with hepatic vein thrombosis:
Evidence of some of the above factors.
Rapidly developing hepatomegaly, with evidence of hepatic failure.
Massive ascites, also rapidly developing.
Jaundice, not too intense.
Splenomegaly and collateral veins in the abdomen, if the patient survives the acute attack, since death is a frequent occurence.

Management of hepatic vein thrombosis:
Anticoagulants.
Surgical approach: portacaval shunt, which has been successful in some cases.

Hyperbilirubinemia Conditions

Having a similar clinical pictures to hepatitis, surgical jaundice, and hemolytic disease are:
Gilbert's syndrome, or constitutional hepatic dysfunction.
Crigler-Najjar syndrome.
Dubin-Johnson syndrome, or familial chronic idiopathic jaundice.
Rotor's syndrome.
Benign intermittent cholestasis.
Recurrent jaundice of pregnancy.

Symptoms of *Gilbert's syndrome* and its management:
Hereditary jaundice.
Asymptomatic and benign.
No treatment needed.

Symptoms of *Crigler-Najjar syndrome* and its treatment:
Hereditary jaundice of neonates.
Kernicterus, characterizing its type I; no treatment available.
Milder cases, constituting type II; may benefit with phenobarbital.

Symptoms of familial chronic idiopathic jaundice, or *Dubin-Johnson syndrome*, and its management:
It is another type of hereditary jaundice, with a non-visible gall bladder and a dark liver seen in biopsy.

The prognosis is good, and there is no need for treatment.

Symptoms of *Rotor's syndrome:*

As above, but the liver is not pigmented, and the gall bladder is visible.

Symptoms of *benign intermittent cholestasis:*

Intermittent jaundice.

Itching and malaise.

Possible life-long persistence, from early youth.

Prognosis very good.

Symptoms of *recurrent jaundice of pregnancy:*

Jaundice begins about the third trimester of pregnancy.

Itching is present.

There are also gastrointestinal symptoms.

Symptoms recur with subsequent pregnancies.

Prognosis is good.

Hemochromatosis

This metabolic disturbance of iron metabolism causes what liver disease?

Hepatomegaly.

Evidence of liver insufficiency.

The clinical traits suggestive of the disease are:

Liver disease.

Diabetes mellitus, for which reason it is also called bronze diabetes.

Slate gray-brown discoloration of the skin, like bronze.

What other symptoms of the disease?

Hemosiderin is deposited in most viscerae of the body, at times developing particular symptoms of heart, adrenals, kidneys, and testes.

Bleeding from esophageal varices may occur.

The disease occurs mostly in mature males.

Management of hemosiderin:

Phlebotomies and the use of deferoxamine.

Treatment also of the concurrent insufficiencies (diabetes, etc.).

Hepatolenticular Degeneration

This disease, also called Wilson's disease, is noted by:

Initial appearance of liver or of neurological symptoms.

Liver symptoms in hepatolenticular degeneration:

They may begin as an atypical hepatitis, in a child.

There are signs of cirrhosis or portal hypertension.

Neurological symptoms in hepatolenticular degeneration:

Rigidity.

Parkinsonian tremors.

Psychotic or behavioral changes (bouts of laughter).

Also, dysarthria, incoordination, open-mouthedness, and drooling.

What is considered a pathognomonic sign of the disease?

The Kayser-Fleischer ring, noted in the cornea, with a brownish or gray-green hue. The ring is not always complete.

Are there more symptoms related to this disease?

Hemolytic anemia is not too rare.

Splenomegaly with hypersplenism may also occur.

Management of the disease:

Treat before damage to the brain occurs.

Remove copper with penicillamine or triethylenetetramine.

Dimercaprol (BAL) may be useful.

Cholelithiasis

The presence of gallstones in the ducts of the liver is a common disease, with the following clinical characteristics:

Asymptomatic in a large number of cases.

Noted in a fortuitous examination done for other reasons.

Discomfort felt in the upper abdomen, more marked at the right side.

Belching and bloating.

Intolerance to some foods (fried foods, some vegetables).

Management of the situation:

Cholecystectomy is the recommended procedure.

Chenodeoxycholic acid has been used to dissolve some stones.

Cholecystitis

The inflammation of the bile ducts is generally expressed by:

Chronic cholecystitis.

Acute cholecystitis.

The symptoms of *chronic cholecystitis* are:

Pain in the epigastrium and right hypochondrium.

Pain continuous or intermittent, with pauses lasting from 15 to 60 minutes.

What are the characteristics of this biliary colic?

The onset of pain is usually abrupt.

It reaches its maximum point in about 1 hour, or less.

It may last about half an hour, but usually lasts somewhat more than 1 hour.

Pain may be referred to the interscapular area, or the shoulder.

Abdominal tenderness on palpation may be diffuse, but is usually marked over the gall bladder area.

The attack usually follows a heavy meal.

It is accompanied by nausea, with or without vomiting, sweating, and extreme activity.

There may be fever in some patients.

Following the attack, jaundice or dark urine may appear.

Management of the biliary colic:

Control the pain with papaverine, morphine, or meperidine.

Use adjunct therapy (distention, dehydration, etc.) whenever necessary.

After the colic is over, discuss surgery.

What are other symptoms of chronic cholecystitis?

Chronic indigestion.

Symptoms of dyspepsia.

Intolerance to certain foods (fried, fatty, etc.).
Bloating, belching, and epigastric heaviness.
Pyrosis, and more or less marked discomfort or frank pain.
Tenderness noted on pressure over the gall baldder area (more marked during inspiration–Murphy's sign).
Jaundice, in some cases.
Note that most of these symptoms may correspond to different diseases; so they are not reliable for diagnosis. X-ray studies may be the best diagnostic approach.

Management of chronic cholecystitis:
Treat symptomatically.
Consider surgery.

Symptoms of *acute cholecystitis:*
Most of them belong to biliary colic, q.v., above.
If not conveniently treated, the pain may last up to 18 hours.
Vomiting is present in most cases.
Fever is present in most instances, not rarely with chills.
There are abdominal distention and jaundice.

What are the most frequent diseases that may mimic acute or chronic cholecystitis?
Perforated peptic ulcer.
Acute pancreatitis.
Appendicitis, or diseases in the hepatic flexure of the colon.
Pneumonia, particularly with pleurisy.
Liver abscess, and hepatitis.
More chronic diseases may resemble chronic cholecystitis (peptic ulcer, chronic pancreatitis, cancer of the abdominal organs, etc.).

Management of acute cholecystitis:
Conservative treatment until subsidence of symptoms.
Thereafter, surgery.

Ascending Cholangitis

What are the essential characteristic of this disease?
Infection of the bile ducts, frequently accompanied by liver abscess.

What are the symptoms of the condition?
Abdominal pain.
Fever, usually intermittent, and with chills.
Jaundice.

Management of ascending cholangitis:
Strict care for symptomatologic treatment.
Surgery.

Sclerosing Cholangitis

Symptoms that may suggest sclerosing cholangitis:
Progressive obstructive jaundice.
Absence of stones, other forms of cholangitis, cirrhosis, and other local problems.

Management of sclerosing cholangitis:
Surgery.

The outcome of the disease will be:
Poor, with a short survival of a few years.

Biliary Stricture

What are the common causes of biliary stricture?
Surgical trauma, the most frequent cause.
Abdominal injury to the biliary area.
Rarely, gallstone erosion.

Symptoms of biliary stricture:
Bile leakage leading to cholangitis, with fever, chills, pain, and developing jaundice.
In complete occlusion, immediate jaundice.

Management of biliary stricture:
Surgery at the earliest possible time.

Postcholecystectomy

When the syndrome may develop:
Usually, 3 or more years after surgery.

What are the common symptoms?
There may be dilatation of the remnant portion of the cystic.
There may be formation of calculi, with the regular symptomatology.
There may be just pain.

Management of this situation:
Surgical repair.

Cancer of the Liver

Symptoms of cancer of the liver:
Not rarely asymptomatic, until the patient begins to deteriorate.
Weight loss and weakness.
Cachexia.
Sudden ascites, frequently with blood, because of thrombosis provoked by the tumor.

Evidence that may be noted on examination of these patients:
Tender hepatomegaly is found.
A mass may be noted.
A bruit or rub on auscultation may be noted on the tumor site; not in all cases.

Management of liver cancer:
Only symptomatic help is possible.

Cancer of the Biliary Tract

Common symptoms of cancer of the biliary tract:
Progressive jaundice, usually the first sign.
Pain in the right upper quadrant of the abdomen, radiating to the back.
Fever and chills, not too rarely.
Anorexia and weight loss.
Once started, rapid deterioration.

As relatively frequent complications, hematemesis or fistulization provoked by the growing tumor.

Evidence that may be obtained by examination of the patient:

A palpable gall bladder (Courvoisier's sign or law states that a dilated gall bladder together with jaundice is most usually due to a neoplasm).

Not rarely, tender hepatomegaly.

Itching and itch-scratching.

Ascites, not rarely.

5. Urogenital Diseases

Acute Urinary Infections

What is the general symptomatology of infections of the upper urinary tract?

- Fever, usually with chills.
- Pain felt in the abdomen and in the costovertebral angle.
- Headache, malaise, and vomiting.
- Tenderness on pressure at the costovertebral angle and the abdomen.
- Urine often containing visible pus (pyuria).
- Dysuria and nocturia, not too rarely.

Do not confuse this situation with:

- Acute abdomen.
- Pneumonia (lower lobe).

Other symptoms that may be present in bacterial infections are:

- Frequency with urgency, and pain of a burning character.
- Generalized muscular pains.
- Flank mass, if renal carbuncle develops.
- Other symptoms of cystitis may also develop.

Characteristics of infection of the kidney:

- See "Pyelonephritis," below.

Characteristics of ureteritis, or infections of the ureter:

- Usually, occurrence together with pyelonephritis or cystitis.
- Long-standing infections because of stasis.

Characteristics of cystitis are:

- Normal temperature, or fever, even with chills.
- Pain noted in the hypogastric area.
- Frequent and urgent urination, at times only a few drops.
- Sensation of bladder fullness after urination.
- Pyuria (pus collected in two glasses).
- Hematuria in cases of hemorrhagic cystitis.
- "Honeymoon cystitis," occurring during the first months of marriage.

Characteristic symptoms of prostatitis:

- See below, in the corresponding paragraph.

Symptoms of urethritis:

- Intense burning pain during micturition.
- Usually pus obtainable by expression of the urethra, in both females and males.

Management of ureteritis:

- Surgery, whenever applicable.
- Antibiotics or sulfas, according to the infective organism.

Management of cystitis:

- Antispasmodics; lavage of the bladder.
- Antibiotics or sulfas, according to the infective organism.

Management of urethritis:

- The specific antibiotic, starting with penicillin or ampicillin.

Chronic Urinary Infection

General symptomatology of chronic urinary infections:

- Possibly, no evident symptomatology.
- Recurrent episodes of acute infection.
- Chronic bacteriuria.
- Symptoms of progressive renal failure, including hypertension.

Management of chronic urinary infections:

- Surgical correction, or specific antibiotic therapy.
- Symptomatic care, particularly when renal failure becomes evident.

Pyelonephritis

Common symptoms of acute pyelonephritis are:

- Very few, or those of an associated disease.
- Sudden onset of fever and chills.
- Headache, nausea, and vomiting.
- Frequency, urgency, and burning on urination.
- Pain, with tenderness on pressure at the corresponding costovertebral angle.
- Pyuria.
- Not rarely, some abdominal rigidity.
- Enlarged, tender kidney may be noted.

Common symptoms of chronic pyelonephritis:

- No symptoms in many instances.
- Fever of varied characteristics, usually intermittent.
- Recurrent symptoms of acute infection.
- Pyuria, not rarely.
- Progressive clinical picture of hypertension or uremia.

Management of acute pyelonephritis:

- Specific antibiotic therapy.
- Symptomatic care.

Management of chronic pyelonephritis:

- Specific antibiotic therapy.
- Adequate care of hypertension and uremia, if they appear.

Tuberculosis of the Urinary Tract

General symptomatology of this situation:
- There may be no or very little clinical manifestation, until late stages of the disease.
- Fever and night sweats are not rare.
- Malaise and asthenia are noted.
- Frequency, nocturia, burning, and tenesmus will occur with cystitis.
- Hematuria is a frequent finding.
- With hematuria there is frequent clot formation, with consequent colic manifestations.
- Pain and tenderness are noted in the costovertebral angle.
- Complications may be noted, such as indurations in testes, epididymis, seminal vesicles, prostate; or draining sinuses in these parts.
- There is persistent pyuria.

Management of this situation:
- Antituberculous treatment with two or three drugs, for at least 18 months.

Parasitic and Fungal Diseases of the Urinary Tract

What are the outstanding symptoms of urinary filariasis?
- Chyluria.
- Elephantiasis, notably of the scrotum.

What are the outstanding symptoms of trichomoniasis?
- Symptoms of urethritis.
- Symptoms of pyelonephritis.
- Symptoms of cystitis.

What is the worst of the urinary complications of schistosomiasis or bilharziasis?
- Cancer of the bladder (carcinoma).

What is the outstanding urinary complication of coccidioidomycosis?
- A not too frequent granulomatous reaction of the prostate.

General management of these infections:

Filaria	Poor results with diethylcarbamazine.
Trichomoniasis	Metronidazole, by mouth; or local furazolidone.
Cancer of the bladder due to schistosomiasis	Cystectomia.
Coccidioidomycosis	Amphotericin B, but results are not always as good as desired.

Acute Glomerulonephritis

Common symptomatology of this condition:
- In some cases, no symptoms, except for urinary changes.
- Hematuria, albuminuria, and urine change of color, to brown or coffee-colored.
- Oliguria; more rarely, anuria.
- Mild tachycardia and hypertension (the latter, rarely high).
- Edema, noted as face puffiness, in the eyelids, in dependent parts, or even generalized.
- General symptoms of fever, headache, asthenia, and flank pain.
- Tenderness in the costovertebral angle.
- Possibly symptoms of cardiac failure.

How these symptoms develop:
- Starting 2 weeks after a streptococcal infection, of the pharynx or tonsils in most cases.
- More rarely following other infections.
- As a reaction to drugs (penicillin, sulfas, etc.).

Management of acute glomerulonephritis:
- Symptomatic.

Chronic Glomerulonephritis

Symptomatology of chronic glomerulonephritis:
- Edema noted in dependent parts of the body.
- Albuminuria.
- Oliguria in some patients.
- Flank pain, in some patients.
- Mild fever and asthenia.
- Symptoms of renal insufficiency, including hypertension.
- Symptoms of the nephrotic syndrome, and final uremia.

Management of chronic glomerulonephritis:
- Symptomatic.

Goodpasture's Syndrome

This acute glomerulonephritis accompanied by diffuse hemorrhagic inflammation of the lungs basically presents these symptoms:
- There is hemoptysis, usually as an opening symptomatology.
- Headache, malaise, and anorexia may also be initial symptoms.
- Dyspnea is rarely absent.
- Symptoms of acute glomerulonephritis rapidly appear.
- In the acme of the syndrome, the acute glomerulonephritis and diffuse inflammation of the lungs with intraalveolar hemorrhage occur together.
- Hematuria and proteinuria are found.
- Symptoms of anemia are commonly present.
- Progressive symptoms of uremia occur.

Management of Goodpasture's syndrome:
- There are high mortality rates in spite of relatively good help with corticoids and immunosuppressive therapy.
- Hemodialysis, with nephrectomy and subsequent transplantation, has helped a few patients.

Prostatitis

Symptoms of prostatitis are, in the acute stage:
- Pain in the perineal area.
- Dysuria, frequency, and urethral discharge.

Fever.
Prostate enlarged, smooth but boggy, with very intense tenderness; at the time of palpation discharge from the urethra increases.

Symptoms of prostatitis are, in the chronic stage:
Pain in the perineal area.
Pain spreading to the lumbosacral area.
Frequency, with dysuria and scanty urethral discharge.
Prostate enlarged, firm, irregular, and mildly tender.

What other diseases may complicate prostatitis?
Recurrent lower tract infections.
Urethritis, epididymitis, and cystitis.

Management of prostatitis:
Use a combination of trimethoprim and sulfamethoxazole.
Erythromycin and other antibiotics effective against the infecting flora may also be used.
Provide general care.
Use massage in chronic prostatitis.

Prostatic Hypertrophy

In case of adenomatous or benign prostatic hypertrophy the symptomatology is:
Slow progress of difficulties in micturition.
Decreased urinary stream, in both force and size.
Hesitancy and straining to initiate urination.
Intermittency of the stream.
Frequency, urgency, and nocturia.
Terminal dribbling, and a sensation of incomplete emptying.
Overflow dribbling.
Hematuria when superficial veins rupture on straining.
Usually, not a complete emptying of the bladder after urination.
Generally, a rapid refilling of urine after micturition.
Enlarged prostate gland (size does not represent actual obstacle).
Distended bladder noted on palpation above the pubic area.
Urine retention may follow delayed micturition, exposure to cold, alcohol ingestion, immobilization, etc.

What are problems related to prostatic hyperplasia?
Urine infection (fever, chills, burning on urination).
Acute urinary retention; possible hydronephrosis.
Progressive renal failure.
Final uremia.

Management of prostatic hyperplasia:
General and symptomatic care.
Surgery.

Urolithiasis

Common causes of urolithiasis:
The majority include obstruction and/or infection (50%).
A good number are metabolic in origin (25%).
Others are of unknown origin (25%).

What conditions antedate calcic stones?
Hyperparathyroidism.
Excessive intake of vitamin D, or milk.
Excessive alkali intake.
Destructive bone disease, or prolonged immobilization.

What condition antedate oxalate stones?
Hereditary oxaluria.
Excessive intake of chocolate, cabbage, spinach, tomatoes, etc.

What conditions antedate uric acid stones?
Gout.
Leukemia, polycythemia vera, etc.

Symptoms of calculi in the renal pelvis or in calyx:
They are asymptomatic in a large number of cases; check for them in patients suffering from any one of the aforementioned diseases.
Hematuria or symptoms of infection may occur.
If there is some obstruction, there is pain in the flank, of a dull character or even a ture colic.
On palpation there are abdominal distention and flank tenderness.
Nausea and vomiting may occur.

Symptoms of calculi in the ureter; or so-called renal colic:
First warning may be an initial vague low back pain.
That pain soon turns into an excruciating pain.
The pain starts at the costovertebral angle and extends downward to the corresponding genital area (penis and teste, or labia majora).
The excruciating pain may reach the thigh.
There may be an accompanying precordial pain.
The pain is intermittent, appearing in a colicky fashion and remaining as a less severe discomfort between the attacks.
In long-lasting crises, the pain becomes more generalized and may suggest an acute abdomen.
Sweating, vomiting, and syncopal symptoms may accompany the colic.

Other symptoms and signs that usually accompany the renal colic:
Dysuria or anuria.
Hematuria, with or without clots.
Fever and chills.
Pain elicited by pressure over the costovertebral angle or the trajectory of the ureter.
Possible expulsion of some sort of solid sediment (sand, calculus) in the urine.

Symptoms of calculi in the bladder:
There is irritability of the bladder, with urgency, frequency, and dysuria.
There is interruption of the urine stream.
With interruption of the stream there is pain in the penis.
Hematuria and pyuria may occur.

Management of urolithiasis:
Treat the cause leading to the formation of stones.
Treat any complication that may arise.

Relieve colic with morphine or similar narcotics.
Perform surgery, whenever needed.

Obstructive Uropathies

Symptoms of chronic hydronephrosis:
- Discomfort is noted at the flank, as intercurrent dull pain.
- There are colicky pains similar to "renal colic" when due to nephroptosis or acute overdistention of the renal pelvis (Dietl's crises).
- A mass in the flank may be noted by palpation.
- Hematuria may occur.
- Symptoms of urinary infection may occur.
- Other vague gastrointestinal symptoms may occur.

Management of hydroephrosis:
- Perform surgery, at the earliest possible moment.
- In some cases, relief may be obtained by removal of the causative factor.

Symptoms of ureteral obstruction:
- Because it may cause hydronephrosis, the symptomatology will be that of this disease.

Management of ureteral obstruction:
- Surgical.

Symptoms of prostatic obstruction of the urogenital tract:
- See in the above corresponding paragraph.

Nephrosis

Diseases that usually cause the nephrotic syndrome:
- Glomerulonephritis.
- Most of the collagen diseases (disseminated lupus erythematosus, etc.).
- Diabetic nephropathy and thrombosis of the renal vein.
- Syphilis, malaria, myxedema, amyloid disease, multiple myeloma, cancer, lymphomas, constrictive pericarditis, and reaction to drugs and other toxins.

What is the outstanding symptom of nephrosis?
- Slow or rapidly forming edema; mildly marked or reaching the proportions of ture anasarca.

Evidence of the edema formation, and other symptoms:
- Taking more or less time, the edema always finally reaches huge proportions.
- Large amounts of edema accumulate in the dependent parts of the body, and striae may develop in the extremities.
- Edema is found in the pleural cavity (hydrothorax) and in the abdominal cavity (ascites).
- Dyspnea (shortness of breath) results from hydrothorax and ascites.
- The abdomen becomes prominent because of ascites.
- Anorexia may become a part of the syndrome.
- Sooner or later, hypertension is an important symptom.
- Ocular manifestations of hypertension are common.

Management of nephrosis:
- Treat vigorously syphilis or heavy metals poisoning, if one of these is the cause.
- Provide general care, and treatment of the causative disease.
- Use corticoids at an early stage of the disease.

Nephrosclerosis

Clinical forms in which nephrosclerosis is usually manifested:
- The greater number of patients present a benign form.
- There is a form of malignant nephrosclerosis associated with malignant hypertension.

Symptoms of the common form of nephrosclerosis:
- It is asymptomatic for long periods of time.
- Most symptoms are laboratory findings, such as proteinuria, hematuria, and uremic changes.
- Cardiac failure or brain hemorrhage may be fatal before frank uremia appears.

Symptoms of malignant nephrosclerosis:
- There is a rapidly progressive course.
- Hypertension is elevated.
- Bleeding is a common finding.
- Other symptoms of renal insufficiency rapidly develop.

Management of nephrosclerosis:
- Treat hypertension in benign nephrosclerosis.

Polycystic Kidney

Polycystic disease is usually discovered in clinics by:
- Checking persons with hypertension.
- Or persons with pyelonephritis or renal insufficiency.

Symptoms of polycystic kidney disease:
- Asymptomatic for many years, in a large number of cases.
- Occasional flank pain (hemorrhage into a cyst).
- Abdominal discomfort (intra-abdominal masses).
- Hematuria or urinary infection.
- Hypertension.
- Final deterioration because of hypertension or uremia.

What are the two forms of cystic disease of the renal medulla?
- Sponge kidney, with a benign clinical course.
- Medullary cystic disease, which may become apparent in adolescence.

Management of polycystic kidney:
- Discuss hemodialysis or a transplant.

Other Anomalies

The most common congenital anomalies are:
- Agenesia, usually of the left kidney.
- Ectopic kidney, usually in the pelvis; infections are common.
- Nephroptosis, mostly evidenced by unusual mobility.
- Horseshoe kidney, both organs united by an upper band of tissure, with frequent manifestations of pyelonephritis. Other forms of fusion may occur (one single pelvis of the kidney, etc.).

Malrotation of the kidney; may cause hydronephrosis.
Duplications may occur (kidney, pelvis, etc.).

What are the defects of function of the renal tubules?

Hepatolenticular degeneration, with aminoaciduria (see the corresponding paragraph in the chapter devoted to diseases of the liver).

Congenital cystinuria, with cystine stones.

Aminoaciduria, because of poor absorption of these acids; the clinical evidence is failure to thrive.

Fanconi's syndrome with multiple defects of the tubular function (glycosuria, aminoaciduria, phosphaturia, and renal acidosis; there may also be osteomalacia).

Vitamin D-resistant rickets, and pseudohypoparathyroidism.

Renal glycosuria, with normal glycemia.

Glycosuric rickets, with osteomalacia, bone pains, tetany, glycosuria, and deformation of bones.

Other syndromes such as renal tubular acidosis, potassium wastage syndrome, renal diabetes insipidus, and idiopathic hypercalciuria.

Acute Renal Insufficiency

What causes provoke acute renal insufficiency with the greatest frequency?

Incompatible blood transfusion.

Crushing injuries, burns, shock, surgery (usually on the abdominal aorta), myocardial infarction, and other similar accidents (obstetrics, etc.).

Septicemia, other infectious diseases.

Drugs, other toxic agents, poisoning.

Severe dehydration, glomerulonephritis, and other renal forms of damage.

Symptoms of acute renal insufficiency during the initial oliguric phase:

There is evidence of some of the above inductive causes.

There is drastic reduction of the amount of urine, with proteinuria, red cells, and casts.

Lumbar pain and tenderness may be noted.

If the oliguric phase lasts long enough, symptoms of uremia will be noted (nausea, diarrhea, nervous irritability, convulsions, and somnolence or frank coma).

Also hypertension, retinopathy, heart failure, and encephalopathy may occur.

Watch for potassium intoxication.

Symptoms noted during the diuretic phase of the diseases:

The urine starts to increase daily, from a few ml to 100 ml or more, until a daily amount of about 500 ml is reached; thereafter the increase is more rapid.

There is a slow return of renal function to normalcy.

Symptoms that may indicate insufficiency due to glomerulonephritis:

Complete anuria.

Hematuria and casts composed of red cells.

Moderate to heavy proteinuria.

Symptoms that may indicate insufficiency due to acute tubular necrosis, also known as lower nephron nephrosis or kidney shutdown:

Incomplete anuria; a few ml are left.

Casts hyaline or granular.

Minimal proteinuria; at most, moderate.

Urine specific gravity less than 1.018.

Urinary sodium concentration greater than 20 mEq/liter.

Symptoms that may indicate insufficiency due to obstruction:

Complete anuria.

Large and irregular variation in urine excretion.

Scanty urinary sediment.

Minimal or absent proteinuria.

Do not mistake acute renal failure for:

Profound dehydration.

Ruptured bladder.

What the outcome or acute renal failure will be:

Acute tubular necrosis (lower nephron nephrosis) is reversible and will cure in many instances, with little renal impairment.

Death may occur, due to heart failure, water intoxication, pulmonary edema, encephalopathy, or potassium intoxication.

Management consists of:

Finding and treating the causative factor.

Accurately balancing diet (no protein), water, and electrolytes.

Watching for and controlling complications. Consider potassium intoxication, heart failure, infection, anemia, uremia, and encephalopathy.

Chronic Renal Insufficiency

What causes provoke chronic renal insufficiency with the greatest frequency?

Glomurulonephritis.

Pyelonephritis.

Infectious, toxic, and metabolic diseases with renal involvement.

Other renal diseases, including congenital diseases.

General symptomatology usually found in chronic renal insufficiency:

Headache, progressive weakness and asthenia, weight loss.

Gastrointestinal symptoms, such as anorexia, metallic taste in the mouth, nausea and vomiting, thirst, diarrhea.

Urinary symptoms, such as polyuria, nocturia, and hypertension that may cause retinal changes, heart failure, and a progressive secondary encephalopathy increasing with the final uremia.

Nervous symptoms, such as irritability, pruritus, hiccup, paresthesias, burning sensations, convulsions, myoclonic jerking, evidence of peripheral neuropathy, cerebral hemorrhage; all increasing as uremia develops.

Other symptoms, such as heart failure, pulmonary edema, hemorrhagic tendency, bone pain.

Findings noted during physical examination of the patient:
- Pale and excoriated skin, with purpuric lesions.
- Hyperpnea, with urinous odor of the breath.
- Symptoms and signs of dehydration.
- Hypertension, with cardiac enlargement usually present.
- Retinopathy.
- More or less marked pulmonary edema.
- Signs of peripheral neuropathy.

Characteristic findings in chronic renal insufficiency:
- Azotemia, acidosis, and anemia.
- Diluted urine, with small amounts of protein, cells, and casts.

Management of chronic renal insufficiency:
- Symptomatic treatment.
- Diet, fluids, and electrolyte replacement.
- Dialysis and kidney transplantation to be considered.

Uremia

The symptoms of advanced renal insufficiency, either acute or chronic, are:
- Decreased mental acuity, fatigue, and lassitude.
- Relatively fixed urinary volume (from 1 to 4 liters a day), not related to water intake.
- Urine specific gravity fixed at about 1.010.
- Skin with yellow-brown discoloration, with intense pruritus and possibly urea crystals in the sweat (uremic frost).
- Nervous and gastrointestinal symptoms as in chronic renal insufficiency, q.v., in the above entry; symptoms increasing in intensity.
- Loss of weight because of marked malnutrition.
- In general, all the symptoms of renal insufficiency, becoming more and more marked.

Stone in the Bladder, or Vesical Colic

The usual preceding diseases that cause vesical stones are:
- Urinary stasis.
- Urinary infection in the presence of residual urine.
- Foreign bodies.
- Ulcers and inflammation of the bladder.

Symptoms due to vesical stones are:
- Symptoms of chronic urinary obstruction.
- Symptoms of stasis and infection.
- Suprapubic pain and slow and painful urination (strangury).
- Bladder irritability (dysuria, urgency, frequency).
- Interrupted flow of urine stream, may occur.
- Hematuria and pyuria, not rarely.
- Enlarged prostate or distended bladder.

The final diagnosis may be made by:
- Radiologic examination.
- Cystoscopic examination.

Management of stones in the bladder:
- General management with antibiotics and symptomatic care.
- Surgical removal.

Trauma to the Kidney

Frequent causes of traumatic injuries to the kidneys are:
- External blows to flanks or abdominal walls.
- Penetrating stabwounds or gunshots.

Types of injury resulting from these traumatic insults:
- Contusion, which may cause massive hemorrhage.
- Laceration or fragmentation, which may cause hemorrhage and urine extravasation.
- Disruption of the pedicle, with sudden death.

Outcome of these injuries:
- With a prompt diagnosis and management, the prognosis is usually good.
- Hypertension may be a late complication when there is a scarring.

Trauma to the Ureter

Most frequent cause of trauma to the ureter is:
- A previous surgical procedure in the pelvis.

Symptomatology of traumatic injuries to the ureter:
- There is oliguria or anuria.
- Fistulization may occur.

What are some other types of injury to the ureter, and the symptoms that they may cause?
- Penetrating injuries, causing extravasation of urine.
- Avulsion of the ureter at the renal pelvis produced by hyperextension of the trunk, also causing extravasation of urine.

Alterations of the ureter can be checked:
- By intravenous pyelography.

Trauma to the Bladder

The most frequent cause of traumatic injuries to the bladder is:
- A car accident.

Symptoms resulting from injuries to the bladder:
- Rupture of the bladder occurs at the upper portion, with urinary extravasation in the peritoneum.
- Oliguria or anuria will occur.
- Rarely peritonitis will occur.

Trauma to the Urethra and Penis

Occurrence of trauma to the urethra and penis:
- Rare among women, for urethra.
- Usually, work accident.

Common types of traumatic lesions to the penis or urethra:
- Crushing blows.
- Avulsion of the skin.

Cancer of the Kidney

According to age, what are the frequent types of kidney malignancies?
- During childhood, neuroblastoma, wich may origninate in the adrenal gland, and Wilm's tumor, which is an adenosarcoma in the kidney.
- During adulthood, mostly in males, carcinoma.

Symptoms of *Wilm's tumor* are:
Abdominal mass.
Pain; possibly hematuria and hypertension, which are symptoms of severe impending danger.
Fever, anorexia, nausea, and vomiting.
Management of Wilm's tumor:
Surgery, chemotherapy, and radiation.
Symptoms of *carcinoma of the kidney:*
Hematuria.
Flank pain.
Fever, usually not too elevated.
Palpable mass, frequently noted.
In some cases, hypertension or polycythemia.
Malignant cells in urinary cytology.
Management of carcinoma of the kidney:
First, radiation; followed by radical extirpation and chemotherapy.

Cancer of the Urinary Tract

Symptoms of cancer of the renal pelvis and ureter:
There is hematuria, painless at the beginning.
Colicky pain may accompany obstruction.
Tenderness in the flank may be noted.
There are red cells and clots in the urine.
Malignant cells may be found in urinary cytology.
Management of cancer of the renal pelvis and ureter:
Removal of all the corresponding urinary tract and kidney.

Cancer of the Prostate

Symptoms of carcinoma of the prostate are:
Evidence of prostatic hypertrophy, q.v.
Low back pain, with metastases to the bones of the pelvis or the spine.
Renal damage if obstruction occurs.
Hard consistency of the gland, stonelike; presenting a nodular irregularity, which is almost pathognomonic.
Management of prostatic cancer:
Radical resection, if possible.
Transurethral resection and antiandrogen therapy.

Cancer of the Bladder

Symptoms of cancer of the bladder are:
Hematuria.
Cystitis with dysuria, frequency, and urgency.
Diminished urinary stream.
Symptoms of obstruction and possible infection. Mass may be noted.
Suprapubic pain if the tumor extends beyond the bladder.
Malignant cells in urinary cytology.
Cystoscopic confirmation.
Management of bladder cancer:
Surgery, according to the extent of the lesion.
Thiotepa instillations for superficial epithelial tumors.

Cancer of the Testis

Symptoms of cancer of the testis:
There is slow and progressive enlargement of the affected testis.
The tumor is painless, symmetrical, and firm.
The mass does not transilluminate.
There may be a dragging inguinal pain.
Gynecomastia occurs frequently.
Metastases to the lungs and liver are frequent.
Hydrocele may occur.
Management of cancer of the testis:
Surgical removal.
Radiation and chemotherapy to be considered.

Cancer of the Urethra and Penis

Symptoms of *cancer of the urethra:*
Hematuria.
Local mass, usually friable and bleeding.
Biopsy usually needed for differentiation.
This occurs in both women and men.
Management of cancer of the urethra:
Radical surgery or radiation therapy.
Symptoms of *cancer of the penis:*
Epidermoid lesion in the corona or foreskin.
Management of cancer of the penis:
Partial penectomy in early lesions.
Total penectomy, whenever feasible.

Myoneurogenic Disorders of the Urinary Tract

Symptoms of *neurogenic bladder* are:
There is a complete urinary retention, or incontinence.
In chronic stages urinary infection may be of importance.
Urinary calculi are common.
When does the hypotonic or flaccid neurogenic bladder occur, and what are the symptoms?
In cases of acute spinal cord injuries.
Hypotonic or atonic, distended bladder.
Continuous overflow dribbling of urine.
Management of neurogenic bladder:
Initial help to avoid a distended bladder.
Rehabilitation (surgical, etc.).
What are the characteristics and management of the *megacystis syndrome?*
Usually found in girls.
Large bladders.
Rehabilitation.
Symptoms and management of *enuresis:*
There is consistent bed-wetting during sleep.
Check for abnormalities (meatal stricture, phimosis, etc.).

Check for Lyon's ring (distal urethral stenosis) in girls.
Rehabilitate.

Priapism

Symptoms of priapism are:
- Penile erection, painful and persistent.
- No accompanying sexual desire, or excitation of any kind.

In cases of priapism the patient should be checked for:
- Blood dyscrasias.
- Pelvic tumor hematoma.
- Central nervous diseases.
- Local infections.

Management of priapism:
- Anticoagulants, in early stages.
- Evacuation and irrigation of the corpora cavernosa (recurrences are frequent).
- Surgery (venous shunt).

Peyronie's Disease

The fibrous dysplasia of the cavernous sheath is noted as follows:
- The penis deviates laterally (to the affected side) when erected.
- Erections may become painful, but this does not always occur.
- Some patients will be unable to perform coitus.

Management of Peyronie's disease:
- Radiation has given some results.
- Corticoids have given some results.
- Removal of the plaque is not too satisfactory.

Renovascular Hypertension

Differentiation of renovascular hypertension from other forms of hypertension is made:
- When it occurs in young patients.
- When it appears suddenly in older patients.
- By acute marked and progressive bouts in already established cases of hypertension.
- By evaluation of the renal parenchyma or vasculature by rapid-sequence pyelography, radioactive renogram, angiography, and other assays.

Management of renovascular hypertension:
- Surgery, whenever feasible.

6. Endocrinology

Pituitary Dwarfism

Clinical features of dwarfism, when due to hypopituitarism:
- Retarded growth, maintaining small height.
- Proportions of body segments almost normal.
- Retarded or absent puberty.
- In cases due to craniopharyngioma, symptoms and signs of pituitary tumor (X-ray showing calcifications in the sellar area, possibility of diabetes insipidus, etc.).

Do not confuse it with:
- Prepuberal hypothyroidism.
- Ovarian dysgenesis (Turner's syndrome).
- Primordial dwarfism (in which persons are born dwarfs).
- Disturbed nutrition caused by chronic or severe diseases.

Management of pituitary dwarfism:
- Surgery for special cases of craniopharyngioma.
- Hormone replacement.

Adiposogenital Dystrophy (Frölich's Syndrome)

Symptomatology of Frölich's syndrome:
- Obesity.
- Hypogonadism.
- Frequently, diabetes insipidus.
- The syndrome starts in adolescent boys.
- It is usually due to craniopharyngioma.

Differentiate from:
- Other forms of hypogonadism.
- Other forms of obesity.

Management of adiposogenital dystrophy:
- Surgical whenever feasible.
- Hormone replacement.

Laurence-Moon-Biedl Syndrome

Characteristic of the Laurence-Moon-Biedl syndrome:
- Obesity.
- Hypogenitalism.
- Organic abnormalities, including skull defects, retinitis pigmentosa, and some patients also presenting syndactylia.
- Mental deficiency.

Pituitary Insufficiency of the Adult

Reference is usually made to two different types of pituitary insufficiency, namely:
- Simmond's disease, or pituitary cachexia.
- Sheehan's syndrome, or postpartum pituitary hemorrhage.
- Other forms of pituitary insufficiency should be included here.

Symptomatology of *Simmond's disease:*
- Marked asthenia, and thinness (cachexia).
- Lack of development or regression of function of sex organs and function.
- Lack of resistance to cold.
- Lack of resistance to fasting.
- Lack of resistance to infections.
- Lack of growth if the disease starts early in childhood.
- Loss (or very scanty development) of hair in the body, particularly axillary and pubic.
- Diminished pigmentation of the skin, which is pale and sallow.
- Dimished sweating, with very dry skin.
- Fine wrinkles.
- Hypotension and orthostatic hypotension; sleepy appearance.
- Small heart.
- Visual symptoms in the case of pituitary tumors.
- Abnormal lactation occurring occasionally, in some cases (both sexes).
- Cerebrovascular symptoms, in some instances.

A careful distinction will be made from:
- Pure pituitary dwarfism.
- Frölich's syndrome.
- Laurence-Moon-Biedl syndrome.
- Anorexia nervosa (cachexia is more marked; asthenia is not so intense; usually psychiatric symptoms are also present).
- Addison's disease.
- Myxedema, nephrosis, pernicious anemia.

Management of pituitary insufficiency:
- Hormone replacement.
- Radiation or surgery for tumors, as advisable.

Evaluating the diagnosis of *Sheehan's syndrome:*
- Patient is a woman who had a previous delivery.
- There is a circulatory collapse following delivery.

Symptoms may appear soon or be somewhat delayed after parturition.

Similar symptomatology may appear in patients who have had shock due to cerebrovascular disease.

The rest of the symptomatology is as stated above.

Other causes of pituitary insufficiency are:

Idiopathic (pure Simmond's disease, which is a rare instance).

Lesions to the hypothalamic pathway.

Rathke's pouch cyst, and other cysts and tumors.

Irradiation to the skull or surgical hypophysectomy.

Sarcoidosis, tuberculosis, or fungal infections.

Aneurism of the internal carotid artery.

Help for the diagnosis of pituitary diseases:

Radiology.

Visual fields.

Hormonal assays.

Diabetes Insipidus

The lack of antidiuretic hormone from the posterior lobe of the hypophysis produces these symptoms:

There is intense polydipsia.

There is excessive polyuria.

Involved fluid volume may range from 5 to 40 liters a day.

The urine is pale, with very low specific gravity (less than 1.016).

Fluid restriction will not increase specific gravity.

Fluid restriction may cause rapid dehydration, with weight loss, irritability, headache, asthenia, muscle pains, tachycardia, hypothermia, and final shock.

When the disease is due to a previous disease, its symtoms will also be present (injury, tumors, infection, hemorrhage, etc.).

Clinical traits of diabetes insipidus due to lack of response of the distal tubules of the kidney to the action of antidiuretic hormone:

There will also be polydipsia, polyuria, excessive fluid involvement, and low specific gravity of the urine.

This disease is inherited and is marked by the lack of the symptoms' response to the administration of the hormone, particularly in homozygotic males (heterozygotus females will present only a partial symptomatology).

Some cases, not inherited, will present a previous nephropathy (hypokalemic, obstructive, nephritis), hypercalcemia, or sickle-cell disease.

What is the most important differentiation to make regarding diabetes insipidus?

Distinguish it from potomania, also called by some psychogenic diabetes insipidus, in which there is usually a better sleep (no urgent need to drink), the urine will increase specific gravity after injection of 3% hypertonic saline solution (this will not happen in true diabetes insipidus), and the response to arginine vasopressin radioimmunoassay is almost specific.

Differentiate it from diabetes mellitus, chronic nephritis, hypokalemia, and hypercalcemia.

Management of diabetes insipidus:

Give pitressin (or vasopressin) tannate.

Some cases may respond to X-ray therapy or the administration of diuretics.

Antidiuretic Hormone Insufficiency (Bartter-Schwartz Syndrome)

This form of water intoxication is characterized by:

Frequent association with oat cell carcinoma of the lung, leukemia, porphyria, and disorders of the central nervous system, myxedema, etc.

Usual symptoms are irritability, lethargy, confusion, and seizures.

Urine osmolality is higher than plasma osmolality.

There is hyponatremia, which reaches lower levels when there is a fluid loading.

Some cases may be due to previous ingestion of chlorpropamide, diuretics (of the potassium-depleting type), vincristine, etc.

Management of the antidiuretic hormone defficiency:

Order water restriction.

May try demeclocycline, or lithium carbonate.

Gigantism and Acromegaly

Differentiate the essential features of these forms of hyperpituitarism:

Gigantism will occur if the disease starts before termination of growth.

Acromegaly will occur if it starts during adulthood.

Characteristic of *gigantism* are:

There is excessive growth, usually above 2 meters in height (6'7" or more).

Both length and width of bones increases.

Growth is mostly proportional; occasional traits of acromegaly occur.

Visual field changes are rare.

X-ray findings will give diagnosis (sella turcica, bone epiphysis).

Characteristics of *acromegaly* are:

Periosteal overgrowth and cortical thickening of bones.

Resultant wide hands, broad fingers, similar large feet, prognathic protrusion of the jaw, that is, acromegaly or great extremities.

Enlarged internal organs.

Thickened skin, increased sweating and hypertrichosis, the latter more easily noted among women; acanthosis nigricans may occur.

Loss of libido, galactorrhea, and among women also frequent amenorrhea.

Hoarseness of the voice.

Symptoms of pituitary tumor, may develop (headache, visual field changes–hemianopsia, diplopia, lethargy).

Other hormonal symptoms, such as diabetes mellitus, goiter.
Hypertension, in one-fourth of the patients.
As for gigantism, X-ray findings will help in the diagnosis; hormonal assays will also help in both cases.
Check for acromegaly whenever there is an unexpected enlargement of the size of feet or hands.

Management of gigantism and acromegaly:
Pituitary irradiation, or surgery.

Cushing's Disease

Differentiation of Cushing's disease and Cushing's syndrome:
In Cushing's disease the primary factor is a primary pituitary hyperfunction causing a secondary adrenal hyperfunction.
In Cushing's syndrome the excessive hyperfunction is primarily of adrenal origin.

Symptoms of excessive adrenal cortisol excretion in both Cushing's disease and Cushing's syndrome:
In the case of the disease there will be noted symptoms of pituitary tumor (headache, hemianopsia, diplopia, lethargy, X-ray findings, hormonal assays).
The face is rounded and plethoric ("moon face").
There is obesity, more marked in the trunk and around the shoulders (buffalo type).
The skin is thin, atrophic, with purple striae (some consider these striae as characteristic of the syndrome); hirsutism frequently occurs.
Easy bruising and poor wound healing are noted; also, chloasma and acne.
Extremities and fingers are slender.
Asthenia and muscle wasting occur, with a plethoric appearance.
Hypertension, renal calculi, osteoporosis, and particularly glycosuria will be noted.
There are sexual symptoms, as amenorrhea in women and impotence in men.
Lability of mood or true psychosis may develop.

Diagnostic problems in Cushing's syndrome:
Obesity (if accompanied by diabetes, amenorrhea, and hirsutism).
Adrenogenital syndrome.
Excessive administration of corticoids.
Good help for diagnosis is given by hormonal assays and radiography.

Management of Cushing's disease or syndrome:
Surgery or radiotherapy.

Galactorrhea-Amenorrhea

Clinical manifestations of the galactorrhea-amenorrhea syndrome:
It may constitute the Forbes-Albright syndrome, with a chromophobe adenoma of the pituitary.
It may constitute the Chiari-Frommel syndrome, which occurs after pregnancy.

Clinical characteristics of the galactorrhea-amenorrhea syndrome:
A psychic trauma may precede the syndrome.
Symptoms of pituitary tumor may be present in the Forbes-Albright syndrome.
Persistent amenorrhea with galactorrhea may follow a previous pregnancy.

Goiter

Different manifestations of goiter:
Simple goiter.
Endemic goiter.
Nodular goiter, nontoxic.
Other forms with altered function, either hypo- or hyperfunction.

Clinical manifestations of simple or nodular (nontoxic) goiter:
There is smooth enlargement of the gland, in simple and endemic goiter;
Multiple nodules and cysts may appear, usually at a later stage.
Nodules and cysts seem to be independent of the gland.
The enlarged gland follows the movements (deglutition) of the pharynx.

Management of goiter:
Perform surgery in the case of large goiters.
Give iodine or thyroid extracts.
A try may be made with bismuth injections.

Thyroiditis

What are the frequent clinical types of thyroiditis?
Infectious thyroiditis due to tuberculosis, syphilis, viral or pyogenic varieties.
Acute or subacute nonsuppurative De Quervain's thyroiditis.
Hashimoto's thyroiditis.
Riedel's thyroiditis.

Symptoms of *De Quervain's thyroiditis:*
There is more or less marked thyroid swelling, appearing like a goiter.
There is painful thyroid, in acute types; less painful or painless, in chronic types.
Pain radiates to the jaws, chest, and arms; also to the ears.
Painful swelling may start in one lobe and extend to the other.
There may be dysphagia.
There may also appear symptoms of hyperthyroidism (q.v.).
There may or may not be a fever.
The untreated disease may persist for a few weeks.

Symptoms of *Hashimoto's thyroiditis:*
There is insidious enlargement of the gland.
The thyroid appears painless, is firm, and shows multiple nodules.

Thyroid function may be altered, mostly late in the disease, either with hypofunction or with thyrotoxicosis ("hashitoxicosis").

Needle biopsy will help the diagnosis.

Symptoms of *Riedel's thyroiditis:*

There is irregular, asymmetrical enlargement of the gland.

Thyroid is stone-hard, firmly attached to neighboring surroundings, thus suggesting cancer.

Hoarseness, dysphagia, and dyspnea are common symptoms.

Considerations for differential diagnosis:

Other forms of goiter.

Thyroid cancer.

Use of needle biopsy for more accurate diagnosis.

Management of thyroiditis:

Surgical for Riedel's struma; rarely needed for other forms of thyroiditis.

For suppurative thyroiditis, antibiotics and drainage.

Corticoid therapy for subacute thyroiditis and Hashimoto's struma.

Thyroid hormones for subacute and Hashimoto's thyroiditis.

Thyroid Cancer

Clinical evidence of thyroid cancer:

The thyroid may appear enlarged or show a nodule.

The nodule is usually firm, or very hard.

The thyroid gland or the nodule is not painful.

First symptoms may come from thyroid metastases to a lymph node, the lungs, or a destructive bone lesion.

In long-standing cases, there are signs of pressure (or invasion) to the neck.

Rare medullary carcinoma will produce excess calcitonin, with hypocalcemic signs and symptoms.

Hardness, irregularity, and fixation of the gland suggest cancer.

X-ray studies with radioiodine will help in the diagnosis.

Management of thyroid cancer:

Surgery, at the earliest possible time.

Radioiodine therapy.

The most frequent form of thyroid cancer:

Papillary cancer (follicular cancer is only second).

The most frequent forms of invasion:

Justanodal in papillary and amyloidic solid cancer (some anaplastic).

To the blood vessels in anaplastic and follicular cancer (some amyloidic solid).

To distant sites, anaplastic and follicular.

Situations that are mostly suggestive of thyroid cancer:

History of previous irradiation.

Hoarseness, vocal cord paralysis.

Nodule that is firm, and the only one.

Enlarged lymph nodes and metastatic lesions.

Hyperthyroidism

What differentiates the varied forms of hyperthyroidism?

Graves' disease characterizes the toxic diffuse goiter with exophthalmos.

Toxic nodular goiter represents one or more nodules together with hyperthyroid reaction.

In Plummer's disease there is an adenomatous goiter with hyperthyroidism.

Add to this list two other forms: apathetic Graves' disease, found in the elderly, with little sign of hyperthyroidism and evident refractory heart disease; and malignant exophthalmos, when it is progressive and resistant to therapy.

There is a rare form of struma ovarii, with characteristic symptoms of hyperthyroidism.

Symptoms of hyperthyroidism are:

Goiter, either diffuse or nodular. A bruit usually heard over the gland.

Tachycardia, frequently accompanied by palpitation.

Nervousness, more or less marked trembling (evidenced by a paper placed over the extended hand), restlessness, and asthenia.

Skin changes: excessive sweating and heat intolerance, making the skin warm and moist; it is thin, and so is the hair, which appears silky.

Excessive appetite, but with weight loss.

Eye signs: exophthalmos characterizing the exophthalmic variety of goiter; bright, stare eyes; lid lag and periorbital edema; diplopia or lack of accommodation.

Dyspnea, in some cases.

Increased frequency of defecation, with or without diarrhea, wich is one of the most frequent symptoms in tropical countries.

More or less frequent findings of increased skin pigmentation or of vitiligo, spider angiomas, cardiovascular manifestations (fibrillation, heart failure, a harsh pulmonary systolic murmur), gynecomastia, enlarged lymph nodes and spleen, wasting of bones and muscles, and more rarely nausea, vomiting, fever, and jaundice.

Mental changes, from mild to severe, which are relatively common.

Pretibial edema, possible in severe forms.

Hormonal studies very helpful for diagnosis.

Do not confuse hyperthyroidism with:

Anxiety neurosis.

Other forms of thyroiditis, with hyperthyroid symptoms.

Hypermetabolic conditions (anemia, leukemia, and the like).

Pituitary tumor with high amounts of thyroid stimulating hormone.

Other diseases, such as cardiac diseases, myasthenia gravis, orbital tumor, etc.

Management of hyperthyroidism:

Surgery, whenever advisable.

Use of antithyroid medication.

Radioactive iodine.
Special measures for general care and the care of complications.

Thyroid Storm

Essential features of this complication of hyperthyroidism are:
A previously existing hyperthyroid state.
Intercurrent occurrence of infection, surgery, emotional stress, or parturition.
Aggravation of hyperthyroid symptoms, particularly extreme tachycardia, vomiting, and diarrhea.
Other symptoms, such as marked delirium and marked dehydration.
Fever a frequent occurrence, mostly very high.
Management of thyroid storm or crisis:
Give large doses of rapidly acting corticoids.
Also give large amounts of propylthiouracil and propanolol.
Treat dehydration.
Use plasmaphoresis and give cholestiramine in other cases.

Hypothyroidism and Myxedema

Characterization of adult hypothyroidism and myxedema:
Practically all body tissues are affected by hypothyroidism.
The severity of hypothyroidism ranges from almost unrecognized to intense myxedema. In newborns it causes cretinism.
A goiter may or may not be present.
Initial symptoms usually are a very dry skin with pallor and lately thickness, coarse thin hair, also thin and brittle nails, asthenia, intolerance to cold, nervousness, and possible lethargy.
Symptoms of well-established hypothyroidism and myxedema:
The former symptoms, more marked.
Lack of sweating and developed myxedema.
Myxedema showing peripheral edema with puffiness of the face and hands, protruding eyelids, and yellowish skin with rosy cheeks.
Myxedematous enlargement or true effusions occurring in the pleura, peritoneum, and pericardium (enlarged myxedematous heart).
Slow speech, with deep-toned voice, slow thinking, and drowsiness.
Decreased appetite, and, in spite of it, weight gain. No true obesity.
Large, thickened tongue, with decreased sense of taste (also smell).
Slow digestion and constipation.
Dyspnea, aches and pains (including anginal pain), loss of muscular strength, slow relaxation of tendon reflexes.
Bradycardia; blood pressure variable; low pulse pressure.
Loss of hair, particularly the outer half of the eyebrows.
Among women, amenorrhea if it starts before puberty, and menorrhagia if starts after.
In some patients, deafness.
Hormone assays helpful in diagnosis.
Do not confuse hypothyroidism with:
Nephritis.
Heart failure (when it does not respond to digitalis).
In the initial stages of hypothyroidism, a large number of diseases.
Symptoms of myxedema coma that may appear in severe cases are:
Evidence of respiratory acidosis (drowsiness leading to coma) and marked hypothermia.
Respiratory insufficiency that may require tracheostomy and assisted respiration.
Management of hypothyroidism:
Thyroid replacement.
Symptomatic care in some instances (myxedema coma).

Cretinism

When and how cretinism will be suspected:
The sooner it is diagnosed, the better; try to diagnose it before the third month, when symptoms and signs are well developed.
There is a characteristic face, with open mouth, large tongue, and drooling.
The face also shows enlarged lips, the nose is flat, and its traits are grossly broad.
The skin is thick and wrinkled, very dry, yellow, and cold (hypothermia).
Hands are puffy and spade-shaped; feet are also puffy.
Dullness, apathy, and constipation are almost the rule.
Infants may be large at birth, but development is unusually slow.
Symptoms of established cretinism:
The above symptoms are more marked.
There is mental retardation, from relatively mild to intense.
Retarded growth results in dwarfism.
Patients are pot-bellied, with umbilical hernia.
Patients have a deep voice; some patients may develop deafness.
Mental torpor or frank retardation in most cases, apathy, and poor muscle activity are found.
There is delayed skeletal maturation, with delayed teething.
Symptoms of myxedema usually are noted.
The thyroid gland may be absent, of relatively normal shape, or goitrous, even reaching enormous proportions.
Help for diagnosis will be given by:
Radiologic studies showing retarded skeletal development (notably, absent femoral epiphyses).
Hormonal studies.

Management of cretinism:

Hormonal replacement, to be started as soon as possible and prolonged through life.

Hypoparathyroidism

Symptoms of hypoparathyroidism:

There is increased neuromuscular irritability.

Irritability causes special reflexes.

Chvostek's sign shows the increased reflex of the facial nerve when tapped near the angle of the jaw, causing contraction of muscles: Chvostek I includes eyelids, nose, and mouth; Chvostek II, only nose and mouth; Chvostek III, only the mouth.

Trousseau's sign shows carpopedal spasms after inflation of an applied cuff.

The skin is dry and scaly, may be infected with candidiasis; there is loss of hair (mostly eyebrows); and the nails are thin and brittle.

Not too rarely cataracts are present.

If the disease starts in childhood, there will be defective teeth (enamel poorly developed).

Hypoparathyroidism may be accompanied by mental troubles and ectodermal disorders.

Symptoms of acute hypoparathyroid crisis:

There is a tetanic crisis with muscle spasms (carpopedal, with ankle or wrist flexed and the phalanges extended), frequently painful, and lasting for about one hour; but duration may vary. Circumoral paresthesia may start the crisis.

Other symptoms may accompany the tetanic crisis: convulsions; stridor, wheezing, and dyspnea caused by laryngospasm; abdominal cramps; photophobia and diplopia; urinary frequency.

For diagnostic help check for early development of cataracts, prolonged Q-T intervals in the electrocardiogram, dense bones and basal ganglia calcifications, and the characteristic changes of blood calcium (low) and serum phosphate (high).

Do not confuse hypoparathyroidism with:

Other forms of tetany (metabolic or respiratory alkalosis, rickets, osteomalacia, pancreatitis, renal failure, hyperaldosteronism, etc.).

Epilepsy, choreoathetosis, brain tumors, and even asthma.

Management of hypoparathyroidism:

Provide calcium replacement.

Use dihydrotachysterol, calciferol, other calciferol metabolites when available, and even parathyroid hormone (this only for 1 week).

Phenobarbital and phenytoin may serve as valuable adjuncts to therapy.

Also, vitamin D may be used.

Pseudohypoparathyroidism

Additional symptoms that change the diagnosis of hypoparathyroidism into pseudohypoparathyroidism:

All symptoms listed for hypoparathyroidism, more or less marked.

Short stature and round face.

Short metacarpal bones, with absence of knuckles for the 4th and 5th fingers when making a fist; also, short metatarsals.

Ectopic soft tissue calcifications.

Mental retardation, which is mostly present in these cases.

No response to the use of parathyroid hormone; no increase in urinary phosphate (Ellsworth-Howard test).

Treat as a regular case of tetany.

What distinguishes pseudopseudohypoparathyroidism?

The symptoms are the same as in pseudohypoparathyroidism, but there are no abnormal blood chemistry findings.

Hyperparathyroidism

Are the clinical manifestations always patent in hyperparathyroidism?

There are cases with very few manifestations, which are discovered accidentally after performing blood chemical analysis.

Clinical manifestations in well-developed hyperparathyroidism:

There are three principal groups: urinary, skeletal, and general manifestations.

Polydipsia and polyuria are early manifestations.

Deposition of calcium salts will occur in the urine in the form of sand, gravel, or true stones.

Symptoms of obstruction may occur; also infection.

Nephrocalcinosis and renal damage may occur, sometimes leading to uremia.

The skeletal manifestations characterize osteitis fibrosa cystica or von Recklinghausen's disease.

Initial bone changes are noted by subperiosteal resorption of the cortex of phalanges (also other bones), a later loss of dental lamina dura, and final bone cysts.

An epulis of the jaw ("brown tumor") may be the first symptom.

Bone changes will result in back pain, painful shins, joint pains, and final fractures. Hyperextension of joints is very frequent.

Fractures will occur in the long bones, the spine, and the ribs, resulting in shortening of height, deviations of the spine, and clubbing of the fingers.

The most important general manifestations are: polydipsia, anorexia, nausea, and vomiting.

Other general manifestation are: hypertension, intractable peptic ulcer, asthenia, anemia, constipation, and weight loss.

Nails become strong and thick.

Paresthesias, depression, and even psychosis may occur.

Calcium may precipitate in tissues (band keratopathy around the cornea, around the joints, in the tubules—nephrocalcinosis).

A short Q-T interval in the electrocardiogram is noted.
Hypercalcemia is diagnostic.

In acute hyperparathyroid crisis the symptoms are:
Evidence of dehydration.
Hypercalcemia and azotemia.
Disorientation and collapse.

Differentiate hyperparathyroidism from:
Idiopathic hypercalciuria.
Sarcoidosis, vitamin D intoxication (response to cortisone).
Osteoporosis, and others.

Management of hyperparathyroidism:
Perform surgery, whenever possible.
In other cases, force fluids; give phosphate preparations; try furosemide or ethacrynic acid.

Rickets

Clinical characterization of rickets:
It will occur during infancy or childhood.
There is a history of deficient ingestion of vitamin D.
The infant will lack hair on the occipital side of the head because of constant movements due to poor rest and sleep.
The infant will present notably delayed activity for sitting, crawling, or walking.
Fontanels close late. They are wide, as are the sutures, in an abnormally soft skull (craniotabes, which is an early symptom).
Long bones show enlarged epiphyses, notably the rachitic rosary in the costochondral junctions.
Long bones may also be deformed (pigeon breast, bowlegs, etc.).
X-ray studies will help for an early diagnosis.

Do not mistake rickets for:
Chondrodystrophy, osteogenesis imperfecta, hydrocephalus.
Cretinism, Fanconi's syndrome, etc.

Management of rickets:
Vitamin D replacement.

Osteomalacia

Clinical characterization of osteomalacia:
It will occur in adulthood.
Symptomatology runs from mild to very severe.
There is bone pain, particularly long bones and ribs.
Symptoms of sprue may become apparent (glossy tongue, anemia).
Muscular weakness is observed, more marked in severe cases.
Listlessness will be apparent in advanced cases.
Bowing of long bones will take place in advanced cases, also.
In acute cases there may be a rapid course of symptoms, including tetany; but when compensation takes place, tetany disappears.
Demineralization occurs mainly in long bones, those of the lower extremities, pelvis, and spine; fibrous lamellas become visible, and fissurelike incomplete fractures will be noted.

Do not mistake osteomalacia for:
Hyperparathyroidism.
Osteoporosis of the senile or menopausal type, or other endocrine types (hyperthyroidism, pituitarism).
Multiple myeloma.
Atrophy due to disuse.

Management of osteomalacia:
Vitamin D replacement.

Milkman's Syndrome

Characteristics of this special type of osteomalacia:
There are multiple transparent stripes of absorption in bones, both long and flat.
These are multiple, symmetrical, bilateral, and appear as pseudofractures.
There is severe bone pain, which may impede walking.
Occasionally spontaneous fractures occur.
Diagnosis depends on X-ray films.

Management of Milkman's syndrome:
Vitamin D replacement.

Osteoporosis

This most common bone disease in the United States is due to:
Lack of estrogens in women, particularly early deprivation.
Low calcium intake.
In the elderly, possibly deficient intestinal lactase.
Lack of activity (bed rest, splints, etc.).
Secondarily, a previous disease, such as Cushing's disease, acromegaly, nutritional disturbances, etc.

Symptoms of osteoporosis:
There is initial pain in the weight-bearing vertebrae, particularly from eighth thoracic vertebra to fifth lumbar vertebra.
Pain is localized in the vertebra with no radiation.
Spontaneous fractures may occur; then bones may be painful; with fractures loss of height will result.
Demineralization occurs mainly in the spine and pelvis.

Differentiate osteoporosis from:
Osteomalacia, and hyperparathyroidism.
Bone metastasis, from breast or uterine cancer.

Management of osteoporosis:
Diet, with calcium and vitamin D.
Maintenance of activity as much as possible.
Specific treatment in all other cases.

Polyostotic Fibrous Dysplasia (Albright's Disease)

Essential characteristics of polyostotic fibrous dysplasia:
There is painless swelling of bones, particularly the skull, femur (upper end), tibia, hands and feet, ribs, and pelvis.

The bones present cysts or hyperostotic lesions.

Lesions may be single, but most frequently they are multiple and in segmental distribution.

Many patients will show a brown pigmentation in the skin over the diseased bones.

What does the brown pigmentation of the skin mean?

Most frequently it appears in females with true precocious puberty and rapid growth.

In this instance it indicates Albright's disease.

Osteitis Deformans (Paget's Disease)

Symptoms characterizing Paget's disease are:

Bone pain may start the symptomatology. There may also be headache.

The bones become soft, allowing easy bowing of legs and spine.

Fractures are relatively frequent, even with slight traumas.

Waddling gait is a common occurrence.

The skull may become notably enlarged, mainly noted in the forehead.

The skin is warmer over the affected bones.

X-ray films will show dense and expanded bones.

Management of Paget's disease:

Use calcitonin, mithramycin, or diphosphonates (if available).

Acute Pancreatitis

General symptoms common to all types of pancreatitis:

There is a sudden onset of the disease, with high fever, 38°-39°C (101°-102°F).

There are tachycardia and hypotension (leading to shock).

The outstanding symptom is severe abdominal pain.

The abdominal pain locates at the epigastric area, radiates to the back (may also radiate to right or left), and is steady.

The pain increases lying supine and improves by sitting, and leaning forward.

The abdomen is tender and distended.

There are nausea, vomiting, and constipation (more rarely, diarrhea).

There may be sweating, anxiety, and severe prostration.

The skin is pale and cold, and may be jaundiced.

How are the different types of acute pancreatitis characterized?

Edematous acute pancreatitis	Usually represents the earlier stages of the disease.
Hemorrhagic acute pancreatitis	Focal or generalized hemorrhages are noted, in the form of ecchymoses in the umbilical area (Cullen's sign), the groin, or the flank (Grey Turner's sign). A mass may be palpated in the epigastric area.
Necrotic acute pancreatitis	A mass is palapted in the epigastric area.

Do not mistake acute pancreatitis for:

Perforated peptic ulcer.

Common duct calculus.

Acute mesenteric thrombosis, or dissecting aortic aneurism.

Renal colic, acute cholecystitis, or intestinal obstruction.

Management of acute pancreatitis:

Careful symptomatic attention.

Chronic Pancreatitis

Symptomatology of chronic pancreatitis:

Not rarely there is a previous episode of acute pancreatitis.

There is pain, constant or intermittent, mild or severe, centered in the epigastrium, and possibly radiating to the back, the left shoulder, or the hypochondrium.

Pain may be relieved by sitting up.

There are anorexia, nausea and vomiting, constipation, and meteorism.

There may be mild muscle guarding, and perhaps paralytic ileus.

Subacute exacerbations, with jaundice and fever, may last from a few hours to 1 or 2 weeks.

Evidence of intestinal malabsorption may occur, particularly with steatorrhea.

The extent of pancreatic destruction will determine the development of other symptoms, including a frequent diabetes mellitus.

Management of chronic pancreatitis:

Symptomatic care.

Diabetes Mellitus

Conditions that usually favor the development of diabetes mellitus:

Heredity.

Obesity.

Hyperpituitarism.

Hyperthyroidism.

Hyperadrenalism.

Infective diseases.

Pancreatic diseases.

Pregnancy.

What are the main types of diabetes mellitus?

Insulinopenic diabetes	Deficient production of insulin; it affects young patients and nonobese adults.
Insulinoplethoric diabetes	Adequate production of insulin, but deficient response of end organ; it usually affects obese adults.

Most frequent symptoms of diabetes are:
- Polydipsia and polyuria.
- Asthenia.
- Polyphagia, with weight loss.
- Nocturnal enuresis.
- Pruritus in the pudendal area.
- Peripheral neuropathy.
- Visual changes, due mostly to refractive problems, but in more advanced cases, to diabetic retinopathy.

What are the symptoms of juvenile diabetes?
- It follows a severe course (is rare in adults).
- There may be a combination of dehydration, loss of tissue fat, and muscle wasting.
- There are frequent acidotic crises, and comatose states.
- There are frequent hypoglycemic attacks, because of incorrect insulin use.
- There is a relatively rapid occurrence of complications.

What are the symptoms of diabetes of adult onset?
- It is frequently associated with obesity.
- Regular symptoms occur, as stated above.
- Skin changes, in addition to pudendal pruritus, are: frequent chronic pyogenic infections; xanthomatosis; fungal infections (candidiasis), mostly in intertriginous areas (between fingers, axillae, breasts); brown, round, painless, atrophic "shin spots" in the pretibial area; vitiligo, which represents a polysyndrome and not a mere coincidence of diseases; and a rare necrobiosis lipoidica diabeticorum.
- Visual changes: refraction alters frequently, cataracts develop more or less rapidly, and the retinopathy is characterized by microaneurisms, hemorrhages, and exudates. Cases may develop retinal detachment and blindness.
- Occlusive vascular disease to the lower extremities, coronary arteriosclerosis, cerebral arteriosclerosis, and hypertension may develop in a relatively substantial number of patients.
- Perpheral neuropathy is almost constant in late stages, but may appear earlier in some instances. Males may show neuropathic impotence, which shows no remittence. Absence of reflexes (knee, ankle, etc.) may be noted.
- Intercapillary glomerulosclerosis will be present in a large number of patients with long-standing diabetes (Klimmestiel-Wilson disease).

Symptoms of diabetic ketoacidosis:
- There is a more or less insidious onset.
- Polydipsia and polyuria usually increase 1 or 2 days earlier.
- Also asthenia, nausea, and vomiting increase.
- Mental stupor will appear in the course of ketoacidosis, increasing in intensity until frank coma takes place.
- There are symptoms of dehydration, including hypotension and tachycardia.
- The breath will smell of acetone (a fruity odor).
- The diagnosis is made because of massive glycosuria, elevated glycemia, and low plasma bicarbonate.

Symptoms of lactic acidosis:
- There is marked hyperventilation, accompanying a rapid onset.
- There is mental stupor, which increases until complete coma develops.
- There are no symptoms of dehydration; blood pressure and heart rate are normal.
- Symptoms of tissue hypoxia or vascular collapse may show in some cases, not always related to diabetes.
- The diagnosis is confirmed by finding an elevated concentration of plasma lactic acid.

Symptoms of nonketotic hyperglycemic coma are:
- It usually follows surgery, infections (pneumonia), burns, or the use of certain drugs (diuretics, glucocorticoids, diazoxide, etc.).
- Onset is very insidious in most cases.
- Increased asthenia, polydipsia, and polyuria are found.
- Marked symptoms of dehydration develop.
- Mental stupor progresses to convulsions and coma.
- Diagnosis is suggested by intense dehydration, with lethargy or frank coma, and the lack of Kussmaul respirations.

Do not confuse diabetes with:
- Renal glycosuria.
- Lactosuria.
- Diabetes secondary to other diseases, particularly due to endocrine glands.

Management of diabetes:
- Diet alone.
- Diet with insulin.
- Diet with oral hypoglycemic drugs.
- Management of complications.
- Management of comatose conditions (insulin).

Hypoglycemia

Main causes of hypoglycemic conditions are:
- Hyperinsulinism.
- Extrapancreatic tumors.
- Effects of insulin or other oral hypoglycemic drugs.
- Fasting states. (Delayed ingestion of food, particularly after hypoglycemic drugs.)
- Gastrectomy, increased vagal tone.
- Chemical or occult diabetes.

Symptoms of hyperinsulinic hypoglycemia are:
- A feeling of disinterest or detachment from surroundings, with asthenia and slurred speech.
- Behavioral changes, including anxiety, aggressiveness, or frank psychosis, all ending in confulsions and/or coma.
- Blurred vision, diplopia, headache.
- Moist and pale skin, ending in profuse sweating. This is an important evidence differentiating hypo- from hyperglycemic conditions.

Palpitations, which may be noted in late stages.

Progression to irreversible brain damage, if not duly corrected.

For the final diagnosis of hyperinsulinism consider: a history of frequent hypoglycemic attacks, blood glucose of 40 mg per 100 ml (or less), and a rapid recovery after administration of glucose.

Symptoms of extrapancreatic tumors are:

Knowledge of existence of one of these tumors, namely, adrenocortical carcinoma, retroperitoneal sarcoma, hepatoma, etc.

Fasting hypoglycemia together with low insulin levels.

Other regular symptoms of hypoglucemia.

Symptoms of hypoglycemia due to administration of hypoglycemic drugs are:

Injection of insulin or administration of oral drugs before the attack.

Insuffient food intake following antidiabetic medication; or unduly delayed intake.

Sudden onset of hypoglycemic symptoms.

Rapid recovery after glucose administration.

Regular symptoms of hypoglycemia always noted.

Symptoms of fasting hypoglycemia:

They are not related to administration of antidiabetic medication.

They are occasionally related to hyperparasympathicotonia with early emptying of the stomach and early hyperinsulinism.

Regular symptoms of hypoglycemia will appear.

Other symptoms have been related but do not always correspond to true hypoglycemia, namely, fatigue, tremulousness, behavioral changes, headache, poor concentration, hunger, etc.

Symptoms of postgastrectomy hypoglycemia are:

History of previous surgery.

Also related to hypersympathicotonia.

Regular symptoms of hypoglycemia.

Symptoms of chemical or occult diabetes hypoglycemia are:

Frequent family history of diabetes.

Hypoglycemic symptoms appearing quite late after ingestion of glucose.

Patients frequently phlegmatic and obese.

Management of hypoglycemia:

Glucose administration as soon as possible.

Surgery for tumors.

Special diets, in other cases.

Cancer of the Pancreas

Symptoms of cancer of the head of the pancreas:

There is abdominal pain, in its upper parts, vague and diffuse.

Pain will be more severe and will radiate to the back, in late stages of the disease; it will also become more persistent.

There are weight loss, anorexia, vomiting, and constipation (rarely, diarrhea).

There is jaundice, accompanied by a palpable gall bladder (Courvoisier's sign or law), which may be painful.

Some patients will develop thrombophlebitis, with swollen legs.

In a few patients the tumor will be noted as a hard, fixed, and possibly tender mass.

X-ray films will aid in the diagnosis.

Symptoms of cancer of the body and tail of the pancreas:

There is upper abdominal distress.

There are anorexia and weight loss.

Distress becomes true epigastric pain radiating to the left lumbar area.

A mass will be palpated in the epigastrium.

Some patients will develop thrombophlebitis, with enlarged legs.

Management of cancer of the pancreas:

Surgical.

Addison's Disease (Adrenal Insufficiency)

Characteristic findings leading to the diagnosis of Addison's disease are:

Intense asthenia, limiting light efforts, and even noted in the morning before leaving bed.

Melanodermia, starting in knuckles, genital areas, and the gums (upper lateral incisive teeth). Easy pigmentation after sun exposure or after irritation.

Fully developed melanodermia diffusely covering the whole body, particularly the exposed parts, pressure points, nipples, genital and perineal areas, recent scars; and increase intensity and number of freckles.

Loss of weight.

Hypotension.

Other frequent symptoms also noted in Addison's disease are:

Anorexia, nausea, and vomiting.

Diarrhea, not too rarely.

Irritability, both nervous and mental; but this occurs together with apathy.

The patient easily fainting, notably after missing meals; there may be other symptoms of hypoglycemia.

Vitiligo, relatively frequent in these cases.

Small heart.

Enlarged lymph nodes.

Scant or absent axillary and pubic hair (more frequent among females).

Scant or absent sweating.

Frequent and severe dental caries.

Stiffness of the cartilages of the ear, or Thorn's sign.

In some patients, tenderness of the costovertebral angle (Rogoff's sign).

Less frequently noted symptoms in Addison's disease are:

Muscle atrophy.

Mood changes.

Tendinous reflexes diminished or absent.
Rare cases of bulimia, instead of anorexia.
Rarely, hemorrhagic stomatitis.
Symptoms of hypogenitalism, both in men and women, not too rarely.

Elements for the diagnosis of Addison's disease are:
Very low amounts of adrenal hormones in blood and urine.
Special tests (8-hour intravenous corticotropin, response to ACTH, water excretion, insulin tolerance test—this rarely used now).

Management of Addison's disease:
Hormone replacement.
Care of complications (tuberculosis, overdosage, etc.).

Adrenal Crisis (Acute Adrenal Insufficiency)

Causes of these crises:
Deprivation of medication, or insufficient administration of hormones.
Trauma to the adrenals, including overwhelming sepsis causing massive hemorrhage in the Waterhouse-Friderichsen syndrome.
Unusual stress or fasting in a patient with latent adrenal insufficiency.
Pituitary necrosis.
Thyroid or insulin administration to a patient with panhypopituitarism.

Symptoms of adrenal crisis are:
High fever, with hypotension.
Headache, nausea, vomiting, and frequently diarrhea.
Asthenia.
Pain and tenderness in the costovertebral angle.
Abdominal pain.
Confusional state, which may lead to coma.
Symptoms of dehydration.
Increased melanodermia.
The skin possibly also showing cyanosis, petechiae (meningococcemia), and sparse hair.
Enlarged lymph nodes.
Eosinophilia, with low sodium and elevated potassium in blood, a good help for diagnosis.

Do not confuse adrenal crises with:
Diabetic coma.
Hypoglycemic coma.
Cerebrovascular accident.

Management of adrenal crisis:
Treat shock, and give hydrocortisone.

Adrenocortical Hyperfunction (Cushing's Syndrome)

Symptoms characterizing Cushing's syndrome:
Are the same as those characterizing the disease, but without any evidence of pituitary tumor.
Good help for diagnosis is given by hormonal assays and radiography.
For more details, consult Cushing's disease.

Management of Cushing's disease or syndrome:
Surgery or radiotherapy.

Adrenogenital Syndrome

Age of occurrence of the adrenogenital syndrome:
Intrauterine, infancy, or childhood.
Adulthood.

Symptoms of females with adrenogenital syndrome starting at early age:
Pseudohermaphroditism, with enlarged clitoris, urogenital sinus formation, and hirsutism. When there is urogenital sinus formation, labia may appear fused.
Accelerated growth, with advanced skeletal maturation.
Final growth results short because of early closure of epiphyses.
Normal female sex chromosomes.
Excessive muscle development.
Possibility of adrenocortical failure.

Symptoms of females with adrenogenital syndrome during infancy:
Only enlarged clitoris and hirsutism; no other symptoms of pseudohermaphroditis.
More frequently occurring adrenocortical failure.

Symptoms of adult females with adrenogenital syndrome:
Enlargement of the clitoris, but not so much as when it occurs at earlier stages. Atrophy of breasts and genitalia.
Hirsutism, including a tendency to baldness.
Hypo- or amenorrhea.
Excessive muscle development (feminine contours are lost).
Enlarged thyroid cartilages ("Adam's apple"), with hoarseness or deepening of the voice.
Skin changes, showing acne, roughening of the voice, and odorous sweat.

Symptoms of males with adrenogenital syndrome starting at early age:
Macrogenitosomia praecox.
Other symptoms, as for females of the same age.

Symptoms of males with adrenogenital syndrome during infancy:
Precocious virilization.
Other symptoms, as for females of the same age.

Do not confuse adrenogenital syndrome with:
Testicular tumors.
Lesions of the hypothalamus or the pineal gland.
Sex chromosome abnormalities.
Ovarian hirsutism.
Very rarely other causes will be involved.

Management of the adrenogenital syndrome:
Surgical removal of the existing adrenal tumor.
Corticoids for adrenal hyperplasia.
Also, estrogen-progesterone therapy to be considered.
Cosmetic surgery frequently needed.

Hyperaldosteronism

Forms of hyperaldosteronism usually differentiated:
- Primary hyperaldosteronism, also known as Conn's syndrome.
- Secondary hyperaldosteronism, this seen in cardiac failure, cirrhosis with ascites, nephrotic syndrome, obstructions of the renal artery.

Usual symptoms of primary hyperaldosteronism are:
- Hypertension.
- Polydipsia and polyuria.
- Muscular weakness, possibly with transient paralysis.
- Tetany, in some instances.
- Paresthesias.
- Headache.

Usual symptoms of secondary hyperaldosteronism are:
- Similar to the above, plus the symptoms of the causative disease.
- Edema may be present; or more marked hypertension, instead.
- Serum sodium tends to increase (in primary hyperaldosteronism the tendency is to decrease).
- Plasma-renin activity is increased (decreased in primary cases).

Diagnosis is given by:
- Elevated plasma and urinary aldosterone levels.

Do not confuse hyperaldosteronism with:
- Excessive intake of licorice or laxatives.
- Periodic paralysis.
- Hypopotassemia.

Management of hyperaldosteronism:
- Surgical, for most cases of primary hyperaldosteronism.
- For secondary hyperaldosteronism, treatment of the cause.

Pheochromocytoma

Clinical evidence of pheochromocytoma shows:
- Paroxysmal attacks of hypertension, with tachycardia and palpitation.
- Paroxysmal attacks, coincident with hypertension, of headache, sweating, pallor or flushing of face and extremities.
- Also, attacks of pain (anginal or abdominal), dyspnea, nervous irritability, blurred vision or actual blindness, aphasia, nausea and vomiting, and, on rare occasions, loss of consciousness.
- Loss of weight, regular hypertension in a number of patients (together with postural hypotension and tachycardia), enlarged heart, febricula, and abdominal or flank tumor palpated in a few patients.
- Rarely: retinal hemorrhage, papilledema, or thyroid enlargement.
- Elevation of catecholamines and special tests helpful in diagnosis.

Do not confuse pheochromocytoma with:
- Other forms of hypertension.

Management of pheochromocytoma:
- Surgery.
- Phentolamine, phenoxybenzamine.

Adrenal Cancer

The existence of an adrenal cancer will be suspected in:
- Diseases with hyperadrenalism, particularly Cushing's syndrome.
- Cases presenting hypercalcemia.
- Cases presenting hypoglycemia.
- Cases with polycythemia.

Management of adrenal cancer:
- Surgery, at the earliest possible stage.

Precocious Puberty

What are the common causes of sexual precocity?
- Constitutional (most cases of true sexual precocity, usually in females).
- Other cases due to lesions of the hypothalamus, the pituitary, encephalitis, tumors of the testis or the ovary, and adrenal tumors.
- Also to be considered, polyostotic fibrous dysplasia (mostly in girls) and some cases of hypothyroidism; rarely it is due to hormonal administration.

What are the common symptoms of precocious puberty?
- Premature development of sex characteristics.
- Pubic and axillary hair (beard in males).
- External genitalia of the adult type; also breasts, in females.
- Spermatogenesis and ovulation in neurogenic or pituitary cases; but not in those due to gonadal or adrenal induction.
- Sex hormones excreted in normal amounts in neurogenic or pituitary cases; in excessive amounts in gonadal cases.
- Initial rapid growth, but results in smaller stature because of epiphyseal closure.

Management of precocious puberty:
- Perform surgery.
- Consider the initial cause.

Hypogonadism

General symptoms of hypogonadism are:
- Lack of sex changes at due age.
- Striking long legs and arms with a relatively shorter trunk.
- High-pitched voice.
- External and internal genitals (prostate, uterus) underdeveloped.
- Skin soft and pale; tans very little.
- Body hair not developed (pubic area, axillae, beard).
- In males no temporal recession of hair in the head, nor the usual development of thyroid cartilages ("Adam's apple").

If the problem starts postpubertally, a normal previous development followed by regression of sex characters (external genitalia, internal genitalia, hair, libido).
Lack of spermatogenesis in males; lack of menstruation in females.
Management of hypogonadism:
Hormonal replacement.

Klinefelter's Syndrome

What characterizes this genetic abnormality?
There is usually an extra X chromosome, that is, XXY instead of the regular male XY. There is, naturally, a positive buccal smear.
Symptoms noted in Klinefelter's syndrome are:
Regular symptoms of hypogonadism.
Gynecomastia, and small firm testes.
Female escutcheon.
Prostate and penis possibly normal, even with some potency and ejaculation (but azoospermia).
Muscular and skeletal development, usually close to normal.
In most patients, mental retardation.
Hormonal and chromosomal studies will clarify the diagnosis.
Management of Klinefelter's syndrome:
Hormonal replacement, if needed.
Plastic surgery, if needed for gynecomastia.

Reifenstein's Syndrome

What characterizes this variant of Klinefelter's syndrome?
Normal karyotype, and also buccal smear.
Symptoms of hypogonadism present, including eunuchoidal proportions.
Hypospadias mostly present.
Gynecomastia rarely absent.
Management of Reifenstein's syndrome:
Hormonal replacement.
Plastic surgery, when applicable.

Turner's Syndrome

What characterizes this genetic abnormality?
There is a karyotype with only one X chromosome, lacking the other sex chromosome, either X or Y; reports read XO.
There are cases presenting the same phenotype, with the same symptomatology, naturally, but with a normal karyotype; these will be males, or if females, they will be referred to as Noonan's syndrome.
Symptoms of Turner's syndrome are:
At birth, lymphedema in the dorsa of hands and feet, and in the back of the neck.
Underdeveloped genitals, and lack of hair.
Amennorrhea and underdeveloped breast, when of age.
Short stature, stocky shield chest, increased carrying angle of the arms, osteoporosis, skeletal abnormalities (short metacarpals, etc.), and very frequently webbing of the lateral folds of the neck.
Frequent cardiovascular disorders, of the congenital type.
Not too rarely, eye disorders.
Nevi relatively common, as well as thyroiditis and diabetes.
Premature senility.
Mental retardation of very slight to more profound character.
Karyotypes will back the diagnosis.
Management of Turner's syndrome:
Hormonal replacement.
Special education, if so needed.

Turner-Mongolism Polysyndrome

What characterizes this genetic anomaly?
The karyotype will show both XO and trisomy 21.
Symptoms of Turner-mongolism polysyndrome are:
The greater majority of symptoms of Turner's syndrome.
The greater majority of symptoms of mongolism.
More or less marked mental retardation.
Regarding external genitalia, the clitoris may be normal or even of an increased size.
Management of Turner-mongolism polysyndrome:
Hormonal replacement.
Special education.

Other Sex Chromosomes Aberrations

What other sex chromosome aberrations may be diagnosed?
There is the superfemale or XXX syndrome, with three X's in the chromosomes and two Barr bodies in the buccal smear. Most cases are retardates.
Cases with more than three X's in the chromosome have been found, XXXX, XXXXX; the great majority are also mental retardates.
The XYY syndrome has been noted in relatively normal males, but the great majority of cases have been found among known criminals, most of them with slight mental retardation.
Other conditions may be true hermaphroditism or the so-called testicular feminization.

Climacterium

Give the exact meaning for both words: climacterium, also called climacteric; and menopause:
Climacterium or climacteric is the final stage of reproductive activity in the female, and of normal diminution of sex activity in the male, with the accompanying symptoms of this period.
Menopause is the cessation of menstruation in the female.

At what age do the climacterium and menopause occur?
- Normally, the climacterium will occur between 45 and 55 years of age; exceptionally, before or after.
- Normally, menopause should occur at about the same time as the climacterium, but even more frequently the climacterium may occur before or after menopause.

What are the symptoms related to menopause?
- Strictly speaking, only one, which is the cessation of menses.
- It cause could be added, that is, the lack of ovulation.

What symptoms are better attributed to the climacterium?
- Menstrual derangements, particularly uterine hemorrhages.
- More or less marked changes of a masculine character, such as hitsutism, exaggerated libido, aggressivity, etc. More rarely, the opposite.
- A more or less elevated hypertension, and vasomotor instability.
- Hot flushes, which may have a more or less marked relationship with the circulatory system; they will rarely be noted in the normal woman.
- A tendency to gain weight; less frequently, to lose it.
- Not rarely, rheumatic pains.
- Nervous symptoms of tension, fullness of the head, instability, depression, exhilaration, lassitude, insomnia, sadness, or other fears.
- Symptoms of a coincident or latent disease will become apparent.
- Among males, the climacterium is much less important than in females; there are only depression, forgetfulness, decreased sexual activity and potency, and perhaps the initiation of other symptoms pertaining to involution, of which the climacterium is a preceding phase.

Do not confuse the climacterium with:
- Any coincidental or latent disease.

Management of the climacterium and menopause:
- Hormonal replacement.

What is important to consider regarding the climacterium?
- It is a transient phase in the life of the person.

Amenorrhea

What is primary amenorrhea?
- The lack of menstruation in a female who has reached about 18 years of age.

What is secondary amenorrhea?
- The lack of menstruation in a woman who already started this function.

Causes of primary amenorrhea:
- Any serious organic illness.
- Hypothalamic dysfunctions.
- Pituitary lesions.
- Uterine malformations, including unresponsive or atrophic endometrium.
- Hermaphroditism, or other forms of hypogonadism.
- Imperforate hymen; other obstructions to the outflow.
- Adrenogenital syndrome and other forms of adrenal influence.

Causes of secondary amenorrhea:
- Pregnancy, and lactation (if prolonged, it is the Chiari-Frommel syndrome).
- Menopause.
- Post-contraceptive medication.
- Pituitary tumors, particularly those tumors secreting prolactin (and prolactin insufficiency).
- Anemia, and malnutritional states.
- Emotional stress.
- Endocrine diseases interfering with ovarian function.
- Polycystic ovaries, and other ovarian dysfunctions.
- Other causes mentioned for primary amenorrhea.

Management of amenorrhea:
- Depends on the causative factor, which will be corrected.

Polycystic Ovaries (Stein-Leventhal Syndrome)

Characterization of the polycystic ovary syndrome:
- Occurrence only in young women.
- Obesity, but not in all patients.
- Mild hirsutism, insidiously progressive. Pubic hair of the male type.
- Acne.
- Menstrual disorders, particularly oligo- or amenorrhea.
- Bilateral polycystic ovaries that may be palpated.

Management of the Stein-Leventhal syndrome:
- Wedge resection of the ovaries.

Intersexual States

Symptoms of intersexual states:
- Patients presenting mixed male and female characteristics.
- Patients presenting different chromosomal karyotypes.

Causes of intersex conditions:
- Turner's syndrome.
- Klinefelter's syndrome.
- Reifenstein's syndrome.
- True hermaphroditism.
- Adrenogenital syndrome.
- Cryptorchidism.
- Congenital absence of one or several of the genital organs.
- Diagnosis helped with karyotyping, X-ray studies, and even surgical procedures and biopsy.

Management of intersex conditions:
- Surgery or hormonal replacement, depending on the cause.

Testicular Feminization

Symptoms of testicular feminization syndrome are:
- Feminine phenotype.
- Normal vulva and shortened vagina; normal or enlarged clitoris.

Absent uterus.
No axillary or pubic hair.
Primary amenorrhea.
Barr buccal smear and karyotype masculine.

Management of testicular feminization:
Removal of testes (high risk of malignancy), which is usually followed by hot flushes.
Estrogen therapy.

Tumors of the Testis

Symptoms of testicular tumors:
Usually the scrotal mass is palpable.
Most of them are hyperfunctional.
There is a high incidence of malignancy.

Symptoms of *seminoma:*
No endocrine manifestations.
Tumor noted after 30 years of age.
High levels of follicle stimulating hormone.

Management of seminoma:
Radiation.

Symptoms of *choriocarcinoma:*
Gynecomastia.
Pregnancy test positive.

Management of choriocarcinoma:
Early removal (invasive and metastisizing).

Symptoms of *Leydig cell tumor:*
May be bilateral.
Is virilizing. Precocious puberty.
17-ketosteroids are elevated.

Management of Leydig cell tumor:
Removal.

Symptoms of *teratoma* of the testicles:
Appearance early in life.
No endocrine symptoms.
Invasive tumor.

Management of teratoma of the testicles:
Removal, as early as possible.

Hypergonadism

Symptoms of hypergonadism in the male:
Precocious puberty, in childhood.
Symptoms of testicular tumor, as above.

Symptoms of hypergonadism in the female:
Precocious puberty, in childhood.
Menstrual changes, particularly menorrhagia, rarely amenorrhea.
Sterility.
Symptoms of metropathia hemorrhagica.
Symptoms of feminizing tumors, such as granulosa and theca cell tumors.

Management of hypergonadism:
Remove the cause, whenever possible.

7. Metabolism and Nutrition

Obesity

What is the guideline for determining ideal weight for a given person?

- The height of that person, which will indicate the accepted standards, as found in special tables. Age also plays a role.
- The deviation from these standards will indicate obesity or leanness, if it is 10% in excess or deficit.
- Actually, an excess of only 10% may be considered overweight and not frank obesity, which starts above 20%, without any doubt.

Symptoms of obesity are:

- Excess weight in relation to height and age.
- Excessive fat deposition in tissues, which increases body volume.
- Symptoms of the causative factor for weight increase.

Factors useful in evaluating obesity due to *excessive food intake:*

- History of feeding habits of the person.
- History of the regular physical activity of the patient.
- No other symptoms usually noted, except those directly related to the burden of excessive weight, that is, tiredness, lack of agility, and the like.

Evaluating obesity due to *psychologic factors:*

- True obesity factors are the same as for excessive food intake.
- There will be added a history and symptomatology of psychologic frustrations; or the need for overprotection.
- A vicious cycle of psychologic factor-overeating-psychologic factor is frequently established.

Evaluating the *Pickwickian syndrome* of obesity-hypoventilation:

- There is excessive obesity; the weight index (weight found divided by ideal weight) comes close to 2.
- The respiratory muscles are weak, and the chest walls show low compliance.
- Patients usually show somnolence, polycythemia with cyanosis, hypoxia with hypercapnia, and periodic breathing.
- In long-standing cases they may have crises with respiratory acidosis, pulmonary hypertension, right ventricular hypertrophy, and heart failure.

Evaluating obesity due to *hyperpituitary* function:

- Symptoms of Cushing's disease.
- The Achard-Thiers syndrome of hyperpituitaric women with excessive growth of facial hair and diabetes (the bearded diabetic women).

Evaluating obesity due to *hypopituitary* function:

- Symptoms of adiposogenital dystrophy or Frölich's syndrome.
- Symptoms of the Laurence-Moon-Biedl syndrome.

Evaluating obesity due to *hypothyroidism:*

- It is rarely encountered; it mostly is a myxedematous infiltration.
- Hypothyroid patients will more easily develop obesity when it occurs due to other, concomitant factors, either exogenous or endogenous.

Evaluating obesity due to *adrenal* causes:

- Cushing's syndrome may be the original factor.
- Obesity is a frequent symptom of most kinds of adrenal symptoms, together with excessive muscle development.

Evaluating obese *diabetics:*

- Family history of diabetes is usually positive.
- There is evidence of occult or chemical diabetes, or frank diabetes.
- Hunger may increase during the hypoglycemic phases, before treatment is advised.

Evaluating obesity due to *hypogenitalism:*

- Symptoms of the hypophysary adiposogenital syndrome with congenital abnormalities (Laurence-Moon-Biedl syndrome).
- Symptoms of Frölich's syndrome.
- Absence or removal of gonads.
- Not rarely, together with climacteric symptoms.

Evaluating obesity due to *other* causes:

- There are symptoms of diseases of the central nervous system, such as hypothalamic lesions, tumors, infections, etc.
- Obesity may occur in patients with hypertension, gall bladder diseases, coronary arteriosclerosis, and gout.

Management of obesity:

- Advise a hypocaloric diet, adequate to the patient and the stage of the disease.
- Treat the causative factor, whenever present.

Jejuno-ileal shunt has been widely performed, but is not advisable.
Appetite supressants may work for only a limited time. Recommend exercise.

Thinness and Cachexia

Symptoms of weight loss are:
- Decreased weight that is more than 10% below the normal for height and age.
- Lack of fat deposition in tissues, which decreases the body volume.
- Wrinkles noted in the face and body; also muscles and vessels more easily seen.
- In some cases, hypotension, tiredness, irritability, or depression.
- Symptoms of the causative factor for weight loss.

Symptoms of *anorexia nervosa:*
- Females are more frequently affected (7:1) than males.
- Patients are affected in their teens or early twenties.
- Amenorrhea is an early and thereafter relatively persistent symptom.
- There is intolerance to cold.
- Fine dawny lanugo may give a hirsute appearance.
- Other symptoms of malnutrition (vitamins, minerals, etc.) will occur.
- In males the symptoms are the same, but instead of amenorrhea there will appear some deficiency of testicular activity.
- Characteristic of the disease are the complex psychologic factors leading to refusal of food.
- Efforts will be made to differentiate anorexia nervosa from hypopituitary cachexia (Simmond's disease): in the first instance the patient will be more cachectic and will present lanugo giving a sort of hirsutic appearance; in the second there will be loss of axillary and pubic hair.

Symptoms of *marasmus* are:
- Atrophy of tissues, with subcutaneous fat absent or minimal.
- Skin changes, including rash, desquamation, ulceration, pigmentary changes, but with no edema.
- Cheilosis, stomatitis, conjunctivitis, muscular wasting.
- Hair sparse or depigmented.
- Anorexia and vomiting, hepatomegaly, diarrhea.
- Irritability and apathy.
- Symptoms of the causative disease, particularly mental retardation, cystic fibrous disease, diarrhea, and also prematurity.
- Retarded growth when affecting infants or children.

Symptoms of inadequate protein intake or *kwashiorkor:*
- Similar to marasmus, above.
- Edema of the tissues, always.
- More often present in weanling infants, but may occur at any age.
- More often in underprivileged families.
- Hepatic enlargement; resembles portal cirrhosis.
- Cases may present only partial symptomatology.

Symptoms of loss of weight due to *endocrine* causes:
- Pituitary cachexia or Simmond's disease, will present a rich symptomatology.
- Symptoms of hyperthyroidism.
- Symptoms of hypoadrenalism (Addison's disease).
- Symptoms of diabetes, particularly of the juvenile type.

Symptoms of *cachexia strumipriva* are:
- A very severe case of hyperthyroidism.
- The patient presenting a good appearance until the cachectic stage.
- Very marked weight loss, with a deteoirated general condition.
- Intense anorexia.
- Anemia.

Symptoms of weight loss due to *infections:*
- Symptoms of an acute infection, such as typhoid fever, tuberculosis, typhus or other rickettsial diseases, etc.
- Symptoms of chronic infection, such as syphilis, chronic septic conditions, gastroenteritis and other gastrointestinal diseases, etc.

Symptoms of weight loss due to *parasitic* infestations:
- Symptoms of malaria.
- Symptoms of ancylostomiasis.
- Symptoms of trichocephalus infestation.
- Symptoms of any of the tapeworm infestations.
- Symptoms of amebic dysentery.
- Symptoms of lambliasis.
- Symptoms of schistosomiasis or bilharziasis.
- Symptoms of leishmaniasis (kala-azar, American leishmaniasis).
- Symptoms of trypanosomiasis.
- Symptoms of toxoplasmosis.

Symptoms of weight loss due to *intoxications* are:
- Those symptoms corresponding to the causative disease, namely, alcoholism, nicotinism, addicting diseases, etc.

More frequent causes of weight loss due to *gastrointestinal diseases* are:
- Pyloric stenosis, and other forms of gastrointestinal stenosis.
- Gastritis, mainly due to anachlorhydria, peptic ulcer, or gastric cancer.
- Resection of the stomach.
- Symptoms of pancreatic or liver disease.

Evaluation of *other* diseases that may cause loss of weight:
- Any psychotic condition may be the cause; the symptoms will be evident.
- Any neurotic condition may also be the cause; the symptoms will also be evident.
- Menière's paroxysmal labyrinthine vertigo may cause weight loss.
- Involutive weight loss may occur; not rarely, transient.
- Any form of cancer may cause weight loss.

Management of weight loss and cachexia:
- Treat the cause aggressively.

Advise a balanced diet with a caloric surplus.

Try a psychologic approach by experienced people for anorexia nervosa; a trial with corticoids may be given.

For marasmus and kwashiorkor give a surplus of high value protein diet, with vitamins, and adequate care for hydration and other factors.

Lipodystrophia Progressivia (Barraquer-Simons Disease)

Evaluation of this mixed form of partial weight loss in the upper parts of the body, and obesity of the lower parts:

It is much more frequent among women than among men.

The fattening of the lower parts of the body is always notable.

The leanness of the upper parts of the body may be less marked; but it also is notable in advanced cases, with disappearance of the fatty ball of Bichat.

In advances cases the face has the appearance of a denuded skull.

Complete deprivation of fat tissues may occur in the upper parts of the body, from the hips upward.

From the hips downward, there is fat accumulation, even with large pads in hips, buttocks, and thighs. Feet remain normal.

If the patient receives a hypercaloric diet, the only result will be further fattening of the lower parts of the body; if a hypocaloric diet, further weight loss of the upper parts.

Management of lypodystrophia progressive:

Some cases may respond to corticoid therapy (in hypercorticalism there is a tendency to accumulate fat in the upper parts of the body), with an adequate caloric diet.

Dehydration

Symptoms of dehydration are:

History of a cause for water loss.

Increased thirst, and notable oliguria.

Decreased skin turgor; flushed skin.

Dry mucous membranes, shrunken and corrugated tongue.

Weight loss.

A soft eyeball, noted at touch.

Tachycardia and postural hypotension.

As dehydration becomes more severe, hyperpnea, weakness with lethargy, confusion with hallucinations and delirium, all of it ending in shock and coma.

Symptoms of the causative factor.

What are the causes that provoke dehydration?

Inadequate fluid intake, or unusual losses through sweating, etc.

Hot environment or fever.

Vomiting or diarrhea.

Polyuria, due to diabetes, kidney disease, etc.

Hypercalcemia or hypopotassemia.

Hypercorrection of obstructive uropathy, or excessive use of diuretics.

Management of dehydration:

Water replacement; intravenous administration of 2.5% glucose, or electrolyte infusions.

Overhydration

Causes of overhydration are:

Intake over excretory capacity.

Excessive infusions given therapeutically (?).

Acute or chronic impaired renal excretion.

Heart failure, liver disease with ascites, or hormonal causes.

Symptoms of water intoxication:

Headache.

Nausea and vomiting.

Abdominal pains of a crampy nature.

Weakness, and possibly convulsions.

Stupor leading to coma.

Management of overhydration:

Water restriction; hypertonic saline infusions may be given.

Respiratory Acidosis

Causes that may induce respiratory acidosis are:

Depression of respiratory centers by anesthesia, drugs, or organic disorders.

Weakened muscles of respiration, as in Pickwickian syndrome, polio, myasthenia gravis, drugs, etc.

Decreased pulmonary function, as with bronchiectasis, pneumonia, pneumothorax, emphysema, laryngeal edema, foreign bodies, etc.

Symptoms of respiratory acidosis are:

Drowsiness.

Stupor, leading to coma.

Cyanosis.

Insidious development in the presence of any of the foregoing causative conditions.

Elevated P_{CO_2} and total CO_2, and low pH, in the blood.

Management of respiratory acidosis:

Treat the causative factor, aggressively.

To improve respiration, surgery may be needed, and assisted respiration may be used. Take care with oxygen administration not to make the situation worse.

Metabolic Acidosis

Causes that may induce metabolic acidosis are:

Diabetic ketoacidosis, including lactic acidosis.

Starvation.

Water loss with diarrhea.

Enteric fistulae.
Kidney insufficiency, including tubular defect.
Ingestion of acid salts, and other poisons.
Continuous use of carbonic anhydrase.

Symptoms of metabolic acidosis are:
Possibly few or no symptoms.
Headache, with weakness or malaise.
Pain in the abdomen; also nausea and vomiting.
Hyperpnea.
In ketoacidosis (diabetes), acetone odor of the breath.
Symptoms of dehydration (poor skin turgor, dry tongue, soft eyeballs).
If prolonged or severe, stupor progressing to shock and coma.
In cases of lactic acidosis there may also be, as causative factor, heart failure, pulmonary edema or insufficiency, anoxic or hypovolemic conditions, nonketotic diabetic acidosis, hepatic failure, and the use of phenformin, salicylates, or paraldehyde.
Check for decreased pH, total CO_2, and P_{CO_2}; lactic acid will be elevated in lactic acidosis.

Management of metabolic acidosis:
Treat aggressively the causative factor.
Use bicarbonate infusions.

Respiratory Alkalosis

Causes that may induce respiratory alkalosis are:
Hyperventilation (from neurosis, fever, hypoxia).
Hepatic coma.
Anesthesia or incorrectly assisted respiration.
Salicylate poisoning.
Lesions of the central nervous system.

Symptoms of respiratory alkalosis:
Check for anxiety and hyperventilation.
Lightheadedness and agitation may be noted.
Paresthesias may occur.
In prolonged cases there will be neuromuscular irritability, with tetany and intermittent assumed posture (asterixis).
Syncope may also occur.
Increased pH and decreased total CO_2 and P_{CO_2} are found.

Management of respiratory alkalosis:
Treat the cause; reduce anxiety.
Rebreathe the expired air from a paper (no plastic!) bag.
Some patients need assisted respiration, with 5% CO_2 and 95% O_2.

Metabolic Alkalosis

Causes that may induce respiratory alkalosis are:
Vomiting. Consider also gastric drainage.
Use of diuretic drugs of any kind.
Adrenocortical excess due to disease or therapy.

Symptoms of metabolic alkalosis are:
Irritability.
Neuromuscular irritability, possibly with tetany (with normal calcium).
Weakness or ileus, in a few cases.
Increased pH, total CO_2, and P_{CO_2}.

Management of metabolic alkalosis:
Adequate replacement of water, sodium, potassium, and chloride.

Hypernatremia

Causes of excessive sodium concentration in blood:
Water loss or deficient water intake.
Fever, heart failure, hepatic cirrhosis, nephrosis.
Diabetes insipidus, or intracranial tumors.
Adrenal hyperfunction (Cushing's syndrome, hyperaldosteronism).

Symptoms of hypernatremia are:
Symptoms of dehydration, usually not well marked.
Confusion and lack of alertness.
Stupor leading to coma.

Management of hypernatremia:
When more than 145 mEq of sodium in blood is measured, give water (by mouth or infusion) and if needed use natriuretic diuretics.
Withhold sodium administration.

Hyponatremia

Causes of deficient sodium concentration in blood are:
Loss of sodium or water retention.
Adrenocortical and pituitary insufficiency.
Renal failure, heart failure, hepatic cirrhosis, nephrosis.
Excessive use of diuretics, loss of gastrointestinal secretions, severe sweating, post-surgery.
Excessive secretion of antidiuretic hormone caused by drugs (vincristine, clofibrate, cyclophosphamide), tuberculosis, aspergillosis, encephalitis, trauma or tumor in the brain, meningitis, lung cancer. Consider the Bartter-Schwartz syndrome.
Hyperglycemia.
Essential hyponatremia or sick-cell syndrome.

Symptoms of hyponatremia are:
Symptoms of overhydration (water intoxication).
Symptoms of the Bartter-Schwartz syndrome, or insufficient antidiuretic hormone secretion.
Sodium concentration in blood below 136 mEq in each 1000 ml; excess of water retention.

Management of hyponatremia:
Sodium replacement.
Restriction of water intake, if that is the cause.

Hyperpotassemia

Causes of excessive potassium concentration in blood are:
Adrenal insufficiency.
Renal failure and severe oliguria.

Release of intracellular potassium in trauma, burns, infarction, severe infections.
Acidosis.
Administration of diuretics that spare potassium, such as spironolactone and triamterene.

Symptoms of hyperkalemia are:
Paralysis of skeletal muscles; generalized weakness.
Dangerous heart effects leading to cardiac standstill, which are noted in the electrocardiogram (peak T waves, to start).
Abdominal distention and diarrhea.
Elevated potassemia.

Management of hyperkalemia:
Withhold potassium; add, if needed, cation exchange resins.
Emergent treatment with glucose infusion with insulin, or with sodium bicarbonate.
Consider hemodialysis.

Hypopotassemia

Causes of defective concentration of potassium in blood are:
Poor potassium intake.
Poor potassium absorption due to vomiting or diarrhea, gastric suction, steatorrhea, regional enteritis. Abuse of cathartics.
Cortical hyperfunction of the adrenals (Cushing's, aldosteronism) or excess of corticoid therapy.
Use of diuretics, tubular disease of the kidneys, diabetes.
Metabolic alkalosis; excessive use of infusions with little potassium.
Burns, freezing.
Familial periodic paralysis.

Symptoms of hypokalemia are:
Muscular weakness and paralysis. Respiratory embarrassment.
Ileus, hypotension (mostly postural) due to smooth muscle weakness.
Polyuria and hyposthenuria.
Cardiac arrhythmias, digitalis potentiation. Final cardiac arrest.
Electrocardiographic changes (lowering or inversion of T waves; prominent U waves).
Decreased potassemia.

Management of hypokalemia:
Potassium replacement.
Treatment of the causative factor.

Hypercalcemia

Symptoms of hypercalcemia are:
Symptoms of hyperparathyroidism.
Muscular weakness. Ileus may occur.
Polyuria, with thirst and dehydration.
Anorexia, vomiting, constipation.
Azotemia, and nephrocalcinosis.
Stupor leading to coma.

Management of hypercalcemia:
Treat hyperparathyroidism, bone neoplasm, sarcoidosis, multiple myeloma, vitamin D intoxication, or milk-alkali syndrome.
Enhance calcium excretion with a lower ingestion and the use of sodium infusions and diuretics. Corticoids may be useful in some instances.

Hypocalcemia

Symptoms of hypocalcemia are:
Those of hypoparathyroid tetany, q.v.

Management of hypocalcemia:
Same as for hypoparathyroidism, q.v.

Hypermagnesemia

Most cases of hypermagnesemia are due to:
Excessive intake of drugs containing magnesium (in many instances facilitated by renal insufficiency).

Symptoms of hypermagnesemia are:
Respiratory failure due to muscle weakness. Death from respiratory paralysis.
Other manifestations of muscle weakness.
Hypotension.
Areflexia, sedation, confusion, or stupor.
Electrocardiographic changes (broadened P-R and QRS, elevated T waves).
Magnesemia of 3 mEq in 1000 ml or above.

Treatment of hypermagnesemia:
Intravenous infusion of calcium for respiratory paralysis.
Improvement of renal insufficiency.
Dialysis to be considered in some instances.

Hypomagnesemia

Most frequent causes of hypomagnesemia are:
Alcoholism (with delirium tremens).
Diabetic acidosis. Pancreatitis.
Diarrhea, prolonged gastrointestinal suction, malabsorption, starvation.
Excessive diuresis.
Hyperaldosteronism, hypoparathyroidism, hyperthyroidism.
Administration of large doses of calcium and vitamin D.

Symptoms of hypomagnesemia are:
Nervous and muscular irritability, with athetoid movements and even hypomagnesemia tetany.
Choreiform movements, tremors (jerking, coarse, flapping), nystagmus, convulsions. Positive Babinski.
Confusion, disorientation, restlessness.
Hypertension, vasomotor changes, tachycardia, arrhythmias.
Magnesemia below 1.5 mEq in 1000 ml.

Management of hypomagnesemia:
Magnesium replacement. (Avoid reactive hypermagnesemia).

Iron Overload (Hemochromatosis)

See chapter on liver diseases for information on hemochromatosis.

Copper Overload (Hepatolenticular Degeneration)

See chapter on liver diseases for information on hepatolenticular degeneration.

Hypo- and Avitaminosis A

Symptoms of vitamin A deficiency are:
Night blindness.
Eye symptoms such as conjunctival xerosis (with dryness, thickness, wrinkling, muddy pigmentation, superficial and foamy Bitot's spots on the exposed bulbar conjunctiva). Xerophthalmia.
In final stages, the cornea turning xerotic, with end result of keratomalacia with extrusion and shrinking of eye contents.
Follicular hyperkeratosis with dryness of the skin. Final atrophy and keratinization.
History of inadequate intake of vitamin A.
In infants and children, retarded growth.
Management of vitamin A deficiency:
Vitamin A replacement. Avoid prolonged administration of large doses.

Hypervitaminosis A

Symptoms of hypervitaminosis A are:
History of absorption of large doses of vitamin A.
Anorexia, loss of weight, hepatomegaly, splenomegaly.
Skin changes, such as rough skin, dryness, cracked lips, hair becoming coarse and sparse, and loss of the eyebrows.
Severe headache and marked asthenia; other nervous manifestations.
Hypercalcemia, hyperostosis, periosteal elevation of the bone, bony resorption, arthralgias.
Management of hypervitaminosis A:
Withdraw the vitamin.

Hypo- and Avitaminosis B_1 (Beriberi)

Symptoms of vitamin B_1 deficiency:
Initial symptoms consist of neurasthenic complaints, anorexia, formication, cramps, muscle tenderness (calf), paresthesias and disturbed knee and ankle jerks (first hyper-, and later hypoactive).
Neurological symptoms due to "dry" beriberi consist of paresthesias in the lower extremities (burning toes, crampy pains, diminished vibratory sense), final diminution of knee and ankle jerks, muscle atrophy, all ending in foot- and toe-drop; thereafter, the arms are similarly involved.
Symptoms of cerebral beriberi or Wernicke-Korsakoff syndrome (acute hemorrhagic polioencephalitis) are due to an acute deficiency superimposed over the chronic deficiency: mental confusion, aphonia, paresia of the lateral rectus muscle of the eye leading to complete ophthalmoplegia, and possible death.
Symptoms of late beriberi are cardiovascular (tachycardia, insufficiency, dyspnea, edema or frank anasarca) and nervous (anorexia, polyneuritis, paralyses).
In infants, there are cardiac failure, aphonia, deficient deep tendon reflexes.
Shoshin is an acute form or beriberi with heart disease and metabolic acidosis, noted in the Orient.
Management of thiamine deficiency:
Vitamin B_1, thiamine, replacement.

Hypo- and Avitaminosis B_2 (Ariboflavinosis)

Symptoms of ariboflavinosis are:
Diet with inadequate intake of milk.
Superficial fissuring at the angle of the mouth, with pallor and maceration (cheilosis).
Residual scarring in the angle affected, leaving superficial linear fissures.
The fissuring possibly becoming infected with *Candida*, resulting in a whitish bulky lesion (perlèche).
Oral pallor, conjunctivitis, and photophobia.
Asthenia and weight loss.
Normochromic anemia with erythrocytic aplasia.
Fissuring of the nares, and magenta tongue; also dysphagia.
Seborrheic dermatitis and some edema.
Keratitis, vascularization of the cornea, lacrimation, and in some patients dimness of vision (amblyopia).
Management of ariboflavinosis:
Riboflavin (vitamin B_2) replacement.

Hypo- and Avitaminosis B_6

Symptoms of hypo- or avitaminosis B_6 are:
Anemia with intramedullary hemolysis, normo- or megaloblastic.
Seborrheic dermatosis.
Cheilosis and glossitis.
Peripheral neuropathy; infants may present convulsions.
May help in relieving some symptoms of pellagra.
Symptoms of defective apoenzyme–coenzyme interaction resulting in poor utilization of pyridoxine:
Mental retardation with convulsions and cystathioninuria.
Iron overload anemia, with asthma and urticaria.
Management of these situations:
Vitamin B_6 (pyridoxine) replacement or overdosage.

Hypo- or Avitaminosis B_{12} (Cyanocobalamin)

Symptoms of cyanocobalamin deficiency are:
- Clinical picture of pernicious anemia.
- Insidious onset of asthenia, palpitation, and dyspnea. Anginal pains.
- Soreness of the tongue, because of glossitis. Redness and smoothness.
- Paresthesias of hands and feet, difficult walking, loss of vibratory sense.
- Anorexia, diarrhea, belching and indigestion; abdominal pain and vomiting may also occur. Weight loss will be the consequence.
- A yellow tint to the skin.
- Mild hepato- or splenomegaly.

Do not confuse it with:
- Medullary lesions, because of outstanding neurologic symptoms.

Management of cyanocobalamin deficiency:
- Cyanocobalamin, vitamin B_{12}, replacement.

Folic Acid Deficiency

Symptoms of folic acid deficiency are:
- Symptoms similar to those of pernicious anemia.
- Coexistence of situations favoring it, such as alcoholism, sprue, sickle cell anemia, the use of certain drugs (primidone, diphenylhydantoin, methotrexate, etc.), dietary deficiency, malabsorption, and pregnancy.
- Changes of the tongue, the gastrointestinal tract and the nervous system.
- The finding of hypersegmented polymorphonuclear leukocytes and megaloblastic maturation in the marrow helpful in diagnosis.

Management of folic acid deficiency:
- Folic acid replacement.

Nicotinic Acid and Nicotinamide Deficiency (Pellagra)

Main causes of pellagra are:
- Diets consisting mainly of corn.
- Also, diarrheal diseases, alcoholism, hepatic cirrhosis, Hartnup disease, carcinoid syndrome, and prolonged isoniazid therapy.

Symptoms of cutaneous clinical picture of pellagra are:
- Rough skin (pellagra), erythematous, thick, inelastic, fissured, and hyperpigmented, notably on parts exposed to sunlight.
- Acute forms (actinic trauma) with vesiculation, crusting, and desquamation.
- Intertrigo, which may occur with infection.
- In long-lasting cases, dry, inelastic, and scaly skin (Casal's necklace, or butterfly-shaped facial lesions).

Symptoms of mucosal clinical picture of pellagra are:
- Redness and hypertrophy of the papillae of the tongue (stomatitis, scarlet glossitis, starting at the tip of the tongue and in the neighborhood of Stensen's duct).
- Late edema of the tongue. Also, sore mouth and increased secretion of salive. Possible ulcerations below the tongue and the lower lip and opposite the molar teeth.
- Mucosal changes also in the urethra and the vagina.

Clinical symptoms of gastrointestinal involvement in pellagra are:
- Abdominal distention, diarrhea (a serious sign when it turns bloody), and possibly nausea and vomiting.
- Burning sensation in the mouth, the pharynx, and the esophagus.
- Peculiar uncontrollable suckling reaction.

Clinical symptoms of nervous system involvement are:
- Symptoms similar to the initial neurasthenic complex of beriberi.
- Memory impairment, disorientation, confabulation.
- Or, instead of the former, excitement, mania, and delirium.
- Other patients depressed, or paranoid.
- A few patients presenting the encephalopathic syndrome with clouding of conscience, grasping reflexes, and cogwheel rigidity of the limbs.

Management of pellagra:
- Niacin or niacinamide replacement.

Hypo- and Avitaminosis C (Scurvy)

Symptoms of scurvy:
- Initial symptoms may be asthenia, irritability, pains (arthralgia, myalgia) which are mild and vague, and weight loss.
- Bleeding tendency is characteristic, at distal ends of nails, and from the typical stomatitis, with swollen gums that are purple, spongy, and friable.
- There is also extravasation of blood into fascial layers; there are perifollicular petechiae, ecchymoses in the lower limbs.
- Anemia may occur.
- Poor wound healing, breakdown of old scars may be noted.
- There may be subperiostal hemorrhages, swelling of the joints, muscle discomfort.
- Loosening or loss of teeth, rarefaction of bone tissue may occur.
- Secondary infections and gangrene may develop.

Symptoms of affected infants or children are:
- Bone pains, with swollen ends, because of which the patient keeps motionless.
- Angular enlargement of costochondral junctions, forming the well-known scorbutic rosary.
- Swollen and bleeding gums around erupting teeth.
- Fever, tachycardia, dyspnea, and anemia.
- Other symptoms similar to adult symptoms.

Do not confuse scurvy with:
- Rickets, or osteomyelitis.
- Rheumatic fever, poliomyelitis.

Management of scurvy:
Ascorbic acid, vitamin C, replacement.
Gingival symptoms improve after 72 hours of ascorbic acid therapy.

Hypo- and Avitaminosis D (Rickets, Osteomalacia)

Symptoms of rickets:
See "Rickets" in the chapter devoted to endocrinology.
Symptoms of osteomalacia:
See "Osteomalacia" in the chapter devoted to endocrinology.
Management of Vitamin D, calciferol, deficiency:
Vitamin D replacement.

Hypervitaminosis D

Symptoms of hypervitaminosis D:
Anorexia, with nausea and vomiting.
Polydipsia, polyuria, itching, and asthenia.
Impaired renal function, with albuminuria, casts, and final uremia.
Metastatic calcifications, mostly in the kidneys, and localized osteoporosis.
Failure to thrive, which may be noted in infancy.
Diagnosis confirmed by finding reactive hypercalcemia.
Management of hypervitaminosis D:
Withdraw medication.
May use corticoids, with sodium phytate.

Hypovitaminosis E

Symptoms of tocopherol deficiency are:
Furfuraceous desquamative dermatitis.
Edema in infants.
Short-lived erythrocytes.
Anemia.
Low plasma tocopherol levels, below 8 mg in 1000 ml.
Management of hypovitaminosis E:
Vitamin E, tocopherol, replacement.

Vitamin K Deficiency

Vitamin K deficiency can be observed clinically with:
Administration of nonabsorbable sulfas or oral antibiotics.
Administration of large amounts of mineral oil.
Administration of coumarin anticoagulants.
Biliary obstruction, and malabsorption problems.
Symptoms of vitamin K deficiency are:
Bleeding tendency, which may end in uncontrollable hemorrhages.
Defective coagulation of the blood, with decreased amounts of prothrombin and factors VII, IX, and X.
Management of vitamin K deficiency:
Administration of naphthoquinones with vitamin K activity, such as menadione, phytonadione, etc., provided there is an effective liver function.

Hypervitaminosis K

What may cause hypervitaminosis K:
Administration of large doses of vitamin K equivalents, particularly to infants.
Symptoms of hypervitaminosis K are:
Hemolytic anemia.
Hyperbilirubinemia.
Hepatomegaly.
Possible death.
Management of hypervitaminosis K:
Withdraw administration of these compounds.

v. Gierke's Disease (Glycogen Storage Disease)

What are the symptoms of this type I glycogen storage disease?
Asthenia.
Anorexia, vomiting, and weight loss.
Characteristic hepatomegaly due to glycogen deposition.
Hyperlipidemia, hypophosphatemia.
Hypoglycemia, with ketosis resulting in convulsions and coma.
Glucose levels not responsive to epinephrine.
Management of this disease due to deficient enzyme glucose-6-phosphatase:
Frequent carbohydrate feedings.
Portacaval shunt, nocturnal intragastric feedings, total parenteral nutrition.
With adequate treatment the child may survive.

Other Glycogen Storage Diseases

Characteristic of type II, or *Pompe's disease,* are:
There is glycogen deposition in heart and muscles (glosso- and cardiomegaly).
All movements become impaired.
The deficient enzyme is α-1,4-glucosidase, or acid maltase.
Characteristics and treatment of type III, or *Forbes' or Cori's disease:*
Hepatomegaly.
Milder hypoglycemia, with less severe convulsions.
Mild proximal myopathy.
Deficiency of the debrancher enzyme amylo-1,6-glucosidase.
Treat with a high protein diet.
Characteristics of type IV, or *Andersen's disease,* are:
Hepatomegaly.
Deficiency of the brancher enzyme amylo-(1,4→1,6)-transglucosidase.
Characteristics and treatment of type V, or *McArdle's disease:*
Excessive exercise leads to muscle cramps, and pigmenturia.
Muscles of the limbs are weak and tender, with pain.

In rare instances there is involvement of cranial or respiratory muscles.
Pigmenturia (myoglobin) may cause serious renal damage.
Increase fructose intake before expected increased exercise; the rest of the treatment is only supportive and symptomatic.

Characteristics of type VI, or *Hers' disease* are:
Hepatomegaly.
Deficient hepatophosphorylase.

Hurler's Syndrome (Gargoylism)

Symptoms are:
Mental retardation.
Blindness and deafness.
Saddle nose.
Heart troubles, such as valvular disease, failure, and angina.

Management of Hurler's syndrome:
Symptomatic.

Malabsorption Syndromes

Which are the most frequently found malabsorption syndromes?
Zollinger-Ellison syndrome.
Sprue, both tropical and nontropical.
Whipple's disease.
Also include: deficient bile secretion, gastrointestinal resections, intestinal lymphatic obstruction, and several others.

For information see the chapter on gastrointestinal diseases.

Disorders of Fructose Metabolism

Symptoms and management of *essential fructosuria:*
There are no organic symptoms; it is recognized only by urine containing fructose.
Treat with a diet containing mainly other forms of carbohydrates.

Symptoms and management of *fructosemia:*
Nausea and vomiting, and possible gastric pain (substernal).
Profuse sweating, tremors, and convulsions.
Confusion that may lead to coma.
Possibly hepatomegaly, splenomegaly, jaundice. Cirrhosis may occur.
Mental deficiency also possible.
Most symptoms increased by the ingestion of fructose (sucrose, fruits, sorbitol, intravenous infusions with fructose).
Avoid the ingestion of fructose.

Galactosemia

Symptoms of galactosemia are:
Soon after birth vomiting of milk starts, and thereafter appears hepatomegaly, edema with ascites, diarrhea, and hepatomegaly.
There are symptoms of hypoglycemia, inanition, and growth failure.
Death may occur from malnutrition.
Those who survive will add jaundice, abdominal distention, mental retardation, cataracts, and more markedly stunted growth.

Management of galactosemia:
There is immediate need for diagnosis and treatment, to avoid further damage.
Exclude milk and all food containing lactose or galactose for at least 3 years.

Hyperoxaluria (Oxalosis, Oxaluria)

Symptoms of hyperoxaluria are:
Urolithiais (calcium oxalate).
Nephrocalcinosis.
Frequent urinary infections.
Final renal failure or hypertension.

What are the types of hyperoxaluria?
Type I, or glycolic aciduria (the most common).
Type II, or L-glyceric aciduria.

Management of hyperoxaluria:
Avoidance of oxalates in the diet.
Hydration, pyridoxine.
Also recommended, calcium carbimide and renal transplantation.

Amyloidosis

What are the causes of amyloidosis?
Unknown, for primary myloidosis; all other forms are secondary amyloidosis.
Infections, mostly long-standing ones, such as tuberculosis, leprosy, osteomyelitis, bronchiectasis, ulcerative colitis, etc.
Rheumatoid arthritis, Hodgkin's disease, multiple myeloma; also it may be due to aging.

Symptoms of amyloidosis:
They are dependent on the affected organ or system.
Asthenia, fever, macroglossia, hepatosplenomegaly, weight loss, purpuric symptoms, lymphadenopathy, abdominal pains, neuropathy, nephropathy, and congestive heart failure may characterize primary amyloidosis.
Amyloid tumor formation in the skin, the larynx, or the thyroid may also characterize primary amyloidosis.
In secondary amyloidosis, amyloid may be deposited in the liver, spleen, kidneys, adrenals, and less frequently also in other organs.
Renal amyloidosis starts with proteinuria, which increases to massive levels, with hypoproteinemia and anasarca, thus giving the clinical picture of the nephrotic syndrome.
Cardiac amyloidosis is noted as intractable heart failure, or any form of arrhythmia.

Gastrointestinal amyloidosis is noted by bleeding.
Biopsy is needed for the final diagnosis.
Management of amyloidosis:
Only symptomatic; but if the causative disease can be eliminated, anyloidosis will notably improve.
Surgical excision of amyloid tumors advisable.

Phenylketonuria (PKU, Phenylpyruvic Oligophrenia)

This disease caused by high blood levels of phenylalanine is evaluated as follows:
Check carefully infants with irritability, vomiting, and epileptic seizures, particularly if they are blue-eyed blonds.
Infantile eczema, or dry skin, and fair hue are noted. Excessive sweating may occur.
There is a mousy smell.
Mental retardation is usually the rule in untreated cases.
Symptoms of extrapyramidal involvement may occur, such as tremor, hypertonicity, and ataxia.
Diagnosis must be determined between 6 and 14 days of life (phenylpyruvic acidin the urine or elevated phenylalanine in blood).
Management of phenylketonuria:
Start low-phenylalanine diets before 3 weeks of age, to maintain normal phenylalaninemia.
Established cases should be treated, also, because in some instances some improvement may occur.

Hartnup's Disease

Symptoms of this disease due to tryptophan malabsorption are:
Symptoms similar to pellagra.
Photodermatitis.
Mental retardation and cerebellar ataxia.
Increased amounts of neutral aminoacids in the urine. Renal colic.
Management of Hartnup's disease:
Use nicotinic acid.
Give large amounts of water, to prevent calculi formation.

Fanconi's Syndrome

This syndrome associated with multiple defects of the renal transport mechanism is characterized by:
Spontaneous fractures.
Glycosuria and aminoaciduria. Also proteinuria, and polyuria.
Emaciation, and dwarfism.
Osteomalacia or renal rickets that are resistant to adequate intake of vitamin D.
Symptoms of dehydration.
Hypophosphatemia.
Management of Fanconi's syndrome:
Poor results with hydration, large doses of vitamin D, and alkalinization of the urine.

Lowe's Syndrome

Characteristics of Lowe's syndrome are:
Mental retardation.
Hyporeflexia.
Cataracts or hydrophthalmos.
Alkaline urine.
Elevated amino acids in blood.

Alkaptonuria (Ochronosis)

The lack of homogentisic oxidase to metabolize homogentisinic acid causes the following clinical picture:
There is dark urine, which will stain diapers or underwear.
Older patients will present cartilages (ears) with ochre-like pigments.
The staining may also occur in the nose.
There are symptoms of arthritis, with cartilaginous degeneration due to the deposition of ochre-like pigments.

Maple Syrup Urine Disease

The lack of amino acid decarboxylase needed for the metabolism of essential branched-chain amino acids will cause:
Initial spasticity, opisthotonos, irregular respirations, and difficulties in feeding the infant.
The child's not responding or responding weakly to striking a table on both sides of the body (arms throw out as if embracing, that is, Moro's reflex).
Maple sugar odor of the urine.

Albinism

This defect of tyrosinase, needed for tyrosine metabolism, is noted by:
Absence of pigment in the hairs, which look like canities.
Absence of pigment in the skin, which is white.
Pink (or reddish) iris, and red pupils.
Nystagmus, photophobia, and visual defects.
Management of albinism:
There is no known treatment for the disease, but the patients should avoid exposure to sunlight.

Homocystinuria

This most probably cysteine deficiency is noted by:
Mental retardation. Emotional disturbances.
Ectopia lentis.
Sparse fine, blond hair.
Long thin extremities, genu valgum, shuffling gait.
Thromboses (both arterial and venous).
Management of homocystinuria:
A diet low in methionine and high in cystine, with supplement of folic acid, and large doses of pyridoxine.

Hypervalinemia

This lack of valine transaminase is noted by:
- Mental retardation, hyperkinesis, and hypotonia.
- Nystagmus.
- Vomiting.

Management of hypervalinemia:
- A diet low in valine.

Isovaleric Acidemia

The elevated concentration of isovaleric acid in the blood will cause:
- Mental retardation.
- Episodic attacks of acidosis.
- Unpleasant cheese odor of the body.

Management of isovaleric or isovalerianic acid hyperconcentration in blood:
- A low protein diet.

Hydroxykynureninuria

Symptoms caused by hydroxykynureninuria are:
- Mental retardation.
- Stomatitis and gingivitis.
- Desquamation of the skin.

Management of hydroxykynureninuria:
- Give niacin.

Histidinemia

Symptoms and management of histidinemia:
- Mental retardation.
- Defects of speech.
- Treatment with a diet low in histidine.

Hypermethioninemia

Symptoms of hypermethioninemia are:
- Mental retardation.
- Hypoglycemia.
- Progressive somnolence.
- Bleeding tendencies.

Hyperglycinemia

Symptoms of pure hyperglycinemia are:
- Mental retardation.
- Lethargy.
- Vomiting, with ketosis.

Symptoms of hyperglycinemia plus hypooxaluria are:
- Mental retardation.
- Convulsions.
- No ketosis.

Management of hyperglycinemia:
- A diet low in leucine, isoleucine, methionine, threonine, and valine.

Hypersarcosinemia

Symptoms of hypersarcosinemia are:
- Mental retardation.
- Marked hypotonia of all muscles, including those in the pharynx, thus making swallowing very difficult.

Carnosinemia

Symptoms of carnosinemia are:
- Mental retardation.
- Seizures of the myoclonic type.

Hyperammoniemia plus Ornithine Transcarbamylase Deficiency

Symptoms of hyperammoniemia associated with deficiency of ornithine transcarbamylase:
- Mental retardation.
- Gastrointestinal symptoms, particularly vomiting.
- Stupor, together with crises of screaming.
- May improve with a low protein diet.

Citrullinuria

Symptoms of citrullinuria:
- Mental retardation.
- Vomiting the outstanding gastrointestinal symptom.
- Symptoms of alkalotic crises, and hyperammoniemia.
- May improve with a low protein diet.

Argininosuccinic Aciduria

Symptoms of argininosuccinic aciduria:
- Mental retardation.
- Peculiar facies.
- Brittle hair, and brittle nails.
- May improve with a low protein diet with the addition of arginine.

Lysine Intolerance

Symptoms of lysine intolerance when it is accompanied by ammonia intoxication:
- There is mental retardation.
- Convulsions occur, accompanied by vomiting.
- Muscle tone may show changes.
- The disease may improve with a low protein diet.

Hyperlysinemia

Symptoms of hyperlysinemia:
- There are mental retardation and changes in muscle tone.
- The disease may improve with a diet low in proteins.

Hyperprolinemia

Symptoms of type I hyperprolinemia are:
- Mental retardation.
- Nerve deafness and also convulsions.
- Presence of different congenital renal anomalies.

Leucine Sensitivity Disease

Evaluation of leucine sensitivity disease is as follows:
- It should be checked for in infants who present hypoglycemic crises.
- Flushing and sweating are frequent findings.
- Most of these patients present convulsions.
- Symptoms are mostly due to ingestion of leucine.

Gout

In the case of *chronic gout*, the symptoms are as follows:
- Symptoms of arthritis progress to reach a stage of functional loss and disability.
- Gross deformities will gradually develop.
- Deposits of trophaceous material are noted in joints, tendons, and ear cartilages.
- Tophi may erupt and discharge chalky urates.
- Frequent associations are hypertension, renal stones, and renal failure.

In the cause of *acute gouty attacks*, the symptoms are as follows:
- There is sudden, usually nocturnal, arthritic pain, mainly in the metatarsophalangeal joint of the great toe.
- Other sites may be other joints in the feet, or joints in the ankles, and in the knees; more rarely, the wrists, elbows, etc.
- The pain reaches unbearable proportions, the swollen joint cannot be touched (not even looked at!), and becomes tense, warm, and of a dusky shiny red color.
- At the same time, there will be noted fever, headache, malaise, chills, tachycardia, and anorexia.
- The attack is usually monoarticular, but may also be polyarticular and asymmetrical.
- After the attack there are local desquamation and itching.
- Attacks may occur close to one another, or after long lapses of time.
- The first few attacks last for only a few days; thereafter, they may persist for weeks.

Management of gout:
- The acute attack is treated with colchicine.
- Alternate drugs are ACTH, phenylbutazone, and indomethacin.
- Chronic gout is also treated with colchicine, and with allopurinol, probenecid, and other similar drugs.

Methemoglobinemia

This lack of erythrocyte nucleotide diaphorase, or presence of the abnormal hemoglobin M, will cause the following symptoms:
- Persistent gray cyanosis of the skin, with no other cardiac or respiratory symptoms, excepting the following.
- Dyspnea and tachycardia.
- Easy fatigability and dizziness with efforts.
- Brown venous blood.

Management of methemoglobinemia:
- Methylene blue, given by mouth for prolonged periods.

Porphyria

The different types of porphyria are:
- Erythropoietic porphyria, and
- Hepatic porphyria; this latter divided into
- Acute intermittent porphyria,
- Porphyria cutanea tarda, and
- Variegate porphyria.
- There are also acquired, secondary porphyrinurias.

Symptoms of *erythropoietic porphyria* are:
- Early onset, at birth or infancy; rarely during childhood.
- Red or pink urine.
- Hydroa aestivale developed after sunlight exposure, characterized by vesicles, bullae, scarring, and pigmentation of the skin, not rarely with infection superimposed.
- Hepato- and splenomegaly, with evidence of hemolytic anemia.
- Hypertrichosis, and erythrodontia with fluorescence under ultraviolet light. Also, bones are red (as seen in postmortem examination).

Management of erythropoietic porphyria:
- Avoid photosensitivity irritation; use protective clothes or ointments; also, use antiinflammatory ointments.
- Beta-carotene by mouth is an acceptable oral protection.
- Consider splenectomy in cases with hemolysis.

Symptoms of *acute intermittent porphyria* are:
- Onset occurs between 20 and 40 years of age.
- Urine is of normal color on emission, but darkens when exposed to sunlight or ultraviolet rays.
- Hypertension and tachycardia may be present; fever may occur.
- Other symptoms include: gastrointestinal symptoms—abdominal colicky pain, nausea, vomiting, and constipation or diarrhea; variable blood pressure from time to time, tachycardia, peripheral vasospasm; sweating and bladder symptoms; these thus constituting an autonomic neuropathic syndrome.
- There may be back pain, and paralyses of the cranial nerves together with other forms of flaccid paralyses, thus constituting a peripheral neuropathic form of the disease.

A form of cortical dysfunction is noted by psychic disturbances, convulsions, and coma. Range is from anxiety to true psychoses.

A hypothalamic form is noted by dysfunction of the antidiuretic and the growth hormones, and also of lactation.

Attacks may be precipitated after the use of sulfa drugs, alcohol, barbiturates, infections, traumas, etc.

Do not confuse acute intermittent porphyria with:

Syndromes presenting acute abdomen.

Other syndromes from the central nervous system.

Management of acute intermittent porphyria:

Avoid precipitating factors.

Advise a diet high in carbohydrates and proteins; fluid restriction, if needed.

Chlorpromazine or rauwolfia alkaloids may help.

Symptoms of *porphyria cutanea tarda* are:

Onset occurs in middle-aged patients.

Most patients are alcoholic, may have had systemic lupus erythematosus, or have used estrogens or iron.

There is photosensitivity causing vesicles, bullae, and eczema.

There are also hirsutism, mild jaundice, hyperpigmentation of the skin, sclerosic changes, and other symptoms of abdominal pain or neurologic disturbances.

Uroporphyrin excretion is elevated.

Management of porphyria cutanea tarda:

Avoidance of strong light, alcohol, estrogens, and iron.

Phlebotomy repeated until there is adequate reduction of uroporphyrin excretion.

Symptoms of *variegate porphyria:*

Attacks of photosensitivity.

Combined manifestation of the former with abdominal or with neurologic symptoms.

May be relieved with a diet high in carbohydrates and proteins.

Symptoms of acquired, *secondary porphyria:*

Symptoms of porphyria, which occur after any of the following.

Intoxication with heavy metals (lead, iron, etc.), or with organic or inorganic poisons.

Anemias, liver diseases, and collagen or neurologic disorders.

Type I Hyperlipoproteinemia (Hyperchylomicronemia)

Evaluation of this exogenous hypertriglyceridemia is as follows:

There are very few cases; in younger adults and children.

Check carefully, particularly hepatomegalic children who present recurrent abdominal pain.

Xanthomas appear as yellow or pinkish papular deposits of fat on pressure points and extensor surfaces.

Complicating pancreatitis may occur.

Lipemia retinalis will occur only with elevated triglyceridemia.

There is latescent serum, which increases with fat intake.

Management of this familiar fat-induced lipemia:

Restrict fats in diet; use mainly medium-chain fatty acids.

Type IIA Hyperlipoproteinemia (Hyperbetalipoproteinemia)

Symptoms of hyperbetalipoproteinemia are:

Xanthomas appearing on tendons, and xanthelasma.

Early myocardial infarction a frequent occurrence.

Patients presenting an accelarated form of atherosclerosis.

The serum clear, but hypercholesterolemia will be elevated.

Management of hyperbetalipoproteinemia:

Diet with restricted amounts of fat and cholesterol.

Type IIB Hyperlipoproteinemia (Hyperbeta- and Hyperprebetalipoproteinemia)

Symptoms of this mixed form of hyperlipoproteinemia:

Mild forms are associated with obesity or diabetes.

Severe forms will present same symptomatology as type IIA, above.

In IIA the serum is clear, and there is no triglyceridemia; in type IIB, the serum is turbid, and there is a moderate triglyceridemia.

Management of type IIB hyperlipoproteinemia:

Avoid hypercaloric and hyperfat diets.

Type III Hyperlipoproteinemia (Dysbetalipoproteinemia)

Symptoms of broad beta disease, or tuberous xanthomatosis are:

Palmar and plantar tuberous and eruptive xanthomas, which may be considered almost pathognomonic. Xanthelasma may also be present.

Premature atherosclerosis.

Obesity, hyperuricemia, mild glucose intolerance.

Serum turbid, with elevated concentrations of cholesterol and triglycerides.

Management of type III hyperlipoproteinemia:

Diet with caloric reduction to obtain ideal weight, and also cholesterol and trigyceride restriction.

Clofibrate administration.

Type IV Hyperlipoproteinemia (Hyperprebetalipoproteinemia)

Symptoms of this endogenous hypertriglyceridemia are:

Appearance of eruptive xanthomas.

Obesity, hyperuricemia, and mild glucose intolerance.

Atherosclerosis, with accelerated vascular disease (coronary).

Management of type IV hyperlipoproteinemia:
Restricted caloric and fat intake; use clofibrate.

Type V Hyperlipoproteinemia (Mixed Hypertriglyceridemia)

Symptoms of this form of mixed lipemia are:
Presence of eruptive xanthomas.
Enlargement of both liver and spleen.
Attacks of recurrent abdominal pain.
Frequent association with diabetes mellitus.
Management of type V hyperlipoproteinemia:
Advise restricted caloric and fat intake; use clofibrate. Treat diabetes.

Secondary Hypercholesterolemia

Symptoms of secondary hypercholesterolemia are:
Xanthomas and xanthelasma after prolonged hyperlipemia.
Secondary hypercholesterolemia is frequently associated with:
Diabetes mellitus, and other endocrinopathies such as hypothyroidism, hypopituitarism, etc.
Biliary cirrhosis.
Nephrotic syndrome.
Management of secondary hypercholesterolemia:
Treat the causative factor.

Abetalipoproteinemia (Acanthocytosis)

Symptoms of abetalipoproteinemia are:
Mental retardation.
Growth retardation, in most cases.
Lack of muscular coordination (ataxia).
Retinitis pigmentosa.
Erythrocytes presenting spiny projections (acanthocytosis).
Malabsorption occurring in a number of cases.
Very low concentrations for blood cholesterol and triglycerides.
Management of acanthocytosis:
Diet containing low fat, and medium-chain triglycerides.

Tangier Disease (Familial Alpha Lipoprotein Deficiency)

Symptoms of Tangier disease are:
Orange-yellow hyperplasia of the tonsils.
Enlargement of both liver and spleen; also, enlargement of most of the lymph nodes.
Peripheral neuropathy.
Corneal deposits of lipids.
Low levels of cholesterol and high-density lipoproteins in the blood.

Gaucher's Disease

Symptoms of Gaucher's disease are:
Onset usually during childhood.
The outstanding symptom, a notable splenomegaly. Also hepatomegaly, and in some instances lymphadenopathy.
Pinguecula (also called palpebral blotch).
The skin showing brown pigmentation, jaundice, anemia, and other evidence of thrombocytopenia.
Epistaxis, and other forms of hemorrhage.
Neurologic lesions, and in infants nuchal rigidity and opisthotonos possible.
Skeletal lesions, with pain and bone fractures. Joints may swell.
Most cases appearing in early childhood presenting an acute course and ending fatally; those who reach adolescence may survive.
Reticuloendothelial cells storing large amounts of glucocerebrosides (Gaucher's cells).
Management of Gaucher's disease:
Supportive treatment.
Splenectomy, provided there is hypersplenism.

Sphingomyelin Lipidosis (Niemann-Pick Disease)

Symptoms of Niemann-Pick disease are:
Onset in early infancy, with mental retardation.
Enlargement of both liver and spleen. Also, enlarged lymph nodes.
Convulsions; possibly other neurologic manifestations.
In skin, xanthomas, a cherry-red macular spot, pigmentation, and anemic paleness.
Diffuse pulmonary infiltration, gastrointestinal bleeding.
Thrombocytopenia.
In cells increased levels of sphingomyelin.
Management of Niemann-Pick disease:
Supportive treatment.

Tay-Sachs Disease (Amaurotic Idiocy)

Symptoms of Tay-Sachs disease are:
Mental retardation.
Changes of the macula lutea leading to early loss of vision.
Paralysis.
Onset in infancy or childhood.
Management of Tay-Sachs disease:
Supportive treatment.

Fabry's Disease

Symptoms of this angiokeratoma corporis diffusum universalis are:
Diffuse distribution over the body of spots with thickened epidermis together with telangiectases or with warty growths, angiokeratomas, more frequently noted on the lower trunk.
Other accumulations of the glycolipid involved in the disease, particularly in the form of ocular deposits.

Burning pain in the extremities.
Febrile episodes also, in some patients.
Renal failure a possible terminal episode.

Management of Fabry's disease:
Supportive treatment.

Marfan's Syndrome

Symptoms of Marfan's syndrome are:
- Patients thin and of a tall height.
- Long extremities, in relation to trunk height.
- Long hands and feet, with long and more or less webbed fingers (arachnodactyly); the feet flat or cavus, sometimes with hammer toes.
- Long, narrow, and pointed head (tower skull).
- High arched palate, winglike scapulae, pigeon or funnel chest.
- The eyes possibly showing ectopia lentis, detached retina, myopia, or other ocular derangements.
- Atrial septal defect or other cardiovascular abnormalities, such as complete heart block, dissecting aneurysm, dilation of arteries, etc.
- A complete clinical picture not found in all cases.

Management of Marfan's disease:
Supportive treatment, with special emphasis on cardiovascular care.

Cystic Fibrosis or Mucoviscidosis

Symptoms of cystic fibrosis are:
- Onset frequently occurring early in infancy.
- Meconium ileus, which may be the first manifestation of the disease; it may be associated with volvulus or secondary atresia.
- Very slow gaining of weight in spite of a good appetite.
- Steatorrhea, and malnutrition. Large and frequent foul-smelling feces.
- Protuberant abdomen, rectal prolapse.
- Important respiratory component of the disease noted by viscid sputum, chronic cough with paroxysms that may induce vomiting, barrel chest, intercostal and supraclavicular retraction, bronchitis and repeated pulmonary infections that may lead to pulmonary obstruction or other type of complications.
- Excessive sweating frequently causing heat exhaustion because of loss of sodium and chloride.
- Hypotension, cor pulmonale, heart failure.
- Cyanosis and clubbed fingers, may be present. Poor sleep.
- Sinusitis or nasal polyposis, may occur.
- Lungs overexpanded and irregularly aerated.

Management of mucoviscidosis:

For meconium ileus	Surgical correction; vitamin K.
For hyperviscosity	Mist tent with propylene glycol, bronchodilators, iodides or pancreatic dornase or acetylcysteine, breathing exercise and postural drainage.
For nutrition and pancreatic replacement	High protein and high caloric diet, but low in fats, vitamins, pancreatin and extra salt during hot weather.
For pulmonary involvement	Sulfa or antibiotic therapy, vaccination, avoidance of infections.

Wilson's Disease (Hepatolenticular Degeneration)

See chapter on liver diseases for information on hepatolenticular degeneration.

Hemochromatosis

See chapter on liver diseases for information on hemochromatosis.

8. Musculoskeletal Disorders

Rheumatoid Spondylitis (Ankylosing Spondylitis)

Symptoms of this condition, also called Marie-Strümpell disease, are:

- Onset occurs in young males, around the twenties. Few women are affected.
- The disease starts gradually, with bouts of spinal pain, notably low back pain. Pain may radiate down to the thighs.
- Initial symptoms occur in the sacroiliac joints.
- Progress is made upward, through the apophyseal joints of the spine.
- The lumbar curve is straightened; and the thoracic curve, exaggerated.
- At this time there is calcification of the anterior and lateral spinal ligaments.
- Motion becomes sharply limited, and atrophy of the trunk muscles results.
- Involvement of the costovertebral joints limits chest expansion.
- Some patients will present involvement of peripheral joints.
- Some other patients will also present uveitis (nongranulomatous), and this may be in some instances the presenting symptom.
- Few cases will develop amyloidosis.
- Neurologic symptoms frequently occur (radiculitis, sciatica, etc.).
- The heart may show conduction defects, aortic insufficiency, or cardiac enlargement.
- Some patients will present symptoms similar to rheumatoid arthritis.
- The characteristic "bamboo spine" will be diagnostic in X-ray films.

Management of rheumatoid spondylitis:

- Give salicylates, phenylbutazone, or oxyphenbutazone or indomethacin.
- Order rest (both physical and emotional), and exercise (both postural and breathing).
- Corticoids may be used for the disease or some complications.

Rheumatoid Arthritis

The initial symptoms of rheumatoid arthritis are:

- It is more frequent among women, past 20 years of age. Younger or older cases may also occur (after 40 years of age).
- The onset is insidious in most instances, but may be rapid (trauma, infection, etc.).
- Initial complaints may be matinal stiffness of most joints, particularly small ones of hands and feet, wrists, ankles, and elbow.
- There are also fever, malaise, sweats, and weight loss.
- Vasomotor disturbances, such as Raynaud's phenomenon, and paresthesias are not rare.
- Symmetrical involvement of joints is the rule.

The symptoms of established rheumatoid arthritis are:

- Progression is centripetal.
- Joints are swollen, stiff, warm, and painful, with tenderness when touched.
- Symptoms, particularly pain and stiffness, are worst in the morning and improve during the day, after use.
- After daytime improvement, stiffness and pain may recur following periods of immobility or stenous exercise.
- The outcome is unpredictable: some may improve; some will develop subsequent joint changes (flexion, subluxation, ankylosis, or at least thickening of the tissues around the joint).

Other symptoms usually accompanying rheumatoid arthritis:

- Fever, asthenia, and continued weight loss.
- Mental depression, anorexia, and atrophy of the skin or of the muscles.
- Also possible: rupture of joint capsule, synovial cysts, subcutaneous nodules, palmar erythema, vasculitis (punctate hemorrhages in the nail folds, in the finger pulps, etc.), splenomegaly, and enlargement of lymph nodes.
- Carpal tunnel syndrome, or other evidence of nerve entrapping.
- Sjögren's syndrome usually appearing with rheumatoid arthritis.
- Other eye symptoms also possible: episcleritis, scleral nodules, nongranulomatous iritis, or scleromalacia.
- A search should be done for complications in the respiratory or the cardiovascular system.

The diagnosis of rheumatoid arthritis is backed by:

- Radiologic examinations (joint erosion and juxta-articular osteoporosis).
- Serologic positivity of the rheumatoid factor.

Management of rhematoid arthritis:

Physical and emotional rest, together with adequate exercise within tolerance limits and radiant or moist heat. Cold application will be better for some patients.

Salicylates, phenylbutazone or oxyphenylbutazone, indomethacin, and, for very severe nocturnal pain, codeine.

Also to be considered: corticoids, antimalarial chloroquines, gold salts, and the more recent ibuprofen, tolmetin sodium, or naproxen.

Still's Disease, or Juvenile Rheumatoid Arthritis

Differences of juvenile as compared to regular rheumatoid arthritis are:

Children are affected, considered as persons under 16 years of age.

High spiking fever usually heralds the rheumatic symptoms.

Frequent accompanying symptoms of the heralding complex are enlargement of the liver and spleen, also of the lymph nodes, or a pleuropericarditis; also an evanescent morbilliform rash.

The main point is that large joints are mostly affected, and changes in development and growth will occur (small jaw, with birdlike appearance).

Iridocyclitis will be noted only under slit-lamp examination.

One, a few, or a relatively large number of joints may be impaired.

Cervical vertebrae are most frequently affected.

There is a favorable prognosis, since most cases will show complete remission.

Be sure to rule out leukemia or other infectious diseases.

Management of juvenile rheumatoid arthritis:

Corticoids are perhaps the best choice.

Otherwise, the treatment is similar to that of regular rheumatoid arthritis.

Septic Arthritis

The types and symptoms of acute septic arthritis are:

The main etiological factor is gonococcal, but there also should be considered staphylococcal followed by streptococcal, pneumococcal, meningococcal, *H. influenzae,* or other gram negative bacilli arthritis.

Symptoms are relatively similar in most instances, and the diagnosis will depend on joint aspiration and culture.

There is a sudden onset with fever, chills, and a painful joint.

The joint is swollen, acutely painful, and warm. Most of the patients will present a red, very tender joint usually surrounded by edema.

Migratory arthralgias may initiate the clinical picture.

Most cases are monoarticular, but two or more joints may be affected: large weight-bearing joints, knees, ankles, and also wrists.

In the case of the most frequent, gonococcal arthritis, other symptoms are:

Initial presentation of polyarthritis and tenosynovitis similar to rheumatic fever.

Ulterior suppuration of the affected joint or joints.

Uretritis, prostatitis, or salpingitis usually simultaneously found; at least there is the history of a recent gonococcal infection.

Skin lesions of the type of purpura or vesiculation.

Less frequently throat or anal infections as the initial stage.

Complication of the type of endocarditis, myocarditis, pericarditis, or meningitis observed.

Management of acute septic arthritis:

Give prompt, appropriate antibiotic therapy.

Physical and surgical procedures may be of help.

Symptoms of chronic pyogenic arthritis are:

There is almost always the history of a previous acute arthritis.

Symptoms may be continuous or intermittent.

Most frequent germs are pyogenic cocci or gram negative ones.

There is continued local pain.

There are persistent limited motion and swelling, and increasing deformity.

Care will be taken not to confuse this disease with gout and other forms of rheumatism.

Management of chronic pyogenic arthritis:

Use adequate antibiotic therapy.

Surgical procedures are often needed.

Rheumatic Fever

Common initial characteristics of rheumatic fever:

Usually occurs between 5 and 15 years of age.

May also occur at 4 years until age 50.

Is most common in males.

Usually follows an evident infection located in the tonsils, the middle ear, or the nasopharynx, generally 1-4 weeks after the incident.

Major criteria from which two are to be chosen for diagnostic purposes:

Heart disease (carditis), which may consist of diastolic murmurs (mitral or aortic), pericarditis, congestive failure, or cardiac enlargement. To consider the existence of carditis, check for a change of heart sounds, the existence of a pansystolic apical murmur, prolonged P-R segment, gallop rhythm, or arrhythmias, if the former symptoms are not evident.

Clinical evidence of Sydenhan's chorea, with ceaseless rapid, jerky, but well-coordinated purposeless involuntary movements of the whole body, including the face. These movements disappear during sleep.

Skin symptoms, which are of two different types, namely, erythema marginatum (rings or crescents with clear centers), or subcutaneous nodules (small, firm, painless, and attached to fascia or tendon sheaths).

A migratory gradual or sudden polyarthritis, with regular joint symptoms, each bout accompanied by a rise of temperature. Large joints are frequently affected among juveniles; small, among adults.

Minor criteria, from which two are to be added to at least one major criterion to assure the diagnosis of rheumatic fever:

Fever, either continuous or intermittent (but not of the febricula type that some persons show almost normally).

Arthralgias (not arthritis!), which are considered as "growing pains".

Abdominal pain, which has to be differentiated from appendicitis.

Recurrent epistaxis.

Anorexia, asthenia, and weight loss.

Outcome of rheumatic fever:

Watch for heart damage, particularly valvular disease.

Management of rheumatic fever:

Use salicylates and penicillin.

Give general care; may use corticoids.

Treat cardiac complications carefully.

Sjögren's Syndrome (Keratoconjunctivitis Sicca)

Symptoms that constitute this syndrome:

It was described first as an eye disease, keratoconjunctivitis sicca, with absent tears, viscous secretions, burning, itching, and an extreme dryness of the organ.

There is also extreme dryness of the mouth (xerostomia), also deprived of saliva, not rarely accompanied by difficult speech, swallowing, and eating, and severe dental caries; taste and smell may be lost.

Other mucosae may lack secretions, as the nasopharynx, the larynx, the vagina, the bronchi.

Also, the skin may be dry; the parotid, enlarged.

A large percentage of these cases will present rheumatic symptoms.

Other symptoms may be pancreatitis, pericarditis, vasculitis, neuropathy, purpura, renal changes, and diseases of the lymph nodes.

These patients will present associated autoantibodies.

Check for associated diseases: hepatobiliary, scleroderma, polymyositis, Hashimoto's thyroiditis, etc.

Management of Sjögren's syndrome:

Artificial tears, lubricated mouth, oral hygiene.

Treatment of rheumatic disease present; give corticoids a trial.

Psoriatic Arthritis

Symptoms of psoriatic arthritis are:

Psoriasis usually opens the clinical picture.

Cutaneous lesions recur and relapse together with the rheumatic symptoms.

The distal phalangeal joints of digits are the ones usually affected.

In cases of psoriasis of the nails, the distal joint is almost always affected.

Distribution of these distal phalanges is mostly asymmetrical, few joints are involved, and the patient is not as much crippled as in the case of rheumatoid arthritis (but may be so!).

Management of psoriatic arthritis:

As for rheumatoid arthritis; but do not use drugs that may cause skin reactions (antimalarials).

Reiter's Syndrome

Symptoms that characterize Reiter's syndrome are:

Most cases are young men, who develop the disease 1-4 weeks following sexual intercourse, or a bout of diarrhea.

There is an asymmetric form of arthritis affecting large joints.

There is also a form of unspecific urethritis, with lesions in the urethral meatus and balanitis.

There is also an ophthalmic reaction, of the type of conjunctivitis, or iritis, or both. Less frequently, uveitis may occur.

And finally, there are also mucocutaneous manifestations, including stomatitis, keratoderma blenorrhagica (with crusted, hornlike lesions mostly on hands and feet), highly similar to pustular psoriasis involving skin and nails.

Additional symptoms may occur, such as heart disease, aortic regurgitation, etc.

Recurrences may happen, and permanent joint lesions may be left.

Do not take this disease for gonococcal arthritis, or any other form of arthritis.

Management of Reiter's syndrome:

Symptomatic.

Gout

For information, please see entry in chapter on metabolism and nutrition.

Tennis Elbow (Epicondylitis)

What other activities, besides tennis playing, may cause this condition?

Mechanical work, like using screwdrivers, etc.

Symptoms of epicondylalgia or radiohumeral bursitis are:

Pain is noted in the medial or lateral aspect of the elbow, over the lateral epicondyle of the humerus.

Pain may be more or less severe, and radiates to the outer side of the arm or the forearm.

Pain may aggravated by grasping, or by dorsiflexion and supination of the wrist against resisting force.

The point of maximal tenderness is noted distal to the lateral epicondyle, but will also occur more distally in the muscle bellies.
Dorsiflexion is weakened at the wrist.
Help diagnosis by infiltrating procaine, which will give complete relief of symptoms.

Management of epicondylitis:
Allay pain, use an elastic bandage, infiltrate trigger points, or perform adequate surgery.
A change in bulk of the handle of the instrument used may be of help.

Bursitis

Symptoms of acute bursitis are:
There is exquisite pain at the site of the inflammed bursa.
Swelling and tenderness are usually noted on the affected area.
Limitation of motion of the corresponding muscles occurs.
Recovery will occur in 1-2 weeks, or disease will become chronic.

The usually affected bursae are:

Subdeltoid or subachromial bursa	Pain in the anterior aspect of the shoulder; restricted abduction and rotation of the shoulder.
Trochanteric bursa (deep)	Obliteration of the normal depression behind the greater trochanter, which becomes extremely tender; the leg is held flexed, abducted, and externally rotated.
Iliopectineal-ilipsoas bursa	Exquisite tenderness, and pain anterior to the femoral head; pain on extension, adduction, or internal rotation of the hip.
Prepatellar bursa (housemaid's knee)	Irritation from repeated or prolonged kneeling.
Achilles tendon bursa	Pain and swelling behind the tuberosity of the os calcis, near the insertion of the heel cord.
Olecranon bursa (miner's elbow)	Swelling and tenderness noted over the tip of the olecranon.

Management of acute bursitis:
Rest, relief of pain, diathermia, massage may be helpful.
Local or systemic corticoid therapy is useful if given early.
A surgical approach may be recommended.

Symptoms of chronic bursitis are:
A previous attack of acute bursitis.
Some pain, swelling, tenderness, limitation of motion.
Acute exacerbation after excessive use of the affected part.
Thickened walls easily palpated.
Muscle atrophy possible.
Symptoms of a causative factor possibly also present.

Management of chronic bursitis:
Treat the causative factor.
Give physical therapy, corticoids applied locally, exercise, and surgery when needed.

Scapulocostal Syndrome

The most probable cause of the scapulocostal syndrome is:
Habitual faulty posture.

Symptoms of the scapulocostal syndrome are:
There is dull pain in the posterior cervical region.
Pain may radiate to the occiput, the scapula, the arm or the forearm (ulnar area), or the scapula and the ribs, posteriorly.
Stiffness and diffuse tenderness may occur in related areas.

Management of the scapulocostal syndrome:
Correct postural habits, exercise, and apply physical therapy.

Scapulohumeral Periarthritis (Frozen Shoulder)

Causes of this adhesive capsulitis are:
Not any known cause, or any of the following.
Rheumatoid arthritis, osteoarthritis, or a history of a previous fracture or a dislocation.
The primary type of unknown etiology is frequent among women past 40 years.

Symptoms of scapulohumeral periarthritis are:
Insidious or acute onset of pain.
Pain noted in the shoulder area, aggravated by shoulder motion, worst at night, and intensified by sleeping on the affected side.
Tenderness when pressure is exerted on the greater tuberosity or the bicipital groove.
Initial stiffness; then follows actual restriction of movement.

Management of frozen shoulder:
Analgesia and physical therapy.

Scapulohumeral Calcareous Tendinitis

Patients suffering the disease:
It is the most frequent cause of shoulder pain among men over 30 years of age.

Symptoms of this form of scapulohumeral tendinitis:
Shoulder pain.
Tenderness when pressing over areas of calcium deposition.
Restriction of joint motion.
Evidence of calcium deposition in X-ray films.

Management of the condition:
Local treatment, or surgical evacuation.

Lupus Erythematosus

Symptoms of cutaneous lupus erythematosus are:
Erythematous skin plaques, macular or with scales, teleangiectasia, and atrophy. Similar lesion in the oral mucosa.
Usually, no systemic symptoms; but a very careful search will be made to disclose evidence of systemic symptoms.

Symptoms of systemic lupus erythematosus:
Diagnosis will be considered positive if any four of the following symptoms are noted:

1) Butterfly rash on the naso-malar area.
2) Discoid lupus, anywhere on the body.
3) Alopecia.
4) Photosensitivity, checked on exposed surface of the body.
5) Oral ulcers.
6) Raynaud's phenomenon.
7) Joint involvement, with nondeforming arthritis.
8) Finding of lupus erythematosus cells.
9) False positive serologic tests for syphilis.
10) Neurologic component of psychoses or convulsions.
11) Proteinuria.
12) Cellular casts in the urine.
13) Evidence of serositis.
14) Hypergammaglobulinemia, positive Coombs test reaction, rheumatoid factor, or other hematologic findings.

General symptoms are fever, anorexia, and weight loss, which may initiate the clinical picture, or appear episodically.
Most symptoms reappear or increase during acute episodes.
In addition to the 14 diagnostic symptoms, there may also be noted ocular manifestations (conjunctivitis, photophobia, transient blindness, cotton-wool spots on the retina), respiratory complaints (pneumonitis, pleural effusion or pleurisy, bronchopneumonia), cardiac involvement (pericarditis, arrhythmias, cardiac failure), or abdominal, renal, or other systemic symptoms.
Consider also for diagnostic purposes: Libman-Sacks verrucous endocarditis, glomerulonephritis, thrombocytopenic purpura, splenomegaly or other lymphadenopathies, Hashimoto's thyroiditis, hemolytic anemia.

Management of cutaneous lupus erythematosus:
Start before atrophy occurs.
Avoid sunlight, and use local corticoids or antimalarials.

Management of systemic lupus erythematosus:
Avoid causative drugs, and sun exposure.
Use corticoids or antimalarials.
Treat according to complications.

How drug-induced lupus erythematosus may be diagnosed:
Sex is not a factor; no depressed serum complement and antibodies to native DNA found.
Rarely kidney or neurologic complications occur.
Improvement will take place at withdrawal of the offending drug.

Scleroderma (Progressive Systemic Sclerosis)

Symptoms of scleroderma are:
There is a cutaneous form not associated with systemic involvement: morphea, characterized by localized patches or bands of thickened and hard skin, without normal folds, teleangiectasia, pigmentation and also depigmentation.
Progressive systemic sclerosis presents similar skin lesions, but these are diffusely spread over the body; the face may be immobilized by increased hardness, and appears smooth and shiny.
The diffuse skin changes are symmetrical and centripetal, beginning in hands and feet.
Muscular and articular symptoms consist of myositis or polymyositis, and arthritic derangements due to calcinosis localized periarticularly.
Skin atrophy and musculoarticular involvement may lead to deformities of the limbs. Also, trophic ulcers appear around the joints.

Other forms of systemic involvement are:
Raynaud's phenomenon, which may be an early symptom.
Fever, malaise, and subcutaneous edema.
Ulcers on the fingertips.
Frequent dysphagia.
Hypomotility and malabsorption of the gastrointestinal tract.
Diverticulosis.
Pulmonary fibrosis.
Cardiac symptoms: pericarditis, myocarditis, myocardial fibrosis, and right heart failure.
Uremia with hypertension.

How the clinical picture runs for these symptoms:
Morphea is benign and is not associated with visceral involvement.
There is a slowly progressive, relatively benign CRST syndrome, which consists of calcinosis, Raynaud's phenomenon, sclerodactyly, and teleangiectasia.
The so-called mixed connective tissue disease shows some similarity with systemic lupus erythematosus, myositis, a high titer of extractable nuclear antigen, and usually responds to small doses of corticoids.
A few patients will present a rapidly progressive systemic sclerosis with involvement of vital organs and relatively prompt death.

Management of scleroderma:
Is only symptomatic and supportive of each failing organ.
Antibiotics and corticoids may give some help, and should be tried whenever they seem needed.

Polyarteritis Nodosa (Periarteritis Nodosa or Necrotizing Angiitis)

Symptoms of this necrotizing vasculitis are:
- Young men are more frequently affected.
- Onset is usually abrupt with outstanding evidence of arthritis.
- Other initial symptoms are myositis, fever with chills, and tachycardia.
- Glomerulonephritis and hypertension occur in a good number of patients.
- Skin and mucosal manifestations are noted, particularly livedo, bleeding tendencies, urticaria, and ulcerations.
- Cotton-wool spots develop in the retina.
- Other manifestations may involve the lungs, the gastrointestinal tract, the heart, and also an almost characteristic mononeuritis multiplex.
- Diagnosis is confirmed by biopsy.
- Outcome may be either a rapid recovery or a prompt death.

Management of polyarteritis nodosa:
- Corticoids for long periods of time.
- Symptomatic and supportive measures.

Behçet's Syndrome

Symptoms of Behçet's syndrome are:
- There is arthritis of the seronegative type, affecting mainly the knees and the ankles.
- There are ophthalmic symptoms, namely, uveitis, keratitis, optic neuritis.
- Ocular symptoms may be fulminant and end in blindness.
- Ulcers are recurrent in the oral and genitial areas.
- This is neurologic involvement, namely, mental disturbances, encephalitis, cranial nerve palsies, convulsions, and spinal cord lesions.
- Neurologic symptoms may lead to disability or death.
- There is a chronic course, with exacerbations and remissions.

Management of Behçet's syndrome:
- Corticoids and immunosupressive drugs.

Intervertebral Disk Disease

Symptoms of intervertebral disk protrusion are:
- Low back pain, radiating to the thigh, calf, or foot.
- Pain increased by defecation, coughing, or sneezing.
- Muscle spasm, with a bending to one side.
- Restricted motion of affected muscles.
- Tenderness on the lumbar spines, usually 4th to 5th lumbar, or 5th lumbar and sacral side.
- Tenderness and pain of the sciatic nerve.
- Pain increased with elevation of the straight leg.
- Hyperesthesia and depression of deep tendon reflexes of affected nerve roots.
- Also possible: loss of muscle tone, weakness of the limb, and atrophy.

Management of intervertebral disk syndrome:
- In the acute phase, rest, analgesia, and physical therapy.
- Final physical or surgical treatment.

Low Back Pain

The characteristics of low back pain are:
- As indicated for the above disease, which is one of the varieties of low back pain.

The causes of low back pain are:

The above-mentioned disk syndrome.	
Lumbar-sacral fractures	Trauma, osteoporosis; may cause deformity; diagnosis by X-ray film; treatment is surgical.
Acute sprain	Lumbosacral sprain a result of lifting heavy weights, twisting, or bending over; causes flattened lordosis, and bending to one side; muscles are tense, and motion diminished; treatment is rest, analgesics, and physical therapy.
Disease or inadequacy of the lumbar vertebrae	Due to malformations, infection of the vertebrae (tuberculosis, pyogenic), malignant tumors, osteitis deformans, ankylosing spondylitis, or spinal osteoarthritis of the aged; treatment is rest, physical therapy, or surgery, as applicable in each particular case.

Neurogenic Arthropathy (Charcot's Joint)

Usual causes of neurogenic arthropathy are:
- Tabes dorsalis.
- Diabetic neuropathy.
- Prolonged intra-articular injection of corticoids into the joint.
- Also, pernicious anemia, peripheral nerve injury, syringomyelia, and spinal cord injuries.

Symptoms of neurogenic arthropathy are:
- Diminution or loss of perception of pain, temperature, and proprioception.
- Signs of degenerative joint disease showing an enlarged painless articulation, with X-ray changes.

Management of neurogenic arthropathy:
- Treat etiological factor; avoid further trauma (orthopedic devices); or amputate, if necessary.

Thoracic Outlet Syndromes

What are the best known of these syndromes?

- Cervical rib syndrome.
- Scalenus anticus syndrome.
- Subclavian steal syndrome.
- Costoclavicular, scalenus medius, pectoralis minor, Wright's, and "effort thrombosis" (axillary and subclavian veins) syndromes.

Symptoms common to all these thoracic outlet syndromes are:

- Pain, radiating from the point of compression to the neck, the shoulder area, the arm, forearm, or the hand; at its worst at night or after exercise.
- Paresthesias, notably in 4th and 5th fingers; also worst at night or after exercise.
- Weakness and atrophy of the affected muscles possible.
- Pallor of fingers produced by ischemia caused by elevation of the arm.
- Sensitivity to cold.
- Veno- or arteriography, when there are pulse alterations, may help to disclose the point of occlusion.

Management of thoracic outlet syndromes:

- Try first conservative physical therapy.
- Surgery may be indicated for some patients.

Osteoarthritis (Degenerative Joint Disease)

Symptoms common to both primary and secondary osteoarthritis are:

- There is an insidious start of joint stiffness.
- After a time pain on motion of the affected joint develops.
- Pain increases with articular activity and decreases with rest.
- No deformity will occur, but there will be local bony enlargement.
- There is limitation of motion, but not true ankylosis.
- X-ray films will help diagnosis.

Osteoarthritis of the primary type includes:

- Heberden's nodes of the terminal phalanges.
- Bouchard's nodes of the proximal phalanges.
- Involvement of thumb's joints.
- Cervical and lumbar spine involvement.
- The hip and lower extremity, including the toes.

The secondary type of osteoarthritis includes:

- Intra-articular injury (from articular disease).
- Extra-articular injury (fracture, over-stress, postural, etc.).
- Metabolic diseases, particularly hyperparathyroidism, hemochromatosis, or ochronosis.

Management of osteoarthritis:

- Rest, analgesics, and physical therapy.

Congenital Hip Dislocation

Symptoms of congenital hip dislocation:

- It is more frequently seen in female infants.
- Skin creases on the inner sides of the hips are at different levels.
- The tip of the trochanter of the dislocated hip is above Nelaton's line (from the anterior superior spine of the ilium to the ischial tuberosity).
- The dislocated hip will not abduct as much as the other when this is intended after flexing the leg 90°.
- The slipping of the dislocated hip is noted when pulling and pushing the affected leg.

Management of congenital dislocation of the hip:

- Conservative physical therapy, if started early in life.
- Physical therapy and surgery, thereafter.

Causalgia (Reflex Sympathetic Dystrophy)

Symptom of causalgia:

- There is a history of a previous trauma to the extremity.
- There are, initially, pain, tenderness, and hyperesthesia localized to the injured area.
- The extremity appears dry, swollen, warm, and red or cyanotic.
- The pain presents a burning character in most cases.
- The extremity is held in a splinted position.
- The nails become ridged, and the hair increases in length.

Symptoms of long-standing causalgia are:

- There is more diffuse pain, which is worse at night.
- The limb turns cool and clammy; the skin glossy and atrophic.
- The limb will not tolerate temperature changes; particularly cooling.
- Stiffness increases owing to disuse, and the limb turns useless.
- The patient avoids stimulation of the developing trigger points.

Management of causalgia:

- It is better to treat it early with physical therapy and tranquilizers.
- Otherwise, surgery is indicated (sympathetic block).

Fibromyositis

The common symptoms of the different types of fibromyositis:

- Acute onset of pain occurs.
- Pain is aggravated by motion.
- There is tenderness on affected muscles, and at special trigger points.
- Local spasm is noted frequently.
- Fever may be present; and all symptoms disappear in a few days.

The most frequently affected areas are:

The neck (torticollis)	Sudden onset (on awaking in the morning), or insidious; contraction of the sternomastoid turns the head opposite and bends the neck toward

	the muscle side; the muscle is tender to palpatation; the spasm may be tonic or clonic (with jerky movements); if long-standing, the muscle becomes hypertrophied; rest, physical measures, local treatment (injections), or etiological therapy, plus psychotherapy, etc.
Low back (lumbago)	Local lesions may be causative; pain is continuous or intermittent, aggravated by motion and mitigated by rest and also heat or massage; rest, analgesics, or surgery.
Thorax (pleurodynia or Borholm disease)	Borholm disease is caused by a virus; otherwise, it is a muscle neuralgia, causing decreased respiratory movements due to intercostal neuralgia with swelling and tenderness; check pain.
Thighs (charleyhorse)	Caused by overstrain; the muscles become sore and stiff (quadriceps); usual therapy.

Polymyalgia Rheumatica

Symptoms of polymyalgia rheumatica are:
- Middle-aged women more frequently affected.
- Sudden onset of pain at pelvis and shoulders, accompanied by stiffness.
- Fever, malaise, and weight loss.
- Anemia.
- Self-limited course, lasting 1 or 2 years.
- Check for frequently accompanying temporal arteritis, which may cause blindness.

Management of polymyalgia rheumatica:
- Corticosteroids; small amounts if there are not symptoms of cranial or temporal artery involvement; in the last instances, larger amounts.

Polymyositis

Symptoms of polymyositis are:
- Onset is either sudden or gradual.
- There is muscle weakness of proximal muscles, mainly of the limbs.
- Flexor weakness of the neck is a frequent occurrence.
- The affected muscles are painful, and also show tenderness.
- Joint symptoms may also be present.
- At later stages there will be contractures and atrophy.
- Also affected are muscles of the shoulders, the pelvis, and even the heart itself, causing cardiac failure.
- The muscles become swollen and stiff.
- Polymyositis may be associated with Sjögren's syndrome.
- Gastrointestinal symptoms may occur, particularly dysphagia.
- Other symptoms may be pleural pain, effusions into cavities, retinal exudates, splenomegaly, and lymphadenopathy.
- Check also for inciting or coincidental malignancies.
- There may be fever, and vasomotor disturbances.
- The disease may present repeated acute exacerbations.

Management of polymyositis:
- Give corticoids; also analgesics may be used.

Dermatomyositis

Symptoms of dermatomyositis are:
- All symptoms of polymyositis, as above, plus the dermic component.

The dermic symptoms of dermatomyositis are:
- A rash similar to lupus erythematosus will occur as butterfly erythema of the face.
- The rash will also affect the neck, shoulders, and the upper part of the chest and back.
- The rash is usually accompanied by edema.
- Periorbital edema together with a purplish effusion on the upper eyelid is very suggestive of diagnosis.
- These symptoms may follow an initial scaling and pigmentation of the skin (of little diagnostic value).
- Erythematous and trophic lesions may also appear on extensor aspect of the digits, the elbows, or the knees (Gottron's sign).
- There may be subungueal erythema, Raynaud's phenomenon, teleangiectasia.

Do not confuse dermatomyositis with:
- Scleroderma or lupus erythematosus.
- Trichinosis, or other myopathies.

Management of dermatomyositis:
- Corticoid therapy; a help with physical therapy and analgesics.

Chondrocalcinosis (Pseudogout)

The symptoms corresponding to calcium salt deposition in the joints are:
- There is articular pain, and limitation of motion.
- The disease is familial, and may be associated with other metabolic disorders.
- The diagnosis is made radiologically, and from needle aspirates.
- Acute recurrent symptoms of arthritis of large joints (knee) in patients over 60 years of age constitute pseudogout.

Management of chondrocalcinosis:
- Treat any possible causative disease.
- Use anti-inflammatory drugs, aspirate the joint, and inject corticoids into it.

Carpal Tunnel Syndrome

This compression of the median nerve is noted by the following symptoms:
- Initial acroparesthesia or frank pain in the area of distribution of the median nerve, notably the thumb and the index finger.
- Pain may be constant or intermittent, is exacerbated by activity of the hand, may be noted only at night, and may extend to the forearm or even the shoulder.
- Extreme flexion or dorsiflexion of the wrist intensifies the pain.
- Cases develop during pregnancy or after menopause, frequently.
- Weakness or atrophy of the thumb muscles (abductor pollicis brevis) may appear relatively late.
- Distal tingling on percussion (Tinel's sign) may be positive when done at the site of compression.

Differentiate carpal tunnel syndrome from:
- Other types of cervicobrachial syndrome.
- Other more proximal lesions of the median nerve that may occur in the forearms or in the arm.

Management of carpal tunnel syndrome:
- Early conservative treatment may be of help.
- Surgical division of the carpal ligament may be needed.

Sudeck's Atrophy

This acute bone atrophy is noted in clinics by:
- Occurrence of a previous injury, usually minor, to the bone, mainly the wrist or the ankles.
- Burning pain, which worsens with activity.
- Edema, swelling, and local heat.
- Later changes to coldness, cyanosis, and atrophy, with stiffness and possible secondary fractures.

Management of Sudeck's atrophy:
- Physical therapy may help early manifestations.
- Sympathectomy may be needed in other cases.

Shoulder-Hand Syndrome

This possible combination of Sudeck's atrophy and frozen shoulder is noted as follows:
- It occurs at a mature age.
- Symptoms of frozen shoulder (q.v.) may precede, or may occur at the same time or after the symptoms of Sudeck's atrophy (q.v.).
- Rarely the elbow will be involved; in this case pain and restricted motion will be important symptoms.

Management of the shoulder-hand syndrome:
- Treat the cause, when evident.
- Treat at the same time the frozen shoulder (q.v.) and Sudeck's atrophy (q.v.).

Osteomyelitis

The implantation of the causative infection of osteomyelitis may be:
- Direct, causing primary osteomyelitis.
- Endogenous, carried by the blood in secondary osteomyelitis.

Symptoms of *acute pyogenic osteomyelitis* are:
- Acute onset as for an infectious disease, with fever, chills, sweating, and malaise or prostration; in adults, less acute onset.
- Pain and tenderness of the involved bone.
- After occurrence of pain, redness and/or swelling; finally, the possibility of abscess formation.
- Limitation of motion because of muscle guarding. This symptom is particularly marked when the infection occurs near a joint.
- Radiologic evidence of late occurrence; better rely on recovery of material from the affected side.
- Acute osteomyelitis is frequently prolonged into the chronic stage.

Do not confuse acute osteomyelitis with:
- Poliomyelitis, Ewing's sarcoma, rheumatic diseases, or cellulitis.

Management of acute osteomyelitis:
- Local care, and the specific antibiotic.
- Surgical care whenever advisable.

Symptoms of *chronic osteomyelitis* are:
- There is an insidious onset, or it may follow an acute attack.
- Symptoms are of the same character as for the acute type, but milder.
- Fluctuation may be noted; also effusion may occur into a joint.

Management of chronic osteomyelitis:
- Surgery is needed for removal of dead bone.
- Give local care, and the specific antibiotic.

Symptoms of *osteomyelitis due to infections* with brucella or salmonella:
- There are symptoms of the previous disease.
- Patients have predisposing diseases that facilitate salmonella osteomyelitis, such as sickle cell anemia.
- Brucellosis is more frequent among laborers in the meat or dairy industries.
- In salmonellosis, osteomyelitis will occur relatively late; and the affected sites are the shafts of long bones, but also metaphyses or epiphyses, or even the spine or the ribs.
- In brucellosis the lesions mainly occur in the spine or the sacroiliac joints. The spine may fuse, at times.

Management of these forms of osteomyelitis:
- Treat salmonellosis or brucellosis, accordingly.

Tuberculosis of the Bones

Symptoms of tuberculosis of the skeletal system are:
- There is a known previous tuberculous infection.
- The onset of symptoms is insidious.

The involved area will show swelling, pain, tenderness, and limitation of motion. There is local increased temperature.
Joints are most frequently affected, and there is an effusion in most cases.
There is a sensation of stiffness, more intense at night.
Besides limitation of motion, there may be limping.
Progression of lesions will cause muscle atrophy and deformity, notably gibbus when the thoracolumbar spine is affected.
Diagnosis depends on finding the causative *Mycobacterium* from the affected area.

Management of tuberculosis of the skeletal system:
General care.
Surgery.
Chemotherapy.

Syphilis of the Skeletal System

Symptoms of skeletal syphilis:
In early or late childhood, periostitis and osteoperiostitis are evidence of congenital syphilis.
Lesions are usually symmetrical, and the "saber shin" is a classical and very suggestive manifestation.
In adults gummatous lesions erode the bone, causing rarefaction and frequent occurrence of fractures.
Surrounding sclerosis will be noted, also.
Diagnosis depends on the diagnosis of syphilis.

Management of syphilis of the skeletal system:
Adequate care of the local lesion.
Chemotherapy for syphilis.

Gonorrhea of the Skeletal System

Symptoms of gonorrheal arthritis:
Almost always there exists a previous gonococcal infection.
Joint symptoms will appear about 3 weeks after the initial infection.
At the start, more than one joint seems to be infected; but later symptoms become localized in only one of the large joints.
Symptoms are of the type of a regular arthritis (q.v.).
Final diagnosis depends on the recovery of the infecting organism from the affected joint.

Management of gonorrheal arthritis:
Local care.
Analgesics for pain.
Chemotherapy as for regular gonorrhea.

Osteopsathyrosis (Osteogenesis Imperfecta)

Symptoms of this fragilits ossium or brittle bones:
Manifestations may be noted at birth (osteogenesis imperfecta congenita).
Manifestation may be noted later in life (osteogenesis imperfecta tarda).
The extremities show angular or bow-like deformities.
Repeated fractures will occur.
The spine may be deformed, also, with scoliosis or kyphosis.
The scleras are blue or very clear.
A large number of cases will present otosclerotic deafness.
Ligamentous laxity will allow extreme hypermotility of joints.
There is hyperelasticity of the skin (easy bruising), and hernia formation.
There are defective teeth, with translucent or opalescent appearance at the beginning, which turns to some form of discoloration of the organs (pink, gray, or amber).
Neurological symptoms may occur, due to pressure on the spinal cord or to hydrocephalus.
Diagnosis is suggested by the triad brittle bones, clear scleras, and deafness.

Do not confuse osteopsathyrosis with:
Achondroplasia, Marfan's syndrome, Ehlers-Danlos syndrome, etc.

Management of osteogenesis imperfecta:
Supportive and symptomatic.
Surgery when it appears useful.

Achilles Tendon Contracture

Symptoms of Achilles tendon contracture are:
Restricted dorsiflexion of the ankle.
Pain noted in the metatarsus and along the longitudinal arch.
Symptoms increased by wearing flat slippers, walking barefoot, or using high heels.
Almost always a weak foot, with a short Achilles tendon.

Management of Achilles tendon contracture:
Stretching the tendon gradually.
Surgical lengthening, if so needed.

Temporal Arteritis

See, for information, chapter on cardiovascular diseases.

Wegener's Granulomatosis

See, for information, chapter on respiratory diseases.

Multiple Myeloma

What are the symptoms usually noted in multiple myeloma?
There are initial weakness, ill health, and weight loss; or merely, anemia.
It occurs mostly in the elderly male.
Patients complain of a constant pain in the bones, which increases with motion.
Tenderness is noted particularly on the back.
Spontaneous fractures are not rare in this disease.

Plasma cell tumors sometimes present in the pharynx, or in the skin, or about the spinal cord.
Anemia is mostly noted; at times it is the only complaint.
The weight loss may reach marked proportions.
X-ray films may help in diagnosing the disease, showing punch-out rounded lesions, mottled areas, or diffuse osteoporosis.

Management of multiple myeloma:
General care, supportive and symptomatic.
Irradiation, or melphalan plus corticoids.

Tumors of the Bones

Usual symptoms of bone tumors are:
Tenderness of the affected bone, with pain and swelling.
Some limitation of mobility of that part.
Spontaneous fractures, or fractures due to minimal causes.
Final diagnosis dependent on X-ray films and biopsy.

Symptoms and management of *osteoid osteoma:*
Occurrence is more frequent in younger persons.
Exostoses occur, single or multiple, more often in femur and tibia, but also in spine and pelvis.
These small tumors may be painful, particularly at night.
Prognosis is good, but cartilaginous exostoses may become malignant.
Surgical removal is employed.

Symptoms and management of *giant-cell tumors* or *osteoclastoma:*
Young and mature persons are affected.
Epiphyses of long bones (at knee or wrist), but also pelvis and spine are involved.
The expanded cortex may disturb motility of the nearby joint.
X-ray films show spherical foamlike areas.
Surgical excision is necessary because some may become malignant. Irradiation is used in case of vertebral involvement.

Symptoms and management of *enchondromas:*
Adults are affected; rarely children.
Bones of hands or feet, or flat bones, or metaphyses of major long bones will show tenderness, pain, and swelling, and there may be spontaneous fractures.
At times there are multiple lesions.
Radiolucency with mottling and compartmentalization will be noted radiologically.
Treatment is curettage of solitary nodules; pelvic lesions may become malignant.

Symptoms and management of *chondroblastomas:*
Most patients are male under 20 years of age.
Long and flat bones swell and are painful.
Radiologically ovoid areas will be noted with mottled translucency and demarcating wall of sclerotic bone.
Some cases may become malignant.
Treatment is curettage.

Symptoms and management of *eosinophilic granuloma:*
It occurs mostly in young patients.
There is a solitary lytic lesion.
Treatment is surgical removal of the lesion.

Symptoms and management of *chondromyxoid fibroma:*
It also occurs mostly in young persons.
Long or flat bones and bones of the hands or feet will present swelling with tenderness, and pain.
X-ray films will show focus of rarefaction or multiple foci of osteolysis.
Care is surgical, by curettage or excision.

Symptoms and management of *chondrosarcoma:*
Occurrence is at any age, but most frequent among mature adults.
Any bone may show slow swelling and pain.
Irregular mottling and calcification are seen in long bones when examined radiologically.
Care is surgical, by radical excision or complete amputation, which will almost always give a good prognosis, particularly if done early.
There is a form of primary chondrosarcoma that occurs in youngsters and is highly malignant.

Symptoms of *osteogenic sarcoma:*
Occurrence is below 40 years of age, a little more frequently among men.
Any bone may be involved, but mainly the diaphysis of long bones.
Pain may be the first symptom, followed by swelling.
Locally, there will be tenderness, heat, and venous engorgement.
About half of the cases will occur at the knees.
Anemia and weight loss occur.
Metastasis will occur in the lungs almost always as the first instance.
X-ray films will show almost characteristic bone spicules perpendicular to the cortex.
Diagnosis will depend on radiological studies and biopsy.
In Paget's disease be suspicious of any swelling and pain because highly malignant osteogenic sarcomas may develop.

Management of osteogenic sarcoma:
Surgical approach by radical resection or complete amputation.
Followed by combination chemotherapy with multiple drugs.
Prognosis usually very poor, depending mostly on early diagnosis of small tumors.

Symptoms and management of *fibrosarcomas:*
The incidence is mostly after 30 years of age; but younger cases may be seen.
There may be a history of a previous irradiation.
The clinical picture is entirely similar to osteogenic sarcoma, q.v.
Diagnosis depends only on a biopsy.
Treatment is surgical, by amputation, with or without a previous radiotherapy.

Symptoms of round cell bone tumor or *Ewing's sarcoma:*

- There is a slight male preponderance of young persons, but it may occur at any young age.
- Any bone may be affected, but particularly the shaft (instead of the ends, as in the case of osteogenic sarcoma) of the long bones.
- Tender swelling is noted, and frank pain of single or multiple lesions.
- Other symptoms are fever and anemia.
- The clinical course is usually slow; but there are remissions and exacerbations; and finally metatases to the lungs or perhaps to other bones (or new growths?).
- X-ray films show osteoporosis with lamination ("onion peel"); medullary destruction is noted by rarefaction or mottling.
- Final diagnosis depends on biopsy.

Management of Ewing's tumor:

- Treatment is supervoltage radiation plus combination chemotherapy with multiple drugs.
- Avoid manipulation and surgery.

Symptoms and management of *malignant lymphoma* of the bones:

- Patients are usually persons between 40 and 50 years of age.
- Any bone may show local swelling and pain.
- Other organs may show lymphomatous lesions.
- Spontaneous fractures are common.
- X-ray films show bone destruction even to the complete loss of bone outline.
- Radiotherapy is the best approach.

Symptoms and management of *chordoma:*

- If the chordoma develops at the upper end of the spine, there will be symptoms from the cranial nerves (mostly, eye nerves).
- If located at the lower extremity, pain in the sacrococcigeal area will be dominant.
- X-ray films will help diagnosis, showing destructive bone lesions together with soft tissue masses.
- Chordomas of the suboccipital region may respond to radiotherapy.
- Chordomas of the sacral area should be totally excised.

9. Blood, Spleen, and Lymphatic Diseases

Posthemorrhagic Anemia

Usual symptoms of posthemorrhagic anemia are:

- Evidence of a previous hemorrhagic condition (this may be hidden and not easily known).
- Faintness, and dizziness.
- Sweating, and thirst.
- Weak rapid pulse, and hypotension (may rise initially, then fall).
- Initially deep, then shallow rapid respirations.
- If profuse enough, shock.
- Death if sudden loss of about one-third of the total blood volume occurs (in 24 hours, two-thirds).

Management of posthemorrhagic anemia:

- Stop bleeding.
- Give blood transfusion (plasma if blood is not available).
- Treat shock, if present.

Iron and Copper Deficiency Anemias

Symptoms of *iron deficiency* anemia are:

- Late appearance of symptoms, until microcytic followed by hypochromic changes appear.
- Waxy pallor of the skin.
- Lassitude, easy fatigability, and dyspnea.
- Tachycardia, palpitations, and possible anginal pains.
- Smoothness of the tongue, cheilosis at the angles of the mouth, and dysphagia (late signs).
- Brittle hair; the nails will also be brittle, ridged, and present a concavity (koilonychia).
- Pica, with a depraved desire for unnatural articles of food, particularly lime or paint. Some will show pagophagia, or desire for ice.
- The Plummer-Vinson syndrome, or sideropenic dysphagia, possible, with dysphagia for solids, due to esophageal webs.
- Diagnosis established by hemograms.

Management of iron deficiency anemia:

- Iron therapy.

Symptoms of *copper deficiency* anemia and its management:

- Symptoms are similar to iron deficiency anemia, q.v., together with hypoproteinemia or any form of severe undernourishment, particularly among infants.
- Copper therapy rapidly improves the situation.

Pernicious Anemia

This Addisonian anemia due to lack of vitamin B_{12} will tive the following symptoms:

- There is a very slow evolution of the disease, which may be more severe than the usual symptomatology would indicate.
- A smooth, and sore, tongue will be present, together with anorexia and dyspepsia.
- There are vague abdominal pain, intermittent constipation and diarrhea.
- Weight loss may reach considerable proportions.
- Skin paleness is variable in intensity; there may be jaundice.
- Numbness and tingling of the feet is symmetric and constant.
- Other neurologic symptoms may also occur, such as paresthesias of the upper limbs, loss of vibratory sensations, hyperactive reflexes, positivity of Babinski's sign, loss of sense of position, etc.
- There may be spasticity, ataxia, color blindness (yellow-blue), etc.
- Also, there may be irritability, depression, delirium, and other psychological symptoms.
- Other secondary troubles may be endocrine deficiencies, fever, etc.
- The final diagnosis depends on hemograms and determination of vitamin B_{12} levels in the blood; gastric achlorhydria is present.

Management of vitamin B_{12} deficiency:

- Cyanocobalamin (vitamin B_{12}) therapy.

Folic Acid Deficiency Anemia

Symptoms of anemia due to folic acid deficiency:

- There is a more rapid evolution of the disease in the case of folic acid deficiency than in the case of vitamin B_{12} deficiency.
- There is a frequent history of malnutrition, particularly of the alcoholic type, but also sprue, other forms of anemia, drug therapy (diphenylhydantoin, primidone, methotrexate, triamterene, etc.), and others.
- Symptoms are similar to vitamin B_{12} anemia, but with normal gastric secretions and absence of neurologic signs.
- Diagnosis depends on hemograms and marrow biopsy.

Management of folic acid anemia:
Folic acid therapy.

Other Vitamin Deficiency Anemias

What other vitamin B deficiencies are known?
Deficiency may refer to pyridoxine, riboflavin, or even pantothenic acid.
Usual symptoms of anemia may be present.
Diagnosis depends on hemograms and evaluation of the vitamin blood level.
There is also a vitamin C, ascorbic acid, deficiency.
Again, its diagnosis depends on hemograms and determination of blood levels of ascorbic acid.
Management of these vitamin deficiency anemias:
Replacement of the needed vitamin.

Aplastic Anemia

Symptoms of aplastic (or hypoplastic) anemia:
There is a history of exposure to chemical agents, antineoplastic drugs, or ionizing agents; but half the patients will not have any history.
There is an insidious onset, with pallor and lassitude.
Chronic cases will show brown skin pigmentation.
Bleeding is common; there will be purpura, and fundi hemorrhages.
Tachycardia, fatigue, and infections with high fever may occur.
Scarcity of all blood cells is noted; but there is a pure red blood cells aplasia in which only erythrocytes and their precursors are affected. If congenital, it will be the Blackfan-Diamond syndrome. (See below.)
Hemograms will aid in diagnosing the condition.
Management of aplastic anemia:
Blood transfusions.

Lead Poisoning Anemia

Symptoms of lead poisoning anemia are:
Those of chronic lead poisoning in children, that is, pica, vomiting, anorexia, hyperirritability, apathy and clumsiness, ataxia, lethargy, etc.
Characteristic stippling of red blood cells.
Management of lead poisoning anemia:
If symptoms are mild, particularly among adults, no treatment is needed.
With marked symptoms (encephalopathic or abdominal cramps, for instance) use calcium sodium edetate.
If symptoms are not too severe, use penicillamine.

Pure Red Blood Cells Aplasia

Symptoms of pure red blood cells aplasia:
Usual symptoms of anemia, particularly those similar to aplastic anemia.
Hemograms helpful in diagnosis.

Management of pure red blood cells aplasia:
Search for the causative factor, and treat it, namely, preleukemic leukemia, kidney failure, thymoma, other forms of anemia, malnutrition, certain drugs, and some infections.
Corticoids are favorable among children.
Testosterone, cobalt, vitamin B_2, or chemotherapy with prednisone and cyclophosphamide may be of some benefit.

Anemias Due to Ineffective Erythropoiesis

These anemias, other than pernicious anemia, thalassemia, or folic acid deficiency, are as follows:
Sideroblastic or *sideroachrestic anemias,* with splenomegaly in most instances, and ringed sideroblasts; there are excessive iron deposits.
Refractory normoblastic anemia, with usual symptoms of anemia, mild splenomegaly; frequent among alcoholics and diabetics.
Pyridoxine responsive anemias, similar to those described above among vitamin B deficiencies, which do not have other symptoms of pyridoxine deficiency, but respond dramatically to this substance.
Management of these anemias:
Try pyridoxine.
Use transfusions.

Acquired Autoimmune Hemolytic Anemia

Symptoms of this form of hemolytic anemia are:
Skin paleness, with some tint of jaundice.
Weakness and easy fatigability; also dizziness.
Palpitations and dyspnea.
Fever, with hepatosplenomegaly.
Previous use of penicillin in large doses, a cephalosporin, methyldopa, and other drugs.
A previous disease of the type of leukemia, lymphosarcoma, erythroblastosis fetalis, lupus erythematosus, etc.
Hemogram and electrophoresis good diagnostic aids.
Management of autoimmune hemolytic anemia:
Give corticoids for cases with unknown cause.
Splenectomy may be needed.
Give immunosuppressive agents if former methods do not work.
Withdraw the causative agent, when known.

Spherocytosis

This spherocytic anemia shows the following symptoms:
Skin is pale and jaundiced.
There is splenomegaly. Splenic infarction may cause acute pain.
There are malaise, abdominal discomfort, and possibly hepatomegaly and cholelithiasis.

In some instances, there are leg ulcers and bone changes. Rarely, there is polydactylism or tower-shaped skull.
Acute crisis occurs with intense anemia, fever, abdominal pain.
Hemograms help diagnosis.
Management of spherocytosis:
Splenectomy. For aplastic crises, transfusions.

Ovalocytosis or Elliptocytosis

Symptoms of this inherited trait:
Symptoms are very few, if existent at all: only mild hemolysis and splenomegaly.
The hemogram will show the oval or elliptical erythrocytes.
Management of this disease:
Splenectomy, particularly when there is evident hemolysis.

Acute Hemolytic Anemia

Symptoms of acute hemolytic anemia are:
Sudden onset of symptoms.
Fever with chills; tachycardia.
Nausea, vomiting, abdominal pain (there may be back pain).
The skin pale, with mild jaundice.
Splenomegaly.
The urine red or black.
Pigmented serum will help to differentiate acute hemolytic anemia from infections and acute abdomen.
Emergent treatment will consist of:
Hospitalization, discontinuance of medications used, and a search for the causative factor.
Supportive and symptomatic help.
Corticoids for severely ill patients.

Paroxysmal Nocturnal Hemoglobinuria

Symptoms of the Marchiafava-Micheli syndrome are:
Most patients are adults.
Moderate spleno- and hepatomegaly are found.
Abdominal and lumbar pain may be present.
Patients are prone to develop thrombi, which may cause death.
There is hemoglobinuria, particularly during night crises; these crises are increased by intercurrent diseases.
Management of paroxysmal nocturnal hemoglobinuria:
Give symptomatic care. If transfusions are needed, give them without plasma.
Dextran of high molecular weight will be convenient before transfusions.

Nonspherocytic Hemolytic Anemia

This form of hereditary anemia will show the following symptoms:
Skin moderately pale and slightly jaundiced.
Start in early childhood, in families with similar cases.
Mild splenomegaly.
Hemograms helpful.
Management of the disease:
Give whole blood transfusions.
Discuss splenectomy.

Anemia Due to Glucose-6-phosphate Dehydrogenase Deficiency

Drugs that usually cause symptoms of the disease are:
Antimalarials, sulfonamides, nitrofurans, sulfones, water-soluble vitamin K, antipyretics and analgesics, and uncooked fava beans.
Persons who usually react with the deficiency:
American Negro males, less frequently females; and even less frequently Italians, Greeks, Arabs, Sephardic Jews, Iranians, Chinese, and northern Europeans.
Symptoms of the disease:
There are acute hemolytic crises, with skin paleness and jaundice.
Acute hemoglobinuria and renal failure may occur.
"Bite cells" in the peripheral blood are a very good clue.
Management of the disease:
Withdrawal and future avoidance of the offending drug.

Sickle Cell Anemia

Symptoms of sickle cell anemia are:
Onset will occur mostly in childhood, but may be delayed to adulthood.
Symptoms of anemia may be present, such as pale face, jaundice better noted by mild scleral icterus, and perhaps others.
Recurrent crises occur with fever, pain in the limbs, and abdominal attacks resembling an acute abdomen.
Rare cases will show cerebral thrombosis, with headaches, convulsions, and paralysis.
Patients are blacks, particularly those descending from certain African tribes, but not all.
Symptoms of sickle cell trait:
There are almost none; rarely there are gross hematuria, impaired renal concentration, splenic infarcts on high altitude flights, or other stressing situations that may also cause visceral infarcts.
Check *in vitro* the sickling of red cells.
Management of sickle cell anemia and trait:
Give supportive and symptomatic care.
Painful crises require hydration and analgesics.
Hemolytic and aplastic crises require transfusions; also hydration and care for a contributing cause (infection, or the like).
Partial exchange transfusions may break repeated painful crises.
Treat complications accordingly; and avoid needless nephrectomies in cases of hematuria! (The latter is frequent in heterozygous patients who present only the sickling trait.)

Thalassemia

The usual symptoms of thalassemia major are:

Onset occurring mostly during childhood.

Evidence of severe anemia, with pale skin, severe asthenia and other usual anemic symptoms, including jaundice.

Hepato- and splenomegaly of very large proportions.

Thickening of cranial and malar bones (hemolytic facies); spontaneous fractures may also occur.

Leg ulcers and cholelithiasis, not too rarely.

Cardiac siderosis that may lead to failure.

Blood studies and radiology helpful in diagnosis.

The usual symptoms of thalassemia minor are:

Patients descendants of natives of the Mediterranean shores or southern China.

Anemia mild, but persistent.

Moderate splenomegaly.

Pain in the upper left quadrant of the abdomen, but only occasionally.

Similar findings, including laboratory examinations, in one of the parents.

Usually, over 6 million red blood cells.

Management of thalassemia:

Give spaced transfusions, as few as possible to children.

Discuss splenectomy, these days seen with little favor.

There is no treatment for thalassemia minor, except that during pregnancy transfusions will be given to maintain hemoglobin over 9 g/100 ml.

Associated Anemias

Secondary anemias associated with other causative disease are as follows:

There are anemias caused by *vitamin deficiency,* as discussed above.

Lead poisoning anemia is also discussed above.

Myxedema anemia occurs in primary or pituitary-induces thyroid hypofunction; it is accompanied by thyroid symptoms and responsive to thyroid medication.

Cancer anemia may be a precocious symptom; its fate is closely related to the causative disease.

Chronic infections usually develop anemia among the symptoms; but the disease is evident by itself in the great majority of the cases. The treatment depends on the causative germ.

Liver diseases, mainly cirrhosis, will cause anemia in the regular clinical way, or in the form of acute hemolytic crises particularly related to alcohol intake. Treat the basic disease, and avoid the use of alcohol.

Renal diseases, particularly with uremia, will present anemia. There is a *hemolytic-uremic syndrome* with hypertension and marked hemolysis. Treat the basic renal disease.

Myelophthisic anemia results from space-occupying lesions of the bone marrow. Regular anemic symptoms will be present, together with those corresponding to the causative disease (carcinoma, myelofibrosis, multiple myeloma, leukemia, Hodgkin's disease, etc.). Splenomegaly may be associated with hepatomegaly. The treatment is that of the basic cause.

Transfusion Reactions

Allergic reactions will pose the following problems:

During or immediately after the transfusion, there will be headache, urticaria, dizziness, or other allergic symptoms of a mild nature.

Rarely, more severe symptoms will be present, such as wheezing, dyspnea, urine incontinence, or even anaphylactic shock.

There is a history of known allergies.

Give an antihistaminic before the transfusion; but if a reaction starts, stop the transfusion immediately, and give an antihistaminic intramuscularly in case the reaction is mild, or epinephrine in the muscle or the vein.

Hemolytic reactions will pose the following problems:

During the transfusion there will be fever and chills. Occassionally these symptoms will appear later on.

The patient will complain of discomfort and anxiety.

Dyspnea and chest oppression may occur.

Pain will be referred to the chest, the back, or the abdomen; also it may occur in the neck or the lumbar area; and it may be severe.

There is flushing of the face, and a bursting sensation in the head.

More or less marked symptoms of shock may show at a last stage.

All symptoms may disappear.

There may be hemoglobinuria; temporary oliguria; mild uremia.

There may be perisitent oliguria leading to anuria and uremia, with the danger of death.

For treatment, stop the transfusion immediately, take care of annoying symptoms, and give mannitol intravenously; in severe cases treat as acute renal failure.

Circulatory overloading will pose the following problems:

It may happen to patients with little cardiac reserve and chronic anemia.

Tachycardia, hypotension, tachypnea with shallow respirations, cyanosis, and symptoms of pulmonary edema will occur.

Do not transfuse whole blood to these patients; stop the procedure immediately; apply tourniquets or do a phlebotomy; treat as congestive heart failure.

Post-transfusion disease transmission will pose the following problems:

Viral hepatitis may appear a relatively prolonged period of time after the transfusion.

Syphilis usually occurs after transfusing relatively fresh blood.

Malaria may occur if blood from persons who lived in infected areas is used.

Bacterial infections, particularly with germs of the coli-aerogenes group, may occur and may be very serious.

Polycythemia Vera

This increase of red blood cells (erythrocytosis) causes the following symptoms:

The face showing a frank redness or dusky redness of the skin or at least of the mucous membranes and the conjunctivas; the dusky redness is also noted on fingernails.

Modest splenomegaly (the spleen is palpable).

Itching, particularly noted after bathing with hot water.

Headache, marked asthenia, poor concentration, mild deafness.

Pain noted in digits.

Tortuous and black retinal veins.

Elevated erythrocyte count.

Not rarely, complicating hemorrhages, and thromboses.

Management of polycythemia vera:

Periodic phlebotomies.

Use of radiophosphorus; or chemotherapy with chlorambucil, cyclophosphamide, or similar drug.

Watch for and treat complications.

Other Forms of Erythrocytosis

Other forms of polycythemia will pose problems as follows:

Stress polycythemia is not considered a true polycythemia, the spleen is not enlarged, the plasma volume is diminished, and the total mass of red blood cells is normal. No treatment is needed.

Polycythemia due to anoxia follows a previous Pickwickian syndrome, arteriovenous shunt, or pulmonary fibrosis; also may be due to high altitude; the spleen is normal and the blood oxygen is dimished. Treat accordingly the causative condition.

Hemoglobinopathies with erythrocytosis are diagnosed by electrophoresis.

Other causes of secondary polycythemias are frankly rare, such as those due to uterine myomas, renal tumors and cysts, hepatoma, and other similar conditions. Removal of the cause is curative in some instances.

Thrombocytopenic Purpura

Symptoms of the idiopathic, primary, thrombocytopenic purpura, also called Werlhof's disease, are:

It may occur suddenly, or follow a chronic course.

The acute form is more frequent among children; the chronic form will occur at any age. More cases are seen among females.

There is a history of easy bruising.

Petechiae develop recurrently, particularly over pressure areas.

In the acute form, there is sudden occurrence of petechiae, and bleeding (from the nose, the gums, the vagina, etc.).

Platelet count is always deficient.

Management of purpura hemorrhagica, or idiopathic thrombocytopenic purpura:

Use corticoids, immunosuppressive agents. Vincrinstine seems to be of good use.

Consider splenectomy after 1 year of symptoms.

Thrombotic Thrombocytopenic Purpura

Symptoms of thrombotic thrombocytopenic purpura are:

The disease is more frequent among young adult females.

Symptoms usually involve many organs.

The kidneys are severely damaged by hyaline thrombi in the arteriolocapillary junctions (proteinuria, hematuria, and casts).

Neurologic involvement will also be noted, with drowsiness and other fluctuating symptoms.

There will be fever, jaundice, evidence of hemolytic anemia, and skin purpuric lesions.

The diagnosis is helped with the finding of fragmented red blood cells, and renal biopsy to demonstrate lesions at the arteriocapillary junction.

Management of thrombotic thrombocytopenic purpura:

Poor results have been obtained.

Some response has been obtained with dipyridamole and aspirin; also with corticoids, heparin, and even splenectomy.

Allergic Purpura (Henoch-Schönlein Syndrome)

Symptoms of anaphylactoid purpura are:

The disease occurs more frequently among children.

There are purpuric lesions in the skin (palms and soles) and mucous membranes, which may be itchy.

Blood or plasma also invades subserous surfaces.

There is also erythema or urticaria.

This is fever, and asthenia.

Arthralgia may be outstanding (Schönlein's purpura).

Abdominal pain may be outstanding (Henoch's purpura).

There may be acute glomerulonephritis with hematuria, proteinura, and kidney damage.

Cases may show intussusception or gastrointestinal bleeding.

Management of allergic purpura:

Give symptomatic care. Eliminate possible allergens. Cyclophosphamide has shown some success.

Hemorrhagic Telangiectasia (Hereditary)

The Rendu-Osler-Weber disease or syndrome shows the following symptoms:

It starts in childhood, but the greatest severity occurs after age 50.

Most lesions are seen in the face, nose, mouth, and upper limbs.

Lesions consist of telangiectasias, noted as bright red areas that blanch on pressure. They may also be violet in color.

There may be bleeding of the lesions, such as epistaxis or gastrointestinal bleeding.

Very few patients will show symptoms of pulmonary arteriovenous fistulas.

The diagnosis is suggested by the telangiectasias, recurrent bleeding, and a family history of similar cases.

Management of hereditary hemorrhagic telangiectasia:

Local treatment for bleeding lesions.

Blood transfusions, and iron, whenever indicated.

Systemic estrogens have shown some results.

Other Similar Diseases

Discuss the *primary familial platelet-ADP release dysfunction:*

Adenosine diphosphate is not released endogenously.

Easy bruising occurs.

Two different types have been described, namely, the regular type and the "storage-pool disease."

Discuss *Glanzmann's disease,* or *thrombasthenia:*

It is similar to the former release dysfunction, but more severe.

Diagnosis depends on studies on coagulation.

Discuss the *Gardner-Diamond syndrome,* or *autoerythrocyte sensitization:*

There are spontaneously propagating ecchymoses, which are painful.

Condition may be duplicated by injection of own erythrocytes.

There may be psychoneurotic disorders.

Purpura may also be noted.

Corticoids may be of help; but an underlying disease, if known, should be corrected.

Discuss the *hemolytic-uremic syndrome:*

Most cases are in infants or children.

The outstanding clinical picture is acute renal failure.

The onset is a gastrointestinal disorder.

Symptoms of hemolytic anemia are present.

Also, lethargy, hypertension, and hepatomegaly are noted.

There is proteinuria, together with hematuria.

Prognosis is usually good; but the use of glucocorticoids or anticoagulants has been advised.

Discuss the *Bernard-Soulier syndrome:*

Presence of unusually large platelets is noted.

It may be associated with other diseases (Chédiak-Higashi syndrome, May-Hegglin anomaly).

Hemophilia

Essentials for the clinical diagnosis of hemophilia are:

Recurrent large hematomas occur in the skin, or muscles, mostly painful.

Postsurgical bleedings and bleeding after minor bruises are observed.

Hematuria, gastrointestinal bleeding occur.

Some cases only bleed after minor surgery (tooth extraction).

Patients are male, and there are other similar cases in the mother's family. Symptoms start in childhood.

Both the clotting time and the partial thromboplastin time (PTT) are increased.

Joints may be deformed owing to repeated hemorrhages.

Episodes of bleeding occur at variable intervals.

Differentiation of defective factors in hemophiliacs:

Most cases show a deficient activity of the antihemophilic factor (AHF).

A few patients will present deficiency of the plasma thromboplastin component (PTC) and will present the Christmas disease.

In Christmas disease the symptoms are the same, but notably milder, with normal clotting time and increased PTT.

Deficient plasma thromboplastin antecedent (PTA) occurs in a very few of the hemophiliacs, both male and female Jews, who show a very mild bleeding symptoms.

Another deficient factor may exist.

Differentiation of the defective factor is given by laboratory determinations.

Treatment depends on the administration of the defective factor or of fresh or stored plasma if it is not commercially available.

The lack of factor XII will not present bleeding and will not need any treatment.

Management of hemophilia:

Administer AHF (factor VIII) concentrates.

Use plasma thromboplastin component (PTC) for patients who are in need of this factor IX.

Check bleeding with the basic factor needed. Hematuria may respond to the administration of corticoids.

Hemarthrosis may need aspiration, but rest may suffice.

If the patient develops inhibitors to the anticoagulants, corticoids plus cyclophosphamide may help; inhibitors of factor VIII may be treated with factor IX concentrates.

Vascular Hemophilia (von Willerbrand's Disease)

This angiohemophilia or pseudohemophilia presents the following symptoms:

Several members of the family, both male and female, present similar symptomatology.

There have been frequent episodes of epistaxis since childhood.

Also, there is excessive bruising.

Females will present menorrhagias.

The skin will present ecchymoses rather than petechiae.

Diagnosis depends on the examination of the blood, prolonged bleeding time with normal platelet count.

Management of this condition:
Treat as for hemophilia with the lack of factor VIII.

Vitamin K Deficiency

Information is found in the chapter on metabolism and nutrition.

Defibrination Syndrome (Disseminated Intravascular Coagulation)

Symptoms of this consumption coagulopathy:
There is bleeding, profuse and diffuse, from the skin and the mucous membranes, including generalized ecchymoses.
The clot is small and poor.
The disease is suggested by profuse and disseminated bleeding, a small clot, decreased number of platelets, and prolonged prothrombin time.
Do not confuse it with primary fibrinolysis, usually present together with prostatic carcinoma, liver diseases, and septicemia.
Management of disseminated intravascular coagulation:
Supportive therapy, with platelet concentrates.
Heparin.
Treatment of the underlying disease, if known.

Primary Fibrinolysis

Suggested approach for the diagnosis of primary fibrinolysis:
It may follow major surgery, or complicate cancer of the prostate or pancreas, or liver diseases or septicemia.
Widespread hemorrhages will occur.
Final diagnosis depends on laboratory findings.
Management of primary fibrinolysis:
Aminocaproic acid.
Care of the underlying cause.

Agranulocytosis

The drugs that may induce the development of agranulocytic angina are:
Anticancer drugs of any kind.
Phenothiazines, such as promazine, chlorpromazine, etc.
Sulfonamides and antibiotics, particularly chloramphenicol.
Anticonvulsant drugs, such as diphenylhydantoin, trimethadione, etc.
Antihistaminics and antithyroid drugs.
Aminopyrine, phenylbutazone, dipyrone, and indandiones, such as phenindione.
Arsenicals and gold compounds.
The symptoms of agranulocytopenia:
There is a rapid onset of fever, of the septic type, with chills and prostration.
There is the simultaneous appearance of the agranulocytic agina, with sore ulcerated throat.
Associated pain and dysphagia are noted.
There is a throat exudate of a brown-gray hue.
Ulcers may also appear in the rectum, the respiratory tract, and the vagina.
Regional adenopathy corresponds to the ulcerated areas.
The skin may show maculae and papules.
If the disease is untreated, there is rapid progression to shock and death.
There is a chronic course, with slow progression of the symptoms, particularly those corresponding to the respiratory system, the skin, or the perirectal area.
The diagnosis is given by a reticulocyte count of less than 3,000 with a disproportionate reduction of neutrophils.
Management of agranulocytosis:
Stop the administration of the offending drug immediately.
Give the specific antibiotic, whenever known.
Carbenecillin and cephalothin are an acceptable combination to start therapy.
Give corticoids to patients with severe toxemia, but otherwise it is better to avoid them.
Oxymethalone may help the bone marrow to recuperate.

Alymphocytosis or Lymphocytopenia

The clinical evaluation of lymphocytopenia consists of the following:
There is a lack of any special symptom.
Symptoms belong to the causative disease.
Only the chronic situation may show a reduced size of lymph nodes, tonsils, and the spleen. In some instances, there may be lymphoadenopathy, instead.
The hemogram will give the diagnosis, with less than 1,500 lymphocyte count (3,000 for children), as absolute counts.
Management of this sort of lymphopenia:
Depends on the causative factor; thus consists of marrow transplantation, gamma globulin, corticoids, radiation, etc.

Acute Leukemia

Usual symptoms of acute leukemia:
They may simulate an acute infection, with fever which may be high and accompanied by marked asthenia.
There may be a secondary infection of the mouth or throat, or of the lungs.
Pain is noted in bones and joints. Frequent sternal tenderness is observed.
Anorexia, and possibly mild hepatomegaly occur.
Adenopathy and splenomegaly may occur.
Pallor, petechiae, ecchymoses, and bleeding (mouth, kidneys, nose, or gastrointestinal tract) are noted.
Do not confuse with cases of purpura, mononucleosis, Hodgkin's disease, certain malignant tumors, or rheumatic fever.

Diagnosis depends on bone marrow aspirates with primitive white blood cells.

The diagnosis will be made from laboratory reports, differentiating acute lymphoblastic leukemia, acute myloblastic leukemia, acute monoblastic leukemia, or acute myelomonoblastic leukemia.

Management of acute leukemia:

For acute lymphatic leukemia use prednisone and vincristine (or methotrexate).

If leukemic infiltration of the central nervous system occurs (with headache, irritability, apathy, and blurred optic discs), give methotrexate intrathecally.

For all the other forms of acute leukemia, give a combination of drugs, such as cyclophosphamide, vincristine, cytarabine, and prednisone, commonly referred to as COAP.

Chronic Myelocytic Leukemia

The usual symptoms of this chronic granulocytic leukemia are:

Vague symptoms of fever, asthenia, anorexia, weight loss, and some abdominal discomfort.

Splenomegaly, and very mild adenopathy in some instances.

Anemia, and pallor of the skin.

Sternal tenderness.

Possible purpura, or retinal hemorrhages or exudates.

Possible skin nodules.

Bleeding after small procedures (dentistry, etc.).

A hemogram with elevated white blood cells count will give the diagnosis.

Management of chronic myeloid leukemia:

Busulfan is the drug of choice.

Chronic Lymphocytic Leukemia

Usual symptoms of chronic lymphatic leukemia are:

Paleness of the skin.

Insidious appearance of weakness, hypermetabolism, and adenopathy of the superficial lymph nodes.

Pressure symptoms (dyspnea, etc.), which may be caused by the adenopathy.

Mild spleno- and hepatomegaly.

Skin lesions due to leukemic infiltration.

Hemogram with absolute lymphocytosis will give the diagnosis.

Management of chronic lymphocytic leukemia:

Do not overtreat!

Use radiation, chlorambucil, corticoids.

Malignant Lymphoma

This group of lymphomas may be divided into:

Lymphocytic well differentiated malignant lymphoma.

Lymphocytic poorly differentiated malignant lymphoma.

Histiocytic malignant lymphoma, formerly reticulum cell sarcoma.

Mixed histiocytic-lymphocytic malignant lymphoma.

Stem cell malignant lymphoma (see Burkitt's lymphoma, below).

Clinical aspects of malignant lymphoma:

Adenopathy: the nodes are rubbery, and become matted at a later stage of the disease, noted in neck, nasopharynx, etc.

Internal lymph nodes may cause organic symptoms: mediastinal, retroperitoneal, gastrointestinal (simulating gastric cancer or provoking malabsorption), chylous ascites, pleural effusion, etc.

The clinical picture may start with fever, asthenia, weight loss, and sweating. The adenopathy is multifocal.

Rarely involvement of skin, bones, or central nervous system occurs.

Frequent hepato- or splenomegaly is noted.

Diagnosis is made by lymph node biopsy.

Management of malignant lymphoma:

Radiotherapy for localized disease.

Chemotherapy for disseminated disease. Cyclophosphamide is the drug of choice; also vincristine is useful, as well as doxorubicin.

Combination therapy is preferable (cyclophosphamide, vincristine, and prednisone).

Leukemic reticuloendotheliosis, also called *hairy cell leukemia,* is a variant of malignant lymphoma characterized as follows:

There is splenomegaly, without any lymph enlargement.

The course is relatively benign.

Slides will show the typical "hairy cells," that is, cytoplasmic projections of lymphoid cells.

Chemotherapy is contraindicated, but splenectomy may be of help.

Hodgkin's Disease

Symptoms of Hodgkin's disease:

It is more frequent among young adults.

The disease usually starts with unilateral adenopathy (cervical nodes affected first in most cases).

The nodes are firm, painless, and nontender.

The size varies for each node.

Nodes may adhere to deep tissues, but the skin remains free.

Mediastinal nodes will cause dyspnea.

Later symptoms are fever, sweating, asthenia, and itching.

Fever occasionally presents elevations lasting for a few days alternating with lapses of normal temperature (Pel-Ebstein pattern).

Bone involvement may cause pain, rarefaction, or compression (vertebral); but fractures will occur rarely.

Symptoms of spinal compression may occur (Horner, paraplegia, paralysis, voice problems, etc.).

Also, jaundice, cyanosis, edema (face or legs), and other symptoms are possible.

In advanced disease, infectious complications are not rare.

The disease is classified in stages, namely:

I. One single abnormal node.
II. More than one node, only on one side of the diaphragm.
III. Nodes on both sides of the diaphragm.
IV. Involvement of other sites than the nodes, that is, bones, lungs, liver, skin, nervous system, etc.

Management of Hodgkin's disease:

Radiotherapy, or radiotherapy together with combination chemotherapy.

Burkitt's Lymphoma

Symptoms and management of this undifferentiated lymphoblastic lymphoma are:

It is more frequent in other countries (Central Africa) than in the United States. Children are mostly affected.

Initial symptom is the involvement of the jaw.

There is further involvement of organs below the diaphragm, namely, the gonads and the kidney.

In a last stage, there is involvement of the bone marrow or the central nervous system.

Cyclophosphamide is the advised drug for initial stages.

There is no treatment for involvement of the bone marrow or the central nervous system.

Heavy Chain Diseases

Symptoms and management of *IgG heavy chain (gamma-chain) disease are:*

Very few cases known, affecting elderly patients.

Fever, anemia, recurrent infections.

Enlarged lymph nodes, liver, and spleen.

Frequent edema of the palate.

Diagnosis dependent on electrophoretic and immunoelectrophoretic findings (chain fragments of IgG).

Only symptomatic care can be given.

Symptoms and management of *IgA heavy chain (alpha-chain) disease are:*

This Mediterranean lymphoma occurs in young people living in the Middle East.

There is a malabsorption syndrome, q.v.

There is diffuse abdominal lymphoma.

Diagnosis depends on immunoelectrophoresis (free alpha-chains).

Some results have been obtained from radiotherapy, cyclophosphamide, corticoids, and antibiotics.

Symptoms and management of *IgM heavy chain (mu-chain)* disease are:

Symptoms are similar to chronic lymphocytic leukemia (q.v.), with involvement of abdominal lymph nodes, spleen, and liver.

Diagnosis depends on laboratory findings.

Do not overtreat; use radiation, chlorambucil, corticoids.

X-Linked Agammaglobulinemia

This infantile hereditary disorder gives the following symptomatology:

During the second year of age, there are repeated pyogenic infections, mostly furunculosis, pneumonia, and meningitis.

There are frequently chronic sinusitis, bronchitis, and arthritis (mainly large joints).

Do not confuse with rheumatoid arthritis.

Diagnosis depends on the finding of low blood levels of IgG, IgA, and IgM.

Management of this Bruton's syndrome:

Intramuscular administration of gamma globulin.

Fresh-frozen plasma, and antibiotics.

Selective Immunoglobulin Deficiency

Symptoms of this Janeway type 3 dysgammaglobulinemia are:

It is perhaps the most common of immunodeficiency disorders.

It may be asymptomatic (absence of serum IgA may be found in otherwise normal individuals).

A syndrome similar to sprue, with steatorrhea, may occur.

Other cases may show bronchitis, or sinusitis.

Management of this condition:

Do not use commercial gamma globulin; use instead fresh-frozen plasma.

Thymic Hypoplasia

Symptoms of DiGeorge's syndrome are:

A disease of very young infants.

Neonatal tetany.

Hypertelorism, antimongoloid slanting, low-set ears, and other abnormalities.

Great susceptibility to infections, which may be viral, fungal, pneumocystis, or bacterial infections.

Infectious bouts very severe; may end fatally.

Management of DiGeorge's syndrome:

Implantation of human fetal thymus tissue has proved to be very successful.

Severe Combined Immunodeficiency

Symptoms of severe combined immunodeficiency are:

A disease of young infants; death may occur before 2 years of age.

Watery diarrhea (salmonella or coli infections).

Pulmonary infections (psudomonas and pneumocystis).

Candidiasis (in mouth and diaper areas).

Usual infant viral diseases commonly fatal.
Diagnosis dependent on laboratory findings.
Management of this condition:
Fresh-frozen plasma, transfer factor, bone marrow transplantation.
Poor results with passive administration of gamma globulins.

Immunodeficiency plus Thrombocytopenia and Eczema

Symptoms of Wiskott-Aldrich syndrome are:
A disease of children, who rarely survive above 10 years of age.
Skin lesions, namely, eczema and thrombocytopenic results, such as petechiae, purpura, and even gastrointestinal hemorrhages.
Recurrent viral and bacterial infections; also fungal infections and those due to pneumocystis.
Increased susceptibility to malignancies, particularly leukemia, lymphoma, sarcoma, etc.
Management of this condition:
Transfer factor, fresh-frozen plasma.
Appropriate antibiotics.

Immunodeficiency plus Ataxia-Telangiectasia

Symptoms of this condition are:
The thymus gland is small.
Symptoms start with ataxia and choreathetoid movements, during infancy (ataxia may be delayed until 4 years of age).
Ophthalmoplegia and muscle weakness and atrophy occur.
There is mental retardation, which is progressive.
At a later stage, telangiectasias will appear in the conjunctivas, eyelids, face, arms.
There are recurrent sinopulmonary infections.
There may be gonadal dysgenesia, testicular atrophy, and diabetes mellitus (this with marked hyperglycemia and absent glycosuria).
There is increased susceptibility to malignancies, particularly leukemia, Hodgkin's disease, gastric cancer, frontal lobe glioma, etc.
Management of immunodeficiency plus ataxia-telangiectasia:
Fresh-frozen plasma.

Immunodeficiency plus Sarcoidosis

Symptoms of this condition are:
Evidence of immunodeficiency appearing in patients presenting the clinical picture of sarcoidosis.
Nonreactivity to intradermal injections of common antigens.

Immunodeficiency with Hodgkin's Disease

Symptoms of this condition are:
Patients already presenting evidence of the clinical symptomatology of Hodgkin's disease.
Frequent infections with cryptococcus, and also herpes zoster.
Lesser frequency of reactivity to skin tests for mumps, candida, or trichophyton.

Immunodeficiency plus Thymoma

Symptoms of this immunodeficiency with thymoma are:
There is a gradual onset of symptoms.
At an earlier or later stage of the disease, the thymus mass will be evidenced by X-ray findings. It may cause wheezing.
Recurrent infections are common, in the respiratory system or in the skin; septicemia is not a difficult occurrence.
There may be chronic diarrhea (giardiasis).
Infections with pneumocystis and with cytomegalovirus are the usual cause of death.
These patients may show evidence of myasthenia gravis, chronic hepatitis, arthritis, and diabetes mellitus.
Management of immunodeficiency with thymoma:
Use gamma globulin and antibiotics.
Consider thymectomy.

Immunodeficiency plus Short Limbs

Symptoms of this complex of immunodeficiency plus short limbs are:
There are three types of immunodeficiency (T cell, combined B and T cells, and only B cell).
Children will also show achondroplasia-like features.
Skull and spine are normal.
Some may show hypoplastic hair or cartilages; some may have congenital megacolon.
Vaccinia and varicella are the common causes of death.
Management of this condition:
Only patients with type III deficiency (only B cells) will respond to the administration of gamma globulin.

Chronic Granulomatous Disease

Symptoms of chronic granulomatous disease are:
Boys are more frequently affected.
There are repeated infections caused by staphylococci, klebsiellae, aerobacter, escherichiae, pseudomonas, aspergillus, proteus, serratiae, salmonellae, and candida.
Infections result in abscess and granuloma formation (adenitis).
Diagnosis depends on laboratory tests.
Other symptoms that may aid in diagnosis are hepatosplenomegaly, persistent rhinitis, persistent diarrhea, dermatitis, perianal abscess, etc.
Management of this condition:
There are poor results, in most instances.
Try bone marrow transplantation.

Give leukocyte transfusions to the acutely ill.
Always give the specific antibiotic.

Chediak-Higashi Syndrome

Symptoms of this condition, and its management are:
- Partial albinism.
- Severe recurrent infections of the pyogenic type.
- Pancytopenia and giant inclusions in peripheral leukocytes.
- A familial pattern.
- Symptoms help with antibiotics and leukocyte transfusions.

Hypersplenism

Evaluation of hypersplenism:
- Basically, it consists of an enlarged spleen (splenomegaly).
- Congestive splenomegaly is the most frequent form, due to cirrhotic portal hypertension, thrombosis, stenosis, atresia, aneurysm of the splenic artery, cysts, etc.
- There is spleen infiltration, as in the case of tuberculosis, Boeck's sarcoid, Gaucher's disease, Niemann-Pick disease, Letterer-Siwe disease, and perhaps others.
- There is frequent bleeding, in the form of gastrointestinal hemorrhages or esophageal varicosities.
- Purpura may be observed, in some cases.
- There is modest abdominal discomfort, in the case of a too-large spleen.
- In cases with primary splenic leukopenia, there will be fever and pain on the splenic area.
- There are laboratory reports of pancytopenia and active marrow.
- Evaluation of symptoms and signs of the basic causative disease, particularly laboratory findings in hemograms, blood chemistries, bone marrow, splenic studies, lymphangiography, etc., is helpful.

Management of hypersplenism:
- Essential therapy is that of the underlying disease.

Banti's Syndrome

Evaluation of this form of congestive splenomegaly:
- Regular symptoms of hypersplenism (see above paragraph).
- Regular symptoms of hepatic cirrhosis, thrombosis of the portal or the splenic vein, or malformations of the portal blood vessels.
- Worsened bleeding from esophageal varicosities.

Management of Banti's syndrome:
- Surgical shunting for venous problems, or medical management of cirrhosis.

Felty's Syndrome

When Felty's syndrome is said to occur:
- When splenomegaly with leukopenia occurs in patients with rheumatoid arthritis.
- When there are frequent infections.

Management of Felty's syndrome:
- Splenectomy will help only half of the total number of patients.

Primary Splenic Neutropenia

Symptoms of this rare disease are:
- Vague complaints of asthenia, or chronic ill health.
- Pain in several joints.
- Recurrent infections, either mild or severe.
- Other causes of granulocytopenia have to be ruled out.

Management of this condition:
- Consider splenectomy.

Ruptured Spleen

Symptoms of rupture of the spleen:
- A previous traumatic injury, which may be mild in the case of a previously abnormal spleen. Symptoms of internal hemorrhage.
- Easy rupture of spleen when rapid enlargement occurs, as in the case of infections.

Management of ruptured spleen:
- Emergent splenectomy.

Spleen Aplasia

Evaluation of spleen aplasia in the infant:
- Suspicion should arise when septicemia and meningitis start before 2 years of age, and the child remains susceptible to repeated very severe infections.
- Most cases are due to meningococci, pneumococci, hemophilus, and coli bacilli.
- Rule out other immunodeficiency syndromes.
- Radioscanning will not show the spleen.

Management of splenic aplasia:
- Prophylactic penicillin is recommended.
- Treat aggressively any infection.
- Postsplenectomy will be treated as splenic aplasia.

Tumors of the Spleen

General considerations about tumors of the spleen:
- They are rare, and may be benign or malignant.
- Most frequent tumors are hemangiomas or lymphangiomas; also abscesses and cysts may be noted as masses in the spleen area; malignant types may also occur.
- The clinical picture is splenomegaly without the blood and marrow findings that accompany other spleen processes.
- Splenectomy is the logical approach for spleen tumors.

Macroglobulinemia

Waldenström's macroglobulinemia shows the following symptoms:

There is difficult aspiration of the bone marrow; its biopsy will show diffuse infiltrate with lymphoid and plasma cells.
Excessive production of IgM characterizes the disease.
Symptoms usually start after 50 years of age.
The so-called hyperviscosity syndrome may be apparent, with dense blood within the vessels, congestion of organs, increased heart work, plethoric appearance, and the risk of thrombosis.
Hemorrhagic phenomena may occur (ecchymoses, petechiae), including bleeding from the mucosae.
Anemia will be noted because of paleness and asthenia.
Fever and weight loss occur.
There is peripheral neuropathy, which may be an early finding.
Headache and drowsiness are noted.
There is modest splenomegaly or lymphadenopathy.
The optic fundi may give a very suggestive finding; namely, the veins show alternating bulges and constrictions.
Recurrent infections may complicate the clinical picture.
Erythrosedimentation rate is very high.

Management of macroglobulinemia:

Use chlorambucil or melphalan.
Plasmaphoresis may control hyperviscosity.

Cryoglobulinemia

Symptoms of precipitation of serum globulins on cooling are:

Raynaud-like symptoms on exposure to cold weather.
Bleeding from the nose or mouth.
Bleeding of the skin, namely, petechiae or purpura.
Constriction or hemorrhage of the retinal vessels.
Other skin symptoms of the type of urticaria, ulcerations, gangrene or necrosis, etc., mostly noted on dependent sites.
There may be symptoms of a basic causative disease, such as the former macroglobulinemia, lymphomas, glomerulonephritis, lupus erythematosus, myeloma, and the like.

Management of cryoglobulinemia:

Prevent coldness, and treat the underlying disease.

Myelofibrosis

Symptoms of myelosclerosis or agnogenic myeloid metaplasia are:

Almost always splenomegaly; at times also hepatomegaly; but no adenopathy.
Asthenia and weight loss.
Bone pain and abdominal discomfort.
Evidence of anemia, which may be severe.
The hemogram quite helpful in diagnosis.

Management of myelofibrosis:

Only treat marked anemia (androgenic steroids and transfusions), and splenomegaly (busulfan, or radiotherapy).

Lymphangitis

Symptoms of lymphangitis in its acute phase are:

Rapid onset, with fever, usually with chills, malaise, headache, and generalized pains over the body; marked tachycardia.
Following the path of lymphatic channels, patchy areas of inflammation, that is, red streaks going from the area of a wound or of cellulitis toward the regional lymph nodes.
Most of the cases occurring in the limbs, going from the infected site toward the regional lymph nodes in the form of linear red streaks.
Tender and painful lymphadenitis.

Symptoms of chronic lymphangitis are:

There is a slow clinical course.
A firm cord is noted, more or less deep under the skin.
It is usually tender, and may show abscesses, ulcers, or scars along its course.
The cord goes from the initial infection to the site of the corresponding lymph nodes.

Management of lymphangitis:

Watch for bacteremia, and local reactions. Use local care.
Treat the initial infection.
Use the adequate antibiotic.
Residual lymphedema (q.v. below) may require surgery.

Lymphadenitis

Symptoms of lymphadenitis are:

A node or a group of nodes become enlarged.
Enlarged nodes may be tender and painful; and the corresponding site of the skin, inflammed.
Pain may restrict motion of the corresponding muscles.
A bout of acute lymphangitis or a previous stage of chronic infection usually precedes this condition.
Cellulitis or even abscess may follow lymphadenitis.
The final stage may be complete or almost complete resolution of lymphadenitis; or the chronic stage of persistent, firm, mostly nontender nodes.

Management of lymphadenitis:

Provide local care, and the adequate antibiotic.
Surgery may be required for formed abscesses.

Lymphedema

Causes and symptoms of lymphedema are:

The lymph flow may be impaired by congenital abnormalities, malignancies, infections (most importantly filariasis), trauma, surgery, or radiation.

There is partial or total swelling of a limb.
The covering skin is not affected.
Swelling of the scrotum is not too rare, due to filariasis, venous compression in the abdomen, cirrhosis with ascites; or it may be idiopathic (Milroy's disease).
A secondary lymphedema due to infection is accompanied by fever, chills, redness, and hot skin, besides the usual symptoms of lymphedema.

Management of lymphedema:
Poor results with physical, diuretic, or surgical therapy; or antibiotic care for secondary infection.

Mycosis Fungoides

Symptoms of this primarily skin lymphoma are:
It starts with skin symptoms.
Lesions mimic eczema, seborrhea, psoriasis, erythroderma, or any other form of a severely itching rash, or a tumor.
Eventually, lesions disseminate, spreading over the body, and become nodular or ulcerate.
In the course of the disease the spleen and the lymph nodes become involved and enlarge; there is also hepatomegaly.
Adenopathy with itching is suggestive of the disease.
The disease is mostly diagnosed late from the onset, in adults over 40 years of age.

Management of mycosis fungoides:
Electron beam radiation of the whole body surface.
Nitrogen mustard, or other similar drugs.
Topical treatment with sunlight, and with steroids.

Hand-Schüller-Christian Disease

This form of histiocytosis presents the following characteristics:
Onset occurs in early childhood; rarely in adults.
There are osteolytic lesions of flat bones principally, but also large bones.
Lungs are also involved, and frequent respiratory infection may occur.
The skin may show eczema, eczematoid dermatitis.
Enlargement of spleen and lymph nodes, also hepatomegaly may occur.
Exophthalmos, and otitis media may be noted.
Diabetes insipidus may also occur.
Diagnosis made by biopsy.

Management of this type of histiocytosis:
Radiation, or chemotherapy (vincristine, prednisone).
Lung involvement treated with corticoids.

Letterer-Siwe Disease

This second type of histiocytosis gives the following symptoms:
Onset occuring mostly before 3 years of age.
A more or less marked cachectic state.
Spleno- and hepatomegaly; also, adenopathy.
The skin showing maculopapular lesions.
Recurrent infections frequent.
Involvement of bones and lungs common; the marrow is filled with histiocytes.
A bad prognosis; but when it starts after 3 years of age, results are somewhat better.

Management of Letterer-Siwe disease:
Prednisone, or some of the antimetabolites.

Eosinophilic Granuloma

Evaluation of eosinophilic granuloma:
A bone will show a solitary osteolytic lesion.
Rarely, this lesion will cause pain, swelling, or a fracture; and in a very few instances it will be tender.
Bones more frequently involved are pelvis, head, ribs, and the spine.
About 20% of the patients will present lung infiltration.
In some instances, the lung infiltration will be the only evidence of the disease.
The disease is seen in children, adolescents, and young adults.

Management of eosinophilic granuloma:
Try curettage, excision, or radiation.
It may recur in a different site.

Mastocytosis

This hyperplasia of mast cells, also called systemic mast cell disease, is characterized by the following features:
There is usually an associated disease, namely, leukemia, myeloid metaplasia, myelosclerosis.
The outstanding symptom is urticaria pigmentosa (macules or papules of a brown color, and dermographia).
Flushing may accompany the skin lesions, but it is episodic.
There may be also a few cases with fever, tachycardia, headache, asthenia, rhinitis, bone pain, and weight loss.
Some patients will show spleno- and hepatomegaly, together with adenopathy.
X-ray studies will show lytic bone lesions, cystic osteoporosis, or sclerosis.
The diagnosis is made by biopsy.

The best care to be given to these patients consists of:
Symptomatic treatment.

10. Allergy

Migraine

The accepted cause of migraine attacks is:

It is the result of vascular changes rather than true allergenic phenomena.

The essential migraine features consist of the following:

It may start at any age, but most frequently in early youth, affecting more women than men. It may improve after 50 years of age.

The outstanding symptom is a throbbing, usually very intense headache.

The headache is mostly unilateral (hemicrania), but it may also be generalized.

The headache may start over one eye, and then spread over the corresponding side, or over all the head.

The pain will last for hours; rarely, days. Adequate treatment will shorten the attack.

The periodicity of attacks varies from patient to patient; attacks may occur daily, or only after months.

Each patient shows a particular pattern, except that unilateral attacks may change side.

The other migraine features include:

Attacks are heralded by irritability or depression, gastrointestinal symptoms, or more rarely paresthesias or paralysis.

Ocular symptoms may announce, or mix with, the migraine attack; these symptoms are photophobia, blurred vision, or hemianopsia.

Scintillating scotomas are not rare; it is said that they may substitute for actual migraine attacks.

During the attack the limbs are cyanosed and cold, and the patient prefers to stay alone in a darkened room.

The diagnosis depends on the family history and the recurrent attacks of headache and gastrointestinal symptoms.

Prophylactic management of migraine:

Give methysergide (may cause retroperitoneal fibrosis), propanolol, or tranquilizers and antidepressants.

A cautious use of ergotamine may be advised; but it is better used to prevent an impending attack.

Management of the established attack of migraine:

Give ergotamine, or dihydroergotamine.

Mild attacks may respond to acetylsalicylic acid or codeine.

Histaminic Cephalalgia

This Horton's cephalalgia, also called cluster headache, presents the following symptoms:

Sudden onset of unilateral pain occurs, involving head, eye, temple, neck, and face.

There is a sudden disappearance of symptoms after a short period of suffering.

Pain may recur several times a day, and is frequent during sleep time.

There is also redness of the eye, edema below the eye, and lacrimation. Also, myosis.

There is stuffiness of the nostril or rhinorrhea.

There is dilation of the blood vessels of the affected side.

The attack can be induced by the injection of small amounts of histamine.

Management of histamine cephalalgia:

Methysergide maleate may prevent the attack.

Desensitization to histamine has been recommended initially.

Try vasoconstrictor drugs or prednisone.

Asthma

For information on asthma, see the chapter on respiratory diseases.

What the allergic skin tests indicate about asthma:

They help in evaluation of causative allergens.

They will detect causative inhalants or other allergens.

They will indicate a possible way to desensitize a patient for a given allergen.

Allergens will be either avoided, or the patient desensitized; if no improvement occurs after 1 or 2 years of this sort of therapy, it should be discontinued.

What is considered the first stage, or mild asthma?

When the patient only shows diffuse wheezes and has a mild dyspnea with adequate air exchange.

What is the second stage, or moderate asthma?

When the patient has marked wheezes, hyperpnea with distress at rest.

What is the third stage, or severe asthma?

Marked respiratory distress with retraction of the sternoclavicular area and worsening of all symptoms.

What is the fourth stage?

The clinical picture of complete respiratory failure, with confusion, lethargy, and similar symptoms.

Therapeutic measures in accordance with the stage:

Stage	Treatment
I, or mild asthma	Epinephrine; aerosol bronchodilator; intravenous aminophylline.
II, or moderate asthma	As above.
III, or severe asthma	Aminophylline; corticoids.
IV, or respiratory failure	Treatment of respiratory failure, with endotracheal intubation and assisted respiration; aminophylline, corticoids, and continuous monitoring in the hospital.

Hay Fever (Pollinosis)

For information see the chapter on respiratory diseases.

Allergic Rhinitis

For information on this perennial allergic rhinitis, see the chapter on respiratory diseases.

Anaphylactic Shock

For additional information see under the heading "Shock" in the chapter devoted to cardiovascular diseases.

The outstanding clinical picture of anaphylactic shock is:

After receiving an injection of the causative agent, the patient develops, after a very short period of time (less than 1 minute to no more then 10 or 15 minutes), a very impressive complex of symptoms.

What is the symptomatic complex of anaphylactic shock?

Initial apprehensiveness and agitation, with a flushed skin.

Almost simultaneously, a generalized urticaria with itching in most instances, throbbing of the ears, palpitations, paresthesias; the urticaria may become frank edema.

The patient appears cyanotic; the pupils dilate; wheezing is obviously heard; there are coughs, sneezes; patient may have nausea and vomiting, and also incontinence, and diarrhea. Fever.

Respiratory distress increases, vascular collapse runs a rapid course, convulsions appear, consciousness is lost, and death may the final event; all the picture happening in an extremely short time.

What is the difference between anaphylactoid reaction and anaphylactic shock?

The anaphylactoid reaction may occur after the first injection of the offending substance.

The anaphylactic shock occurs after an incubation period has elapsed since the injection of the allergenic substance.

How to prevent the anaphylactic reactive shock:

Proceed cautiously when using drugs that may cause hypersensitivity.

Always have at hand a syringe with epinephrine.

Place the patient in a recumbent position, with the legs elevated.

Watch respiration for obstruction (be prepared for intubation, or better tracheostomy).

If epinephrine fails, give diphenhydramine, or aminophylline.

Give a final shot of hydrocortisone.

Keep the patient under observation for at least 24 hours after the accident.

Serum Sickness

When serum sickness is manifested clinically:

It occurs 1 or 2 weeks after injection of the offending substance.

The most frequent offending substance is penicillin.

Other substance may be a foreign serum, such as an antitoxin.

Clinical symptoms of serum sickness are:

Malaise, fever, musculoskeletal pain.

Skin rash with urticaria and adenitis; may be morbilliform or scarlatiniform.

Gastrointestinal symptoms (nausea and vomiting, pain).

Rarely, neuropathy, glomerulonephritis, or other form of vasculitis.

Myocarditis, also rarely.

What special care should be taken in these cases?

Polyarthritis and periarticular edema are not rare; when it affects the temporomaxillary joint, it may simulate tetanus.

In previously sensitized persons the clinical course may be very severe, and even cause death.

In patients who have had severe allergic reactions, or whose family presents a serious incidence of allergic problems, always do a previous test of the drug to be used. If there is a reaction, the patient must be desensitized before the medication is given.

Management of serum sickness:

Most cases are mild and recover in about 2 or 3 days.

Mild reaction are treated with antihistaminics and salicylates.

Moderate or prolonged reactions need epinephrine or corticoids.

Severe cases need epinephrine or better diphenhydramine or aminophylline, plus a final shot of hydrocortisone.

Urticaria (Hives)

What is the outstanding clinical evidence of urticaria?

There is a skin lesion characterized by a wheal, or there are a number of wheals, that is, skin lesions noted by a slightly elevated smooth portion of the dermis.

The wheal is more red or pale than the surrounding skin and usually attended by severe pruritus.

Normally, this basic lesion lasts for less than 2 days.

Severe cases may show bullae (urticaria bullosa).

Rarely, it may be hemorrhagic (urticaria hemorrhagica).

When it lasts longer than usual, it is called urticaria perstans.

The size of the wheal is variable, from a surface of a few square millimiters to a few centimeters. Larger sizes intermix with giant hives that characterize angioneurotic edema.

What other symptoms characterize an attack of urticaria?

Urticaria is usually acute, in both its appearance and disappearance.

There may be a mild fever, and malaise.

Lesions appear on an area of the skin, then disappear while other elements appear somewhere else.

The diagnosis is obvious; usually there is a previous history of ingestion of a particular food, of a streptococcal or viral infection, or some drug.

There is a chronic form of urticaria, lasting 3 or more weeks, mostly due to the administration of a drug, or of some food.

In the case of food allergens, nausea is a frequent accompanying symptom.

Management of urticaria:

Try to avoid ingestion of the offending factor.

Active laxatives may remove the offending cause.

Stop all medications.

Use an antihistaminic for mild or moderate cases, such as diphenylhydramine; hydroxyzine has also been recommended. Corticoids, also.

For chronic urticaria, use antihistaminics.

Angioneurotic Edema

Symptoms of angioedema or giant hives are:

Lesions are similar to the regular urticarial hives, but of a considerably larger size, in surface and depth.

This form of diffuse swelling affects the loose tissues of the mucous membranes (particularly the upper respiratory tract, including the larynx), and of the dorsum of the hands and feet, the genitalia, and the eyes and the lips.

In cases involving the respiratory tract there will be stridor or wheezing (which may be mistaken for asthma), or alarming signs of respiratory distress.

There may be also a previous history of exposure to an offending substance, drug, or food.

Management of angioneurotic edema:

Epinephrine will be the first choice.

Give additional epinephrine in aerosol form in case of laryngeal involvement, and be prepared for respiratory assistance (intubation or tracheostomy).

When there is hypocalcemic irritability, the use of calcium may help.

Hereditary Angioneurotic Edema

Symptoms of hereditary angioedema are:

There is a family history of similar problems, almost always.

The wheals are unifocal.

The character is not exactly urticarial, but rather indurated and painful instead of smooth and pruritic.

Involvement of the gastrointestinal tract is characterized by nausea and vomiting; and there may also be evidence of colicky pains and obstruction.

Also, evidence of respiratory involvement will be noted by stridor and wheezing, or more serious signs of respiratory failure that may even cause death.

There is frequently a previous history of a viral infection, or of trauma.

Diagnosis depends on immunoassay tests.

Management of hereditary angioedema:

Place a free airway, if there is respiratory obstruction.

Danazol (pre-hypophysis suppresant) seems to be effective.

Aminocaproic acid may be useful (watch for side effects).

Before surgical attempts (dental work, particularly), give fresh-frozen plasma.

Contact Dermatitis (Dermatitis Venenata)

What the personal history of the patient subject to contact dermatitis symptoms may consist of:

Use of strong irritants, such as acids, alkalis, detergents, soaps, etc.

Contact with strong allergenic substances, such as poison ivy, oak, ragweed, etc.

Contact with substances used in the manufacture of shoes, dyes, cosmetics, metal compounds, and other industrial agents.

It is important to recall that some of these agents take years to induce the allergic reaction.

Symptoms of contact dermatitis:

They appear on exposed parts of the body, or those parts in direct contact with the offending substance (dress, or the like).

At a later stage the lesions may spread to other areas.

Symptomatology starts with erythematous macules, papules, and vesicles, which are edematous, itching, and burning, at times severely.

The area with lesions becomes warm, gives off exudates, forms crusts, and may develop secondary infections.

Laboratory tests (patch test) may help in diagnosis; but in instances of relatively severe reactions another test must be performed in a different individual.

How the location of symptoms may help in diagnosis:

Linear streaks suggest poison ivy.

Face involvement (also the hands) suggests soap, creams, etc.

Scalp involvement suggests tints, shampoos, etc.

Neck involvement is as for face, or suggests jewelry.
Fingers suggest fingernail polish or color.
Feet involvement may suggest the shoes.

Management of contact dermatitis:
Avoid re-exposure.
Use corticoids for acute reactions.
For subacute and chronic cases use shake lotions, or hydrophilic, greasy ointments or creams.

Atopic Dermatitis

Evaluation of the clinical features of atopic dermatitis:
It occurs in patients with a personal or family history of some of the known allergic disorders.
It may begin in early infancy.
Itching is the outstanding feature.
First symptoms consist of exudative, crusted lesions on scalp, face, and extremities.
Exacerbations and remissions are almost the rule.
Because of the itching a cycle is established with itch-scratch-rash-itch, which causes lichenified areas.
The lichenified areas are noted on the wrists, eyelids, neck, and also the antecubital and popliteal areas.
Secondary infections and adenitis may occur.
Symptoms may subside by four or five years of age, but they may recur, even in adulthood.

What severe reactions are prone to occur in these patients?
Early appearance of cataracts, usually before 30 years of age.
Kaposi's vericelliform eruption, which may follow the complication of herpes simplex or vaccination, developing a very severe febrile illness.

Management of atopic dermatitis:
Avoidance of all inductive causes.
Local corticoids.
Antihistaminics for severe itching.
Oral corticoids for severe cases.

Allergic Conjunctivitis

What differentiates allergic conjunctivitis from other forms of conjunctivitis?
It may occur together with another allergic syndrome, particularly hay fever.
If it happens to be the only allergic reaction, it will mostly occur in springtime and last until summer.

What are the characteristic symptoms of allergic conjunctivitis?
Itching is the outstanding symptom.
With itching, lacrimation is a common accompanying symptom.
There are edema and hyperemia of the conjunctivas.
A tenacious mucoid discharge may occur (rich in eosinophils).
Bilateral manifestations are the rule.

What are the particular clinical pictures with involvement of the bulbar or the palpebral conjunctiva?
In the bulbar form the conjunctiva around the cornea becomes hypertrophied and of a gray color.
In the palpebral form granulations develop, which are square, flat, hard, and closely packed; the color is pale pink or gray; they mostly appear in the upper eyelid.
A loss of corneal epithelium may occur, thus provoking pain.
The pain due to corneal lesions will provoke photophobia or will increase a previously existing one, which is not a rare symptom.

Management of allergic conjunctivitis:
Avoid all known causative allergens; do not use contact lenses.
Antihistamines are helpful in atopic cases.
Corticoid ophthalmic ointments will help in severe contact dermatitis, and also in vernal conjunctivitis, which occurs in the springtime.

Other Eye Diseases of Allergic Origin

What allergic diseases may occur in the eyelids?
There may be urticaria or angioneurotic edema, contact or atopic dermatitis.
Beware of ophthalmic medications, or of any other substances that may be conveyed with the fingers to the eye.

What allergic diseases may occur in the cornea?
Allergic conjunctivitis may spread to the cornea.
Circumcorneal reaction in uveitis may be of allergic origin.

What other eye diseases should be considered here?
Sympathetic ophthalmia after trauma or surgery, which will develop symptoms in the noninjured eye as well as in the injured one (photophobia, pain, lacrimation, blurred vision).
Endophthalmitis phacoanaphylactica, which occurs after removal of one of the lenses with residuals left.

Management of eyelid allergic reactions:
Treat as for urticaria, angioneurotic edema, contact or atopic dermatitis, or any drug reaction.

Management of allergic reactions of the cornea:
Corticoid ophthalmic ointment in the case of allergic conjunctivitis.
In the case of uveitis, scopolamine and corticoid drops; and systemic corticoid therapy.

Management of sympathetic ophthalmia or endophthalmitis phacoanaphylactica:
In sympathetic ophthalmia, enucleation of the inductive eye may be advisable before sympathetic inflammation develops. Use corticoids.
In endophthalmitis phacoanaphylactica, surgery may also be indicated.

Goodpasture's Syndrome

Information will be found in the chapter on respiratory diseases.

Allergic Bronchopulmonary Aspergillosis

Who are the patients presenting allergic bronchopulmonary aspergillosis?

- Asthmatic patients will present this form of eosinophilic pneumonia as a reaction to a noninvasive infection with aspergillus.

Symptoms of allergic bronchopulmonary aspergillosis are:

- Intermittent febricula, plus the following.
- Wheezing, cough, and dyspnea, as in asthma.
- Tenacious and purulent sputum, with brown plugs.
- Pulmonary obstruction noted by prolonged expiratory sounds.
- Possible atelectasis, caused by mucous plugs.
- Possible bronchiectasis in chronic cases.

How the diagnosis can be established in these cases:

- In addition to the positive culture for aspergillus (which is usually found in men), there are antibodies against it, and the skin tests are also positive.
- Lung biopsy may be needed in some cases.

Management of allergic bronchopulmonary aspergillosis:

- Corticoids and antiasthmatic drugs.

Gastrointestinal Allergy

The usual reactions of gastrointestinal allergy consist of:

- Urticaria or angioneurotic edema, which appears together with the following symptoms.
- Crampy abdominal pains, frequently of a chronic type, and diarrhea.

Reactions of a more severe nature of gastrointestinal allergy consist of:

- Symptoms of anaphylaxis, q.v.
- Violent abdominal pains.
- Nausea and vomiting.
- Diarrhea.
- Burning or itching of the mouth rapidly calls attention to the ingestion of the offending substance.

What is called *eosinophilic enteropathy* refers to:

- A protein-losing enteropathy.
- Developing of eosinophilic infiltrates in the gut.
- Evidence of atopic disease.

Management of gastrointestinal allergy:

- Avoidance of the offensive food or substance.
- Corticoid treatment for eosinophilic enteropathy.
- Treatment of very severe cases as for anaphylactic shock.

Diarrhea

For more information see chapter on gastrointestinal diseases.

Evaluation of allergic diarrhea:

- It follows the ingestion of certain foods.
- Accompanying gastrointestinal symptoms consist of nausea with or without vomiting, borborygmi, abdominal pain, and sometimes fever.
- Evidence of other allergic manifestations is noted.
- Elimination diets will help in diagnosis.

Management of allergic diarrhea:

- As for gastrointestinal allergy, q.v., above.

Membranous Glomerulonephritis

Evaluation of membranous glomerulonephritis:

- Symptoms are those that correspond to a regular nephrosis, q.v.
- Diagnosis is based on biopsy and immunofluorescence studies (IgG and C3 component).
- The disease ends in renal failure in about 10 years.
- There is no known treatment.

Hemolytic Reaction

For information on hemolytic anemia, see the chapter on blood diseases.

When the patient should be checked for hemolytic reactions:

- If symptoms develop after large doses of penicillin are given.
- After the use of quinine, quinidine, or stibophen.
- After the use of methyldopa.
- When suffering from spherocytosis or ovalocytosis, q.v.
- When there is a sudden onset of symptoms of the type of acute hemolytic anemia, q.v.
- When there is paroxysmal nocturnal hemoglobinuria, q.v.
- When patient has hereditary nonspherocytic hemolytic anemia.
- When patient has another form of hemolytic anemia; though in many instances the hemolytic anemias of this kind are due to red cell defects.

Intermittent Hydrarthrosis

Symptoms and management of intermittent hydrarthrosis:

- There are symptoms of joint effusion, noted particularly in the knee.
- The effusion is painless.
- The attacks occur at relatively regular intervals.
- During the intervals the joint appears practically normal.
- Adolescent females present the disease, usually until pregnancy or an older age, when it disappears.
- These patients are prone to develop rheumatoid arthritis.
- Remove fluid and treat symptomatically.

Periodic Leukorrhea

Evaluation of periodic leukorrhea:

- Leukorrhea occurring at relatively periodic intervals and not due to any infection, senility, etc., may be considered of allergic origin.

Treatment will be symptomatic; if the causative allergen is discovered, avoid it, or desensitize.

Physical Allergy

The usual causes of this type of allergy are:

- Sunlight, or photosensitivity.
- Heat.
- Cold.
- Trauma to the skin.

The usual symptoms of physical allergy are:

- Itching is the outstanding symptom.
- Urticaria or angioedema commonly accompanies itching.
- In photodermatitis the skin burning occurs with fever, pain, and gastrointestinal symptoms, and is followed by exfoliation and pigmentary changes; in sunlight allergy there is urticaria or a chronic polymorphous skin eruption.
- Cold allergy will develop after exposure to chilly weather, bathing, or swimming, and will show as urticaria or angioneurotic edema.
- Heat causes some sort of cholinergic urticaria, similar to that due to emotions or stress.
- Also, a cholinergic urticaria will be the base to the allergic reaction caused by trauma to the skin; this will consist of *dermographism* (after scratching or stroking the skin, the lesions following the path of the inciting cause), or of *pressure urticaria* (after the release of the inciting pressure, noted as wheals or angioneurotic edema).

The diagnosis of cholinergic urticaria is confirmed by:

- The injection of a 1:5,000 solution of methacholine in the dermis (0.05 ml), which will induce satellite lesions; normal people will respond with a local urticarial wheal.

Management of cases presenting physical allergy:

- Avoid the inciting cause, with adequate protection.
- For photodermatitis or sunlight allergy sunscreening preparations are of help; try also chloroquine or hydroxychloroquine in resistant patients.
- In cold allergy, itching may respond better to cyproheptadine.
- Cholinergic urticaria usually responds well to hydroxyzine.
- In severe cases, particularly those induced by sunlight allergy, a trial will be given with corticoids.

Drug Allergy

What are the clinical pictures of lesions caused by drug allergy?

- There is typical urticaria, mostly due to penicillin, acetylsalicylic acid, other antibiotics, sera, etc.
- Photosensitization may be caused by griseofulvin, oral hypoglycemics, phenothiazines, chlorothiazides, tetracyclines, sulfonamides, sweeteners, etc.
- Erythematous reactions may be induced by barbiturates, sulfonamides, antihistaminics, atropine, arsenicals, bismuth, etc.
- Any form of dermatosis should be suspected as being caused by any kind of medication, either those mentioned above, or any other drug.

Characteristics of the clinical picture due to drug allergy are:

- Usually an abrupt onset and symmetrical distribution are observed.
- At times, a sensitization lapse will take place.
- Fever, arthralgia, headache, malaise, etc., may be present.
- Bright and very itchy lesions are usually present.
- Leukopenia is a frequent finding; patch tests are useful, especially on patients with contact dermatitis; the final diagnostic test will be given by administration of the offending substance (with care!).

Management of drug allergy:

- Do not use the offending substance again.
- Treat reactions symptomatically, as they arise.
- In severe cases dialysis may speed the elimination of the drug.
- Also, in severe cases corticoids will be given.
- Epinephrine will be used as an emergency medication.

Animal Bites and Stings

The insects that may cause anaphylactic or less important allergic reactions are:

- Bees, wasps, hornets.
- Ants.
- Mosquitoes, and some species of flies.
- Ticks, and mites.
- Fleas, lice, bedbugs, and other similar species.
- Other dangerous animals not only may cause allergic reaction but actual poisoning, such as snakes, spiders, scorpions and marine animals.

Symptoms caused by *bees, wasps,* and *hornets:*

- There are usually local wheals, more or less large, according to the reaction.
- Anaphylactic shock may occur in hypersensitive persons, or in those previously sensitized by a sting.

Management of allergic reaction caused by bees, wasps, or hornets:

- Remove the sting in case it was left in the skin.
- Use an ice cube or an analgesic-corticoid ointment.
- Severe cases will be treated with epinephrine and antihistaminics.
- Known hypersensitive patients should always carry a kit with epinephrine and antihistaminics; and will be desensitized whenever possible.

Symptoms caused by *mosquitoes* and *flies:*

- A local urticarial lesion is present, usually itchy.
- Occasionally there are more severe reactions, even reaching the characteristic features of a swollen, painful ulceration.

There are patients who may show systemic sensitivity reactions, possibly ending in a fatal outcome.

Management of allergic reactions caused by mosquitoes and flies:

Remove the sting or head if left in the skin.

Also, remove the whole body if it has remained attached to the skin.

Cleanse the area; apply a corticoid ointment or lotion.

Severe reactions will be treated as for anaphylaxia.

Symptoms caused by *ticks* and *mites:*

Symptoms are as described above.

These arthropods may also transmit important infectious diseases.

Tick paralysis may be an important reaction; it will be treated symptomatically.

Larvae may induce intense itching ("chiggers"); and the treatment for chiggers will be as for scabies.

Symptoms caused by other arthropods, and their management:

As above for ticks and mites.

Wiskott-Aldrich Syndrome

For information, see the chapter on blood, spleen, and lymphatic diseases.

Hypersensitivity Reactions

Evaluation of *type I reactions:*

These reactions are of the immediate, anaphylactic type (also including atopic and reaginic reactions).

Clinical conditions included are allergic extrinsic asthma; seasonal rhinitis; reactions to insect stings, foods, and drugs; and, most importantly, anaphylactic reactions.

Symptoms due to type I reactions are urticaria, angioneurotic edema, hypotension, and smooth muscle spasm.

The direct skin test is the best diagnostic help; other tests are equally helpful.

Evaluation of *type II reactions:*

These are cytotoxic reactions.

Induced clinical conditions are mostly immunologic, such as thrombocytopenic purpura, leukopenia, systemic lupus erythematosus, hemolytic anemia, etc.

Evaluation of *type III reactions:*

These occur in serum sickness, viral hepatitis, rheumatoid arthritis, reactions to drugs, and others.

Evaulation of *type IV reactions:*

This is the tuberculin type of hypersensitivity reaction.

Induced clinical conditions are contact dermatitis, allograft rejection, some forms of drug sensitivity, thryroiditis, encephalomyelitis following rabies vaccination, and granulomas due to intracellular organisms.

Patch tests are a good diagnostic help.

11. Neurology

Stroke

The common causes of cerebrovascular accidents or strokes are:

- Cerebral embolism.
- Cerebral thrombosis.
- Intracerebral hemorrhage.
- Subarachnoid hemorrhage.
- Intracranial bleeding.
- Vascular malformation.

The basic symptoms of stroke are:

- Premonitory symptoms, such as headache, drowsiness, confusion, etc.
- Premonitory symptoms of a focal nature, which may occur in thrombosis.
- More or less sudden onset of neurologic symptoms (paralysis or only paresthesias, speech defects, convulsions, coma).
- Symptoms corresponding to the affected area of the brain, depending on the lesioned vessel. See the following paragraphs for each one.
- Symptoms may be mild or severe; may be transient or prolonged, even to an indefinite period.

Management of stroke:

- Complete bed rest, better in the hospital.
- Symptomatic treatment for agitation, and for those unable to swallow or to void.
- Further treatment according to the nature of the vascular accident.

How does the onset of symptoms occur in each different vascular accident?

- In cerebral embolism there are no prodromic symptoms, and it occurs in a matter of seconds or, at most, minutes.
- In cerebral thrombosis there is a gradual progression of symptoms in the form of attacks, with some improvement between them.
- In intracerebral hemorrhage there is a rapid occurrence of hemiplegia during hours of activity, usually preceded by headache.
- In subarachnoid hemorrhage the rapid onset of headache is not related to previous activity.
- In intracranial bleeding and in vascular malformations the symptoms occur in younger people, with no previous headache and no relation to previous activity.

What are the most frequent secondary symptoms accompanying each one of the different vascular accidents?

- In cerebral embolism there are usually previous arrhythmias, mostly long-lasting fibrillation, or cardiac infarction, the heart thus being the source of the emboli.
- In cerebral thrombosis arteriosclerotic changes are mostly evident.
- In intracerebral hemorrhage there is a previous evidence of hypertension (cerebrovascular, hypertensive retinopathy, cardiac hypertrophy).
- In the other instances preretinal hemorrhages may be noted.

The particular neurologic symptoms due to the involvement of each individual artery are as follows:

- The middle cerebral artery is the most frequently involved; there are numbness and tingling of the limb nerves, difficult speech, hemianopsia of the side of the lesion and limb paresia of the opposite side; symptoms vary according to the portion of the artery that is closed, that is, the proximal or distal portion.
- Involvement of the internal carotid artery is also frequent; symptoms are similar to those due to the middle cerebral artery, but there may also be dysphagia, mental confusion, personality changes, transient blindness or dimness of vision.
- Involvement of the vertebrobasilar arteries is usually very severe; limb symptoms may reveal mono-, hemi-, or quadriparesis or paralysis; there may also be dizziness, ataxia, dysphagia, dysarthria, diplopia or blindness, and deafness; also difficult gait, mental confusion, and loss of memory and of consciousness.
- Involvement of the posterior cerebral artery will cause scintillating scotomas, hemianopsia, or possible blindness; also hemisensory loss, hemiballism, thalamic pain, and word blindness (alexia).
- Lesions of the anterior cerebral artery are relatively rare; outstanding symptoms are weakness or numbness of the opposite leg, and reflex incontinence; there may also be contralateral weakness of the face and arm, apraxia or aphasia; bilateral occlusion will provoke either euphoria or apathy and final catatonia or spastic paraplegia.

Lesions of the subclavian and the innominate arteries may cause a deficient supply of blood to the corresponding vertebral artery, with the corresponding symptomatology, q.v., above.

Cerebral Embolism

Evaluation of symptoms of cerebral embolism:

There is an almost fulminant onset, with no prodromic symptoms, not related to previous activity or effort.

There may be evidence of other embolic accidents because the usual source is the heart (fibrillation, infarction).

Consciousness is not totally lost in most instances.

Other symptoms depend of the artery involved in the accident, q.v., in above paragraph.

The overall course may soon improve.

Usual tests will help in diagnosis (X-ray, scanning, tomography, echoencephalography).

Management of cerebral embolism:

The usual measures as for cerebrovascular accidents.

Cerebral Thrombosis

Evaluation of symptoms of cerebral thrombosis:

Prodromic symptoms may be dizziness, aphasia, and the like; not related to previous activity or effort.

Patients may be diabetics or present hyperlipidemia.

They may also present symptoms of arteriosclerosis; there may be hypertension.

Consciousness is not totally lost in all instances.

Other symptoms depend on the artery involved in the accident, q.v., in the above paragraph.

The overall course progresses rapidly; at times there is also a relatively rapid improvement.

Usual tests will help in diagnosis.

Management of cerebral thrombosis:

Use the common measures as for other cerebral accidents.

Subarachnoid Hemorrhage

Evaluation of symptoms in subarachnoid hemorrhage:

There is usually a previous asymptomatic aneurysm; but if it is symptomatic, the patient will present effort headache, cranial bruit, and disorder of cranial nerves, ophthalmic (II), oculomotor (III), and trigeminus (V); also the trochlear (IV) and the abducens (VI) may be involved.

Hemorrhage following rupture will be accompanied by a sudden headache not related to an apparent cause.

There is a syncopal state mostly of brief duration, but patients may remain obtunded or in actual coma.

Heacache may be prolonged, accompanied by vomiting and dizziness.

Changes may occur in pulse rate and respiration. Fever may last 1 week.

There may be convulsions, stiffness of the neck, Kernig's, Babinski's Brudzinski's, and similar signs.

Focal neurologic signs may be absent, but preretinal hemorrhage is frequent.

The remaining clot may act as a brain tumor.

Usual tests are helpful; but spinal tap is important.

Management of subarachnoid hemorrhage:

Avoid anticoagulants.

Consider spinal puncture; and particularly discuss the surgical approach to the problem.

Cerebral Hemorrhage

Evaluation of symptoms of intracerebral hemorrhage:

There is a sudden onset, with headache and rapid establishment of hemiplegia and other neurologic deficits.

Rapid progression to coma may occur.

Small hemorrhages will cause symptoms similar to those of involvement of individual arteries, q.v.

Hemorrhages located in the cerebral hemispheres may cause hemiplegia or hemiparesis.

If located in the posterior fossa, symptoms will be conjugate eye deviation, ophthalmoplegia, stertorous breathing, myosis, and coma.

Most patients will also present nausea and vomiting, focal or generalized convulsions, delirium.

The general course may be fatal or may show some improvement of functional powers.

There may also be cardiac hypertrophy, hypertensive retinopathy, and similar hypertensive problems.

Diagnosis is helped by the evaluation of simultaneous or previous hemorrhagic manifestations, particularly in cases of leukemia, thrombocytopenic purpura, aplastic anemia, cirrhosis of the liver, and other similar diseases.

Usual tests are also helpful, particularly spinal puncture (be cautious!).

Management of intracerebral hemorrhage:

Avoid anticoagulants.

Provide care usually given for stroke; consider surgery.

Cerebrovascular Ischemia

Evaluation of symptoms of cerebrovascular ischemia:

Symptoms are the same as those mentioned for cerebral thrombosis or embolism.

Symptoms may be reversible if they last only a few minutes.

Symptoms lasting a longer time may be permanent because of the resultant infarction.

Less frequently than arteriosclerosis, other causative factors should be considered, namely, vascular inflammation, extrinsic arterial compression, fat from bone fractures, air in caisson disease, circulatory insufficiency, anemic conditions, marked hypotension, etc.

Clots from surgical procedures, mainly heart surgery, may also cause cerebral ischemic symptoms.

Management of cerebrovascular ischemia:
In each case proceed as for the basic cause.

Transient Ischemia Attacks (TIA)

Evaluation of symptoms of transient ischemic attacks:
The outstanding characteristic of the syndrome is the sudden onset and brief duration of each attack, just a matter of minutes.
During the attacks there is no loss of consciousness.
After the attack there are no neurologic residua.
Symptoms depend on the involved artery, q.v., above.
"Drop attacks" consist of falling without loss of consciousness, because of sudden weakness of the legs.
Attacks may be repeated daily, or there may be only a few over several years.
Attacks may be prodromic to actual strokes.
What are the usual accompanying features of transient ischemic attacks?
They mostly occur in middle-aged or elderly person, but children with severe cardiovascular disease may also present the syndrome.
They may occur from arteriosclerotic stenosis, embolism, or thrombosis.
Patients may suffer from diabetes mellitus, hypertension, polycythemia, heart disease, etc.
Angiography and other similar tests will help in diagnosis.
Management of transient ischemic attacks:
Treat carefully the underlying disease.
Consider surgery or other type of therapy.

Cerebral Angioma

Clinical manifestations of cerebral angioma are:
There are seizures starting in early youth.
The convulsive symptoms are focal in nature.
The patient may feel a pulsating noise in the head.
A bruit may be heard on auscultation.
Symptoms may be similar to those of aneurysm, namely, effort headache, and disorders of cranial nerves (ophthalmic, oculomotor, trigeminus, trochlear, or abducens).
A ruptured angioma may develop a milder clinical syndrome than a ruptured aneurysm, but that depends on its size and site.
X-ray films with crescent linear calcifications will help in diagnosis.
Management of cerebral angioma:
Discuss convenience of surgical therapy, evaluating the possible future neurologic deficit.

Brain Abscess

In brain abscess the usual clinical symptoms are:
An infection outside the brain, most often otitis media, mastoiditis, septicemia, lung infection.
Headache, usually accompanied by nausea and vomiting.
Hemiparesis, ataxia, convulsions.
Visual field defects, motor and sensory changes.
Aphasia and palsies due to cranial nerve damage.
Fever with chills, if the abscess is not encapsulated.
Increased intracranial pressure (papilledema, slow pulse and respirations; also headache).
Possible meningeal signs (neck rigidity, Kernig and similar symptoms).
Somnolence and sluggishness.
Usual tests helpful in diagnosis.
Management of brain abscess:
Drain pus.
Treat the basic cause of infection.

Encephalitis

Most frequent causes of encephalitis are:
Viral encephalitis.
Encephalitis due to measles, rubella, varicella, or infectious mononucleosis, mostly in children.
Encephalitis following vaccination against smallpox, pertussis, and rabies.
Toxic encephalitis.
Encephalitis due to other infectious diseases, namely, typhoid fever, malaria, pneumonia, influenza, tuberculosis, syphilis, puerperal fever, abscesses, etc.
The symptoms common to most form os encephalitis are:
A paucisymptomatic complex with fever and malaise but no neurologic manifestations; though this is mostly consistent with meningitis.
Fever, malaise, nausea and vomiting.
Sore throat, not rarely.
Stiff neck, usually present.
Course that may progress to stupor, convulsions, and coma.
Neurologic evidence of lesioned upper motor neuron, namely, spastic paralysis, abnormal reflexes (exaggerated deep reflexes, or pathologic ones), absent superficial reflexes.
Usually confusion, personality changes, and paresis.
Evaluation of the clinical features of *herpes simplex encephalitis:*
In the early stages of the disease, there are repeated seizures.
Symptoms point out involvement of the temporal lobe (seizures, olfactory or visual hallucinations, speech disorders, visual changes), or the frontal lobe (mental changes, focal or generalized seizures, hemiplegia, aphasia, and other symptoms).
Diagnosis is difficult because the virus is not easily recovered; it is inferred by a close relationship to a known infection with herpes simplex.
Evaluation of *St. Louis encephalitis:*
It is mainly present in Florida, and the western and central areas of the United States; also present in the Caribbean, Brazil, and Argentina.

Like all arthropod-borne transmitted infections of this class, it refers to mosquitoes; the reservoir exist in birds, even domestic ones.
Urban and rural outbreaks may occur.
The disease affects all ages, mainly young people; but the prognosis is worst among the elderly.

Evaluation of *California encephalitis:*
It is present through all of the United States, not just California.
The reservoir is in small mammals; transmission is by mosquitoes.
Children are affected mainly.
Rural or suburban areas present the disease most often.

Evaluation of *Western equine encephalitis:*
It is present in North, Central, and South America.
Birds are the reservoir, and mosquitoes the transmitter.
Any age may be affected, but the great majority of cases occur in children, and mainly under 1 year of age. Sequelae are left.
Sick horses may be found in the infected area.

Evaluation of *Eastern equine encephalitis:*
Distribution corresponds to the eastern side of the American hemisphere.
Birds and small rodents are the reservoir; mosquitoes also transmit the disease.
Most cases are found among young children and persons over 55 years of age. Also, sick horses will be found in the infected areas.
The mortality is higher than with the Western equine encephalitis; sequelae are left with children under 1 year of age.

General management of encephalitis:
Treat the cause aggressively, if known.
Give supportive treatment, according to symptoms, namely, dehydration (water and electrolyte balance), shock or vascular collapse (plasma expanders, levarterenol, etc.), cerebral edema (mannitol), etc.
Idoxuridine, cytosine arabinoside, and adenine arabinoside are being tried for herpes simplex encephalitis.

Meningitis

Common symptoms of an *acute bacterial meningitis:*
A sore throat or other respiratory illness may be prodromal.
Sudden onset of fever, headache, and vomiting, together with a stiff neck, are highly suggestive of meningitis.
Stiffness of the back, confusion, delirium, convulsions, and positivity of Kernig, Brudzinski, and similar signs may be observed.
Most patients will show a petechial rash in the skin or the mucous membranes.
There is extremely rapid progress of worsening symptoms.
Infants may present the high-pitched cry, bulging of fontanels, irregular respirations, and possibly jaundice.
Among neonates and other infants the diagnosis is extremely difficult and must be suspected in the presence of any unexplained fever (mandatory for a spinal puncture).
Examination of the cerebrospinal fluid is diagnostic (pressure, cells, glucose, and protein contents).

Evaluation of clinical symptoms of *meningococcal meningitis:*
It may occur in epidemics, among the military, in jails and boarding schools; contagion may come from asymptomatic carriers.
Symptomatology is as stated above; there is frequent involvement of joints.
The *Waterhouse-Friderichsen syndrome* may occur in overwhelming infections, due to adrenal hemorrhage; its symptoms are:
Sudden onset, frequently accompanied by child's cry.
Initial paleness, rapidly followed by intense cyanosis.
A few cases paler and less cyanotic.
Increased fever, tachypnea, marked hypotension.
Myoclonus, spasm, stupor, nystagmus, convulsions.
Purpuric rash.
An almost typical clinical appearance of an acute abdomen.
There is an almost typical cerebrospinal fluid (cloudy or purulent, elevated pressure, decreased glucose, increased protein), with the presence of the causative neisseria.
If the patient survives the first day, probably will survive the disease, and the sequelae may not be too severe.

Evaluation of clinical symptoms of meningitis due to *hemophilus infection:*
It most frequently occurs below 6 years of age.
It may start as a respiratory infection.
During this initial stage, meningitis will be suspected because of headache, irritability, and some nuchal and back stiffness; there will be frequent involvement of joints.
The causal germ will be found in the cerebrospinal fluid; and this is the only positive clue to the diagnosis.

Evaluation of *tuberculous meningitis:*
The onset is not sudden, but gradual.
Initial symptoms may be listlessness, anorexia, and irritability.
These are followed by vomiting, headache, convulsions, stiffness of the neck and back, and final coma.
Night cries are frequent, mostly with children.
Behavioral changes may be noted with older patients.
Opisthotonos or paralysis will occur as the disease progresses.
Ocular signs are not rare (paralysis, choroid tubercles).
Evidence of tuberculous infection is found elsewhere in the body.

Evaluation of symptoms in *other forms* of meningitis, namely, pneumococcal, colibacillary, streptococcal, or staphylococcal:

There is almost always a previous infection; check carefully for all sort of infectious foci, namely, ears, throat, skin, and other parts of the body as well.

Management of meningococcal meningitis:

Start penicillin immediately; chloramphenicol as a second choice.

For the Waterhouse-Friderichsen syndrome give plasma expanders and levarterenol; try corticoids.

Management of meningitis due to hemophilus:

Give together ampicillin and chloramphenicol.

Management of tubercuolous meningitis:

Start with isoniazid and ethambutol, streptomycin, and corticoids.

Management of other forms of meningitis:

For pneumococcal meningitis give penicillin.

For colibacillary meningitis give kanamycin.

For streptococcal meningitis give ampicillin.

For staphylococcal meningitis give methicillin or nafcillin.

Other forms will be treated according to the infective organism.

In all instances, give supportive treatment as well.

Lymphocytic Choriomeningitis

Symptoms of lymphocytic choriomeningitis are:

There is an initial prodromic stage similar to influenza, with fever, chills, headache, vomiting, cough, and muscle pains.

The meningitic stage will present a worsening of headache and vomiting, plus lethargy, stiffness of neck and back, positive Kernig and similar signs, and in severe cases paralysis and anesthesia of the skin.

The same viral infection may cause symptoms of encephalitis, orchitis, parotiditis, or hemorrhagic fever.

The source of infection comes from rodents, namely, dust or food that is contaminated.

Patients will present a biphasic course, with the initial influenza-like syndrome, a remission, and then the meningitic picture.

Most cases follow a relatively benign course.

Management of lymphocytic choriomeningitis:

Only supportive.

Coma

Frequent causes of coma are:

Hemorrhages (intracerebral, subarachnoid, intracranial bleeding).

Intracranial masses (hematoma, tumor, abscess).

Head injuries, including surgery.

Central nervous system infections (encephalitis, meningitis).

Ischemic or anoxemic syncope or shock.

Epilepsy or other convulsive disorders.

Increased intracranial pressure.

Metabolic accidents in diabetes mellitus, hypoglycemia, uremia, electrolyte imbalance, hepatic coma, addisonian crises, hyponatremia.

Poisoning with alcohol, barbiturates, morphine, heroin, bromides, tranquilizers and analgesics, carbon monoxide, heavy metals, methyl alcohol.

Physical causes, such as hyperthermia, hypothermia, electric shock.

Anaphylaxis, and severe infections.

Hysteria, catatonia, malingering, and perhaps others.

Evaluation of the clinical picture of coma:

Clues may be obtained from medical history, such as previous disease, an accident, poisoning, etc.

Alcoholic coma is frequent, usually indicated by the characteristic odor of the breath; but always keep in mind that even with an alcoholic intoxication a coma can be due to a different cause.

The outstanding symptomatology of coma consists of complete unconsciousness simulating a deep sleep, from which the patient cannot be aroused.

Evaluation of coma due to a *stroke:*

Patients are middle-aged or elderly.

There is a previous history of arrhythmia (mostly fibrillation), cardiac infarction, arteriosclerosis, hypertension.

Premonitory symptoms may be general or focal.

Neurologic symptoms may occur suddenly, or may be somewhat delayed.

Symptoms of a neurologic nature will depend on the involved blood vessel (see paragraph on stroke, for details).

Symptoms may be mild or severe, transient or prolonged.

There is a flushed or cyanotic, and frequently asymmetric face.

Unequal, inactive pupils are noted.

There is evidence of hemiplegia (puffing of one cheek on respiration; the paralyzed limb will fall heavily when allowed to; it will not react to vigorous stimulation).

Cerebrospinal fluid will be xanthochromic or frankly bloody.

Evaluation of coma due to *cerebral embolism:*

There is a fulminant onset, with probable evidence of other embolic accident.

Coma may not be complete in all instances; and the symptoms depend on the involved artery (see paragraph on cerebral embolism for more details).

The overall course may soon improve.

Evaluation of coma due to *cerebral thrombosis:*

Patients may present diabetes mellitus, hyperlipidemia, arteriosclerosis, or hypertension.

Prodromic symptoms may be present, coma may not be complete, symptoms depend on the involved artery, and the overall course may progress rapidly.

Evaluation of coma due to *subarachnoid hemorrhage:*
- Symptoms of a previous intracranial aneurysm may be present.
- There is a sudden onset with headache, vomiting, dizziness, and other neurologic symptoms (see paragraph on subarachnoid hemorrhage for more details).

Evaluation of coma due to *cerebral hemorrhage:*
- There is a sudden onset with rapid progression into coma.
- Symptoms depend on the area involved (see paragraph on cerebral hemorrhage for more details).
- There will also be vomiting, delirium, convulsions, cardiac hypertrophy, hypertensive retinopathy, etc.

Evaluation of coma due to *cerebral ischemia:*
- Symptoms are the same as for embolism or thrombosis; those lasting only a few minutes may be reversible; those lasting longer will result in infarction.
- Causes of ischemia, other than arteriosclerosis, are clots from surgical procedures, fat from bone fractures, air in caisson disease, and others (see paragraph on cerebrovascular ischemia, for more information).

Evaluation of coma due to *trauma to the head:*
- Evidence or history of injury; but it may be lacking.
- Coma, which may occur suddenly or gradually.
- Bleeding from the ear, nose, or throat; also discoloration behind the ear (Battle's sign) may indicate skull fracture.
- Unequal and sluggish, or actually inactive pupils.
- Slow and irregular respirations; initial tachycardia followed by bradycardia.
- Abnormal reflexes, incontinence, and paralysis.
- Check cerebrospinal fluid, and have a film of the skull.

Evaluation of coma due to *acute alcoholism:*
- Coma is not always complete, the patient looks hyperemic, and the breath smells of alcohol.
- Pupils are equal, and reactive, moderately dilated.
- Deep and noisy respirations are observed.

Evaluation of coma due to *epilepsy:*
- There is sudden coma, with accompanying convulsions.
- Pupils are reactive.
- The tongue may be bitten, and may present scars from previous similar lesions.
- There is a history of the disease.

Evaluation of *other forms* of coma:
- There is a history of an infection in the case of encephalitis or meningitis.
- There is a history of a previous mass within the skull, in the case of tumors, etc., together with the corresponding neurologic symptoms.
- There is a history of anoxemia, increased intracranial pressure, a metabolic disease, poisoning, or a physical cause.
- The immediately previous injection of a drug will suggest anaphylactic shock.
- Other causes will also present a particular history and the corresponding symptoms that will lead to the diagnosis.

Management of coma:
- Coma calls for an emergent treatment, better followed in the corresponding unit of the hospital.
- Maintain adequate respiration.
- Treat shock, and maintain water and electrolyte balance.
- Treat specific cause in each instance, namely, control hemorrhage, inactivate a poison, etc.

Cerebral Palsy

What are the most frequent syndromes encountered in clinics?
- Spastic syndromes, the most frequent.
- Athetoid or dyskinetic syndromes.
- Ataxic syndromes.
- Mixed forms.

Evaluation of *spastic syndromes:*
- The spastic limbs are underdeveloped and the corresponding muscles are hypertonic and stiff, with awkward movements and resistance to stretching.
- The affected limbs may be both on one side (hemiplegia), both legs (paraplegia), similar parts of both sides (diplegia), or all four limbs equally affected (quadri- or tetraplegia).
- There are increased tendon reflexes on the affected limbs.
- There are weakness and tendency to contractures of the affected limbs.
- With affected legs there will be a characteristic "scissors gait" or "toe-walking."
- Dysarthria is common when the movement of mouth organs is impaired.
- Mental retardation only affects those with spastic quadriplegia.

Evaluation of *dyskinetic* or *athetoid syndromes:*
- The affected limbs will present slow, writhing, involuntary movements (athetoid); or the muscle involvement will affect only the proxymal part of the limb but also the trunk (dystonic).
- Choreiform jerky movements may also exist.
- Dysarthria is usually severe.

Evaluation of *ataxic syndromes:*
- They are relatively rare.
- Fine movements are difficult to perform.
- There is a wide-based gait.
- Weakness, incoordination, and tremor are found.

Most frequent *mixed forms:*
- Spasticity with athetosis the the most frequent mixed form.
- There are also cases of athetosis with ataxia.

Other problems that may be shown by these patients:
- Convulsions may occur (notably, if the patient presents hemiplegia).
- Mental retardation accompanies not only those with spastic quadriplegia, but also mixed forms.

If athetosis was due to kernicterus, there will also be deafness and ocular palsies.

Visual defects may occur, most often strabismus.

Management of cerebral palsy:

Re-education.

Treatment of associated symptoms.

Epilepsy

What is the outstanding disorder that qualifies epilepsy?

A paroxysmal, recurrent attack with loss of consciousness, convulsive motor activity, sensory phenomena, or inappropriate behavior, of sudden onset and usually brief duration.

In *petit mal* attacks, jacksonian and psychomotor attacks (particularly in automatism), consciousness may not be totally lost.

Evaluation of symptoms in *major epilepsy*, or *grand mal attacks:*

An aura may announce the episode; it is almost always identical for the same individual in all attacks.

Auras are of different character, namely, gastrointestinal, visual, a memory, sensations of smell or taste, etc.

Following the aura the patient loses consciousness and falls to the floor, emitting a cry.

Convulsions constitute the immediately following stage: initially, they are very strong tonic contractions; thereafter, they are clonic convulsions of all limbs, trunk, and head.

During the tonic attack, dyspnea and cyanosis are usually present.

During the clonic convulsions there may be urinary and/or fecal incontinency, frothing of the mouth, and biting of the tongue.

Symptoms of an inductive cause may coexist (fever, severe pain, metabolic disturbances, and the like).

The whole attack will last 2 to 5 minutes.

Flaccidity of muscles will follow the convulsive stage, together with dilated pupils, absent corneal and deep reflexes, positive Babinski, and a period of deep sleep that usually ends the attack.

During the post-attack stage the patient may complain of sore muscles, confusion, and disorientation; headache is not rare.

Only rarely, there will be focal motor or sensory phenomena.

Evaluation of symptoms of *minor epilepsy*, or *petit mal seizures:*

It will appear before 20 years of age.

The "petit mal triad" consists of myotonic jerks, a brief loss of consciousness (absences or blank spells), and akinetic seizures.

There is no fall, nor are there convulsions.

During the blank spell there is a sudden absence of consciousness with cessation of motor activity and loss of muscle tone, and a very rapid and sudden return to normal activity, usually in less than 30 seconds.

Attacks may occur while the patient is quiet; rarely, during activity.

Some attacks may pass unnoticed; they may be repeated up to 100 times a day.

Some patients are highly intelligent.

Evaluation of *psychomotor attacks:*

The attack is similar to that of minor epilepsy, but lasts up to 1 or 2 minutes.

There is a lack of contact with surroundings, during which stage there are automatic behavior, movements of the head and the eyes, also of the limbs, smacking of the lips, unintelligible speech, etc.

During the attack the patient cannot listen to anybody, and may resist any intention of help.

A confusional state will persist for 1 or 2 minutes more, after the attack is over.

The attacks may start at any age.

Evaluation of *jacksonian epilepsy:*

Consciousness may be retained, or it may be lost when the seizure becomes generalized.

There is a focal seizure, which may stay (waxing and waning in intensity) at the original site, thus constituting the epilepsia partialis continua.

The seizure, which may be motor, sensory, or autonomic, may start in a digit, the face, etc., and thereafter spread over larger areas, marching up the limb, etc.

How the *partial seizures* point out the site of cerebral dysfunction:

Smacking of lips is due to anterior temporal lobe dysfunction.

Flashes of lights are due to occipital lobe dysfunction.

Formed images are due to temporal lobe dysfunctions.

Olfactory hallucinations are due to posterior temporal lobe dysfunction.

Automatic behavior is due to temporal lobe dysfunction.

Evaluation of *status epilepticus:*

Recurrent severe seizures.

Short or no interval between the recurrent seizures.

Consciousness not recovered.

If long-lasting, possible hyperthermia and exhaustion.

The condition may last for hours or for days.

Evaluation of *other forms* of epilepsy:

Infantile spasms occur suddenly with contraction of the whole body musculature, with flexion of the trunk and of the extremities.

Febrile convulsions may occur in the very young.

Epileptic equivalents may appear as abdominal pain, repetitive auras, mental cloudiness, or any other manifestation.

Diagnosis and management of epilepsy:

An electroencephalogram will give accurate information on the different patterns of epilepsy.

During attacks, prevent all sorts of injuries (tongue, etc.).

For grand mal, give diphenylhydantoin.

For petit mal, ethosuximide is preferred.

For psychomotor attacks, also give diphenylhydantoin.
For jacksonian epilepsy, give diphenylhydantoin or phenacemide.
For status epilepticus, give diazepam and phenobarbital.
For infantile spasms, give corticoids or corticotropin.
For epileptic equivalents, give diphenylhydantoin.

Narcolepsy

Evaluation of the symptomatology of narcolepsy:
The outstanding symptom is an uncontrollable need to sleep.
The attacks will be repeated once or several times a day, will occur at inappropriate times, and will last for minutes or hours.
Most patients are males; but the disease is relatively rare.
The sleep seems to be a natural sleep, from which the patient can be aroused as from a normal sleep.
There is a consistent physiologic difference: namely, normal sleep always presents non-rapid-eye movements preceding the rapid-eye movements, while in narcolepsy the rapid-eye movements occur first.
Paralysis can occur immediately after awakening; the patient finds that it is impossible to perform any movement for a while; this can also happen at the time of falling asleep.
Hypnagogic hallucinations at the onset of sleep, auditory or visual, may also occur.
Cataplexy is closely related to narcolepsy, consisting of transient loss of muscle tone that occurs mostly together with emotional reactions; mainly affected are hands (sudden drop of objects) or legs (sudden fall to the floor).
Management of narcolepsy:
May use amphetamine, dextroamphetamine, ephedrine; but methylphenidate is particularly recommended.

Hypertensive Encephalopathy

Clinical evaluation of hypertensive encephalopathy:
This reaction found in patients with severe hypertension.
Severe headache together with drowsiness and confusion.
Rapidly changing neurological abnormalities, such as blindness, hemisensory defects, or hemiparesis.
Nausea, blurred vision instead of blindness, and twitching.
Progress of symptoms leading to stupor, convulsions, and coma.
Differentiation from uremia consists of the finding of a blood urea nitrogen content below 100 mg in each 100 ml.
Management of hypertensive encephalopathy:
Start with diazoxide, together with furosemide or ethacrinic acid.
Other potent antihypertensive drugs may also be used; but there is a need for monitoring the patients carefully.

Brain Tumor

Evaluation of symptoms common to most brain tumors:
Headache, personality changes, vomiting.
Papilledema, which may not be an early sign in all instances.
Convulsive seizures, which may be focal or generalized.
Psychotic episodes, disordered conduct, lethargy, and other neurologic or mental changes.
Most symptoms, particularly the focal neurologic ones, often progressive.
If the tumor is metastatic, symptoms of the primary tumor possible.
Evaluation of focal neurologic changes that may reflect the location of the brain tumor:
Frontal lobe tumors cause disturbed mental state, impaired judgment, defective memory, irritability and mood changes, and convulsive seizures; if located on the left side, aphasia; if in the base, anosmia.
Parietal lobe tumors cause sensory and motor disturbances, that is, focal seizures and contralateral hemiparesis, impaired sensory perception with astereognosis, positivity of Babinski and similar signs, and aphasia when the left lobe is lesioned; denial of sickness is not a rare occurrence.
Temporal lobe tumors may be silent if they locate in the nondominant hemisphere (usually the right); otherwise, there will be seizures, either convulsive or of the psychomotor type, aphasia, and visual defects.
Occipital lobe tumors cause predominantly visual changes following an aura of lights and visual hallucinations; the usual hemianopsia frequently spares the macula; there may also be headache and papilledema, but seizures will almost always be present.
Subcortical tumors will cause contralateral hemiplegia if they invade the internal capsule; contralateral cutaneous sensory impairment, if the thalamus; athetosis or other symptoms as tremors and dystonia, if the basal ganglia; or the regular corresponding symptoms if the corresponding lobes of the hemisphere are invaded.
Cerebellar tumors are noted by disturbances of equilibrium and coordination, increased intracranial pressure, and papilledema.
Pituitary tumors, while not exactly brain tumors, will cause the characteristic bitemporal hemianopsia together with other symptoms due to pituitary impairment.
Pineal tumors, also not exactly brain tumors, are noted particularly among children, and may cause hydrocephalus, papillededma, and changes in the movement of eyes.
Tumors of the fourth ventricle will cause symptoms similar to those already mentioned for the cerebellum.
Evaluation of procedures to diagnose these tumors:
Complete eye and ear examination included as part of the neurologic examination.

All specialized X-ray procedures.
Electroencephalography, plus other electrographic procedures.
Lumbar puncture and diagnosis of the primary site of the lesion whenever needed.

Management of brain tumors:
Surgery or irradiation.
Chemotherapy.
Mixed procedures.
Symptomatic supportive treatment.

Injury to the Head

Evaluation of symptoms of *cerebral concussion:*
Loss of consciousness that lasts for a few minutes to less than 24 hours.
Pupils and their reaction remaining intact.
No evidence of neurologic impairment (paralysis, etc.).
No changes in the cerebrospinal fluid.

Evaluation of symptoms of *cerebral contusion or laceration:*
There is true coma accompanied by the following symptoms. Confusion may substitute.
There are more or less severe surface lesions, and possible skull fracture.
Pupils are unequal, the one on the lesioned side more dilated; they eventually become equally mydriatic and unreactive in advanced damage; nevertheless, pupils will show intense miosis in primary brainstem injuries.
Paralysis will indicate the injured site of the brain; also, rigidity may be noted.
Respiratory symptoms are frequently associated.

Evaluation of symptoms after recovering consciousness:
With mild concussion, complete recovery occurs soon.
In other instances, mental confusion will remain, together with the following.
Hemiplegia.
Neurologic focal signs.
Aphasia, and amnesia.
Personality changes, headache, and dizziness may persist for months (*post-traumatic cerebral syndrome*).

Evaluation of prolonged coma:
Check carefully for signs of hemorrhage, namely, subarachnoid, subdural, cerebral, or extradural.
Check carefully for paralysis.
Check carefully for complications, such as increased intracranial pressure, infectious complications, pulmonary reactions, etc.

Management of head injuries:
If present, treat shock.
Check and treat all accompanying symptoms.
If needed, give sedatives, but avoiding morphine, and antibiotics.
Surgery should always be contemplated.

Parkinsonism

Evaluation of the onset of parkinsonism:
Most cases will start after 50 years of age.
The onset will be insidious, and the progress slow.
Initial symptoms will be tremor, rigidity, or both.

Characteristic symptoms of parkinsonism are:
The tremor of the hand will be of the "pill-rolling" type, involving fingers and thumb.
The pill-rolling movement is mostly accompanied by flexion and extension of the wrist.
This tremor is maximal at rest, worst with emotions and fatigue, and disappears with voluntary movements and with sleep.
The tremor is also accompanied by a rigid and fixed facial expression.

Other symptoms usually noted in parkinsonism:
Movements are slower (smiling, body movements, turning, etc.).
Voice becomes weak, low, and monotonous.
There are stiffness and heaviness of most muscles, particularly those of the limbs.
Stooping position, with diminished spontaneous movements (akinesia), is observed.
Walking is difficult; legs feel very heavy so that it is hard to start to walk, but after starting many patients have to go faster and faster (festination) to avoid falling forward.
On walking, the heavy shuffling steps are not accompanied by the corresponding movements of the arms.
On stopping, some patients are unable to start walking again; and if pushed, they may pitch forward (propulsion) or backward (retropulsion).
Fine movement (adjusting a tie, using a spoon, etc.) may be almost impossible; in any case, they become very slow (bradykynesia).
Eyes become unblinking and staring, and saliva may drool from the corners of a semiopen mouth.
Seborrhea is very frequent.
Hypertonia causes the characteristic findings of "cogwheel" or "lead-pipe" rigidity; in the first case, on passive movements of the limbs they proceed with short intermittent jerks instead of the smooth normal sequence; in the second, as with a too-tight brake.
Oculogyric crises with prolonged fixation of the eyes in one position may occur.
Muscle strength is diminished, and cramps may also occur.

By what other names is parkinsonism also known?
Paralysis agitans.
Parkinson's disease.
Shaking palsy.

What are the essential components of the disease?
Involuntary tremors.
Muscular rigidity with diminished power.
Slow and poor purposeful movements.

What can be the final outcome for many of these patients?
Almost total invalidism.
Depression, or a mild dementia.
Management of parkinsonism:
Consider surgery for some special cases.
Levodopa (alone or together with carbidopa), amantadine hydrochloride, or derivatives of atropine or belladonna can be tried.
Do not stop any drug abruptly once it has been prescribed.

Torsion Spasm (Dystonia Musculorum Deformans)

Evaluate the symptoms of this torsion dystonia:
Onset usually occurs between 5 and 15 years of age.
First symptom may be inversion of a foot.
Progression occurs as involving any muscle.
Positions may become fixed, so distorting growth and normal shape (scoliosis, etc.).
It may have some relationship to spasmodic torticollis.
The mental condition remains normal, but the patient will become severely twisted.
Management of torsion spasm:
Always consider stereotaxic cryosurgery, which may be helpful.
Try levodopa, haloperidol, or both.

Progressive Supranuclear Palsy

Evaluate this Steele-Richardson-Olszewski syndrome:
Usually it starts at middle age, and mostly affects men.
There is opthalmoplegia (vertical plane).
Patient has poor control of oral and pharyngeal movements.
Other symptoms of pseudobulbar palsy are noted, such as dysarthria, and inappropriate emotion.
There are Parkinson-like symptoms, namely rigid face and bradykynesia.
There is progressive neck and trunk rigidity.
Gait is of the spastic-ataxic type.
Dementia is a common occurrence.
Management of progressive supranuclear palsy:
Treat extrapyramidal symptoms, as for parkinsonism, q.v.
Other symptoms will not respond to treatment.

Chorea

What are the symptoms of the classical *Sydenham's chorea,* also known as Saint Vitus' dance?
There is always a close relationship with a previous streptococcal infection (group A).
The disease may start even 6 months after the previous infection.
Very rare cases are not related to a previous known infection.
The disease affects young persons, mostly girls.
Characteristic of the disease are purposeless and involuntary quick and irregular jerky movement of the face (except the eyes), the trunk, and the extremities.
There are a mild hypotonia, incoordination of voluntary movements, irritability, restlessness, and insomnia.
Speech may be impaired.
Difficult gait may also exist.
Excitement and voluntary efforts to move may aggravate the involuntary choreic movements.
Evaluate the symptoms of chronic progressive *Huntington's chorea,* also called degenerative chorea:
It starts in adult life, usually between 30 and 50 years of age.
First notice is given by personality changes and bizarre behavior, which may increase (or be severe from the start) to psychotic episodes or any form of mental deterioration.
Psychic symptoms are accompanied or followed by choreic movements.
Choreic movements consist of the classical involuntary jerky traits, noted in the arms, neck, or face, and finally involving larger areas of the body.
Patients have impaired gait, and impaired fine movements.
Patients may become either euphoric or violent.
Final stage consists of severe mental deterioration (paranoia is common), and increasing invalidism (walking, swallowing, etc.), leading to complete dementia and death about 15 years after the beginning of the disease.
Management of both forms of chorea:
Only symptomatic, supportive treatment can be offered.

Tabes Dorsalis (Locomotor Ataxia)

Evaluation of symptoms of this syphilitic posterior spinal sclerosis:
There is a previous history of syphilis (may be unknown).
Outstanding symptoms are, first, very intense sharp recurrent leg pains, mostly known as lightning pains; and also the inability to walk in the dark.
The onset is insidious and follows a slow course.
There is a wide-based gait.
Argyll Robertson pupils, which accommodate well but react badly to light, are observed.
There are hypotonia and hyporeflexia.
In addition to the repetitive fulgurant leg pains, there are paresthesia, analgesia, extremely acute gastric crises simulating an acute abdomen, and other crises than similarly may start abruptly, last for a few days, and then also end abruptly, in the larynx, urethra, bladder, rectum and anus, and perhaps others.
Trophic, painless ulcers are also characteristic.
The Charcot joint is not rare among these patients.

Some patients complain of a feeling of walking on foam.

Most patients are thin, and show a sad expression.

Management of tabes dorsalis:

Use large doses of short-acting penicillin.

Dementia Paralytica (General Paresis)

Evaluation of symptoms concerning this disease, also called cerebral tabes or syphilitic meningoencephalitis:

There is a previous history of syphilis, which may be unknown.

The onset is insidious, at about 40 or 50 years of age.

First symptoms are decrease of concentration, loss of memory, irritability, headaches, tremor of fingers and lips, and dysarthria.

There is a profound behavioral deterioration, mental symptoms increase, and the general appearance becomes characteristically dirty and shabby.

The patient also becomes slovenly, confused, and irresponsible.

There is also insomnia, or lethargy.

Other symptoms consist of fatigue, emotional instability (outbursts of weeping or of violent temper), depression or delusions of grandeur, epileptic attacks, aphasia, hemiparesis, etc.

Management of general paresis:

Large doses of short-acting penicillin.

Shy-Drager Syndrome (Idiopathic Autonomic Insufficiency)

Evaluate the symptoms of Shy-Drager syndrome:

Orthostatic hypotension.

Dysfunction of the bladder and the bowel.

Impotence.

Tremor, rigidity, incoordination.

Iris atrophy.

Anhidrosis.

Pyramidal tract signs, cerebellar ataxia or muscular atrophy and fasciculations.

Onset in middle aged and young adults.

Management of Shy-Drager syndrome:

Give levodopa, fludrocortisone, tranylcypromine, etc.

Do not use a monoamine oxidase inhibitor together with levodopa.

Damage to the Olfactory Nerve

Evaluation of damage to the olfactory nerve:

Anosmia, or loss of smell, is the only symptom.

It has to be differentiated from anosmia due to diseases affecting the nasal mucosae, either infectious or atrophic rhinitis.

The cause of damage will be an infection, an intracranial tumor, or a trauma.

Damage to the Optic Nerve

Symptoms and management of damage to the end of the optic nerve in the eye, constituting *papilledema:*

An enlarged blind spot will occur, but not damaged vision.

There is a swelling of the blind spot or optic disc.

The disc is hyperhemic; there are tortuous engorged retinal veins, and hemorrhages in the retina.

This situation may be due to tumors, abscesses, and other cerebral diseases, that is, intracranial pressure, and presents bilaterally.

In the case of chocked disc due to hypertension the arteries and blood pressure are affected.

Treat the basic cause.

Symptoms and management of *optic neuritis,* or papillitis:

Most of the cases are unilateral, but this symptom depends on the cause.

Vision is lost, completely or in the form of scotoma.

There are hyperemia and edema of the optic disc.

Vitreous opacities or more marked changes will occur.

Beware of temporal arteritis as the cause of the condition in those patients over 60 years of age.

Treat the basic cause; and use corticoids (systemic or retrobulbar).

Symptoms and management of *retrobulbar neuritis:*

Commonly, a unilateral condition.

Rapid loss of vision.

Pain when the eye is moved in any direction.

Normal fundus in ophthalmoscopy.

Treat the basic cause, and use corticoids, either systemically or by retrobulbar administration.

Symptoms and management of *optic atrophy:*

According to the degree of atrophy there will be a corresponding loss of vision.

Total blindness accompanies unreactive pupils.

Treat the basic cause; but results are always poor.

Evaluate visual changes according to the site of the nerve lesion:

If the lesion occurs before the chiasm	There will be total loss of the corresponding eye.
If the lesion is in the chiasm	There will be bitemporal hemianopsia.
Lesions that occur after the chiasm	Cause homonymous hemianopsia, that is, visual loss on the same side of the visual field.

Ophthalmoplegia

Evaluate extraocular muscle palsies, or ophthalmoplegia:

The outstanding symptom is a recent diplopia.

Diplopia may vary according to the involved muscles and the direction of the gaze.

Divergent strabismus will occur when the oculomotor nerve is affected.

Vertical diplopia corresponds to trochlear nerve damage.
One eye will not be able to abduct beyond the midline in the case of abducens nerve lesion.
Pain and mydriasis suggest a lesion pressing on the oculomotor nerve.
Management of ophthalmoplegia:
Treat the cause.

Trigeminal Neuralgia (Tic Douloureux)

Evaluate the symptoms of neuralgia of the trigeminus nerve:
The outstanding, almost diagnostic, symptom is a sudden attack of lancinating pain, lasting 1 or 2 minutes (may reach 15 minutes), and a burning sensation.
The attack may be repeated several times a day, but in some circumstances is less frequent, occurring only a few times a year.
Not rarely, there will be a trigger zone.
Any of the zones of the ophthalmic, the maxillary, or the mandibular may be affected.
More women than men are affected after reaching maturity.
Management of trigeminal neuralgia:
Use carbamazepine, diphenylhydantoin, vitamin B_{12}.
Alcohol may be injected in the Gasserian ganglion.
Surgery may be contemplated if the above measures fail.

Glossopharyngeal Neuralgia

Evaluate the symptoms of glossopharyngeal neuralgia:
More men than women are affected, after 40 years of age.
The clinical picture is similar to trigeminal neuralgia, but the pain occurs in the posterior pharynx and tonsils, back of the tongue, and in the middle ear. The anterolateral aspect of the neck may also hurt.
The attack may be triggered by talking, chewing or swallowing, sneezing, and similar circumstances. They may not be too frequent.
Pain may start at the base of the tongue, spreading from this site.
Syncopal episodes due to cardiac arrest may occur.
Local application of an anesthetic will eliminate pain (this will not happen if the pain belongs to trigeminal neuralgia).
Pain will last only seconds or at most a few minutes.
Management of glossopharyngeal neuralgia:
Carbamazepine.
Local anesthesia of the pharynx.
Surgery to be considered.

Peripheral Facial Paralysis (Bell's Palsy)

Evaluate the symptoms of Bell's palsy:
It may occur at any age, but more frequently between 20 and 50 years.
It may be provoked by trauma, chill, or other form of exposure.
Initial symptom may be pain behind the ear.
There is sudden paralysis of one side of the face, which appears flat and without wrinkles, the poorly expressive face deviated toward the intact side.
Imperfect closure of the eye occurs in the affected side; lagophthalmia is also noted during sleep.
There is continuous shedding of tears.
Some patients will present hyperacusia, or disturbances of salivation and taste, otalgia, a prickly sensation behind the ear, etc.
When patient closes the eyes, the affected one is directed upward.
All symptoms are more marked when the patient talks, laughs; and the cheek is more inflated than the other side when blowing.
Some patients will refer their complaints toward the intact side rather than the paralyzed one.
Symptoms that distinguish peripheral facial paralysis from central facial paralysis:
Deviated mouth, lagophthalmia, and frequent sensitive symptoms, such as hypoesthesia, paresthesia, painful formication.
Keratitis, which results not rarely.
Peripheral facial paralysis is due to chilliness (a frigore), diabetes mellitus, otic lesions, infections, polyneuritis, injuries, etc.
Management of Bell's palsy:
Protect the eye.
Decompress the facial nerve, at an early stage.
Corticoids are estimated above all other measures.

Central Facial Paralysis

Evaluation of *supranuclear palsy:*
It usually accompanies hemiplegia.
The mouth is deviated, but the eye closes rather well.
There are very few, if any, sensitive troubles.
Only in very extensive injuries will there be more extensive symptomatology.
This form of paralysis is due to the same causes that provoke hemiplegia.
Evaluation of *nuclear* or *protuberancial facial palsy:*
Symptoms are identical with those of peripheral facial palsy.
It more frequently accompanies alternate hemiplegia.
Management of these forms of facial paralysis:
Similar to hemiplegia.

Cerebellar Diseases

Evaluate symptoms due to cerebellar diseases:
Cerebellar ataxia, which is perhaps the most important, presenting a wide-based very marked staggering gait similar to that of a severely intoxicated person. Romberg's sign is negative.

Dysmetria, showing improper measurement of distance in muscular movements, such as reaching the ear instead of reaching the nose when asked to do the latter.

Asynergia of movements associated for a purpose.

Adioadochokinesia, or inability to perform correctly rapid alternating movements.

Other symptoms, such as catalepsy, hypotonic passive movements, tremor, nystagmus, etc.

Evaluate symptoms of *cerebellar tumors:*

Patients are usually young and mature. There are regular symptoms, as above.

There may be a cancer in another site.

Cerebellar angioma may associate with retinal angioma and cystic malformation of the kidney or the pancreas, and in the Hippel-Lindau syndrome. May improve with age.

Evaluate symptoms of *cerebellar abscess:*

It may occur without symptoms; or only show fever.

There is frequently a previous otorrhea; or any other previous infection.

There may be fever, localized cephalalgia, nystagmus with large oscillations (directed to the diseased site), deviation of the head and eyes. Very bad prognosis if nystagmus is directed toward the intact site of the cerebellum.

Management of cerebellar diseases:

Treat the basic cause, whenever known.

Otherwise, the treatment may be symptomatic; rarely surgical.

Evaluate the symptoms of *cerebellar cortical degeneration:*

It occurs in persons subject to severe nutritional deprivation.

Usually, the patient is an inveterate alcoholic.

There is a sudden onset with incapacity to walk.

Incoordination and imbalance occur, due to dysmetria and hypotonia of the lower extremities.

The strength of the affected extremities remains normal.

Cerebellar ataxia is the dominant trait.

Management of cerebellar cortical degeneration:

Abstinence from alcohol, and proper nutrition.

Physical therapy.

Injury to the Spinal Cord

Evaluate symptoms of *contusion* to the spinal cord:

Rapid onset of severe dysfunction.

Thereafter, spontaneous recovery.

Minimal residual disability may remain.

Evaluate symptoms of *hemorrhage* into the spinal cord:

Muscle weakness, and muscle wasting.

Fasciculation, easily seen under the skin.

Loss of tendon reflexes, more or less marked.

Symptoms are more or less permanent.

Evaluate symptoms of *lacerations* or *transections* of the spine:

Immediate onset of paralytic symptoms.

Permanent dysfunction will follow.

Evaluate symptoms of a *complete transverse lesion of the spinal cord:*

There is loss of movement, sensation, and reflexes from below the lesion.

Paralytic paraplegia gradually turns into spastic paraplegia, in a matter of hours or days.

Myotatic reflexes become exaggerated, that is, the reflex contraction response of a muscle to passive stretching.

In a later stage, if the lower portion of the cord is intact, there will be a return of deep tendon and autonomic reflexes; also, there appear spasms of the extensor or flexor muscles.

Evaluate symptoms according to the *level of the cord lesion:*

Most lesions at the thoracic level will cause the symptoms mentioned above, involving both legs.

Below the last thoracic vertebra, the paralysis will be noted only below the knee.

Most lesions to the cervical spine will cause paralysis of respiration; most of them are fatal.

Lesions at the level of the fourth and fifth vertebrae will cause quadriplegia.

Lesions at the level of the fifth and sixth will allow the arms to abduct and flex.

Lesions between the sixth and seventh will allow shoulder and elbow movements, but will paralyze legs, wrists, and hands.

Lesions between thoracic and cervical vertebrae will cause the *Horner's syndrome,* presenting on the affected side:

Miosis.

Palpebral ptosis.

Anhidrosis of the face.

Sinking in of the eyeball.

Narrowing of the palpebral fissure, because the lower eyelid is somewhat elevated.

Lesions to the lower sacral roots will cause complete loss of control of the bladder and the bowel.

Hemisection of the cord will cause the *Brown-Sequard syndrome,* presenting the following features:

Spastic paralysis and loss of postural sense, on the same side of the lesion.

Loss of pain and thermal sense on the opposite side.

Management of the lesioned spinal cord:

Extreme care in moving the patient, not to aggravate the situation.

Rest, traction, or surgery, according to the case.

Spinal Cord Compression

Evaluate symptoms of *subacute cord compression:*

There is back pain.

There may or may not be a radicular distribution of pain.

There is hyperreflexia with positivity of Babinski and similar signs.
After the reflex changes there will be weakness (mostly proximal) of the lower limbs.
Also, there is loss of sensation and of sphincter control.

Evaluate symptoms of *chronic spinal cord compression:*
These are caused by extrameduallary neoplasms, or by bony or cartilaginous masses protruding into the spinal canal.
The symptoms will vary according to the level of the offending mass, that is, whether it is cervical or lumbosacral.

Evaluate symptoms of *cervical disc herniation:*
Pain and paresthesias invade paroxysmally from the back of the neck into arms and fingers.
The distribution belongs mostly to the lower vertebral bodies of the cervical area.
Pain is accentuated by efforts, such as straining, coughing, or sneezing.
There is a decreased mobility of the neck.
There is cervical muscle spasm.
There is weakness (and possibly atrophy) of the biceps or triceps, with diminution of the corresponding jerks.
There is narrow intervertebral space, as seen in X-ray films.

Evaluate symptoms of *lumbosacral disc herniation:*
Most cases (90%) correspond to the discs between the fourth or fifth intervertebral spaces.
There is a change of the normal lumbar curve.
There may be scoliosis directed to the opposite side of the sciatic pain.
There are symptoms of sciatic pain (sciatica); pain on pressure over the nerve, impaired straight-leg rising (Lasègue's sign), radiation of pain along the nerve in efforts (straining, etc.).
There will be mild weakness of extensors to the foot and great toe, diminished pain and touch sensations on the dorsum of the foot and leg, and decreased ankle jerk, which may even be absent.

Management of spinal cord compressions:
Treatment will be according to the causative factor, with emphasis on surgical decompression.

Multiple Sclerosis (Disseminated Sclerosis)

Evaluate symptoms of multiple sclerosis:
It occurs in early adult life; perhaps more women are affected.
An increase of human leukocyte antigen (HLA) has been reported recently.
The course of the disease is very slow, with exacerbations and remissions.
The classic Charcot's triad only appears in late stages, consisting of nystagmus, intention tremor, and scanning speech.
The initial attack, at times also other attacks, may follow:
Acute infections or serum injections.
Vaccination.
Injuries.
Somatic stress.
Pregnancy.
Symptoms will reveal multiple involvement of the central nervous system.
Visual disturbances, paresthesias, and weakness or clumsiness of one of the limbs may be the first symptoms to occur.
Most common visual disturbances might be partial blindness of one of the eyes (retrobulbar optic neuritis, q.v., in the paragraph devoted to the optic nerve, in this chapter), scotomas, dimness of vision, diplopia, weakness or paralysis of ocular movements.
Other initial symptoms might be vertigo, emotional disturbances, and decreased bladder control.

Evaluate the neurologic symptoms of multiple sclerosis:
Increased deep reflexes.
Clonus, Babinski, and other similar findings, which are easily noted.
Ataxic motion, static and intentional tremor.
Weakness and spasticity of muscles, leading first to a stumbling gait, and later to a disabling ataxia.
Spasms due to mild stimuli, as those elicited while in bed.
Paresthesias of the face.
Hemiplegia, which is noted occasionally.
Impotence among men, and sexual anesthesia among women.
Possibly other symptoms due to optic involvement, such as ophthalmoplegia, partial atrophy of the nerve, etc.
Convulsions, in some patients.
Nystagmus and scanning speech, already mentioned, which will appear in long-standing cases.

Evaluate the mental symptoms noted in multiple sclerosis:
Emotional instability.
Inattention and apathy.
Poor judgment.
Depression, in some patients, due to the condition.
Sudden laughter or weeping.
In later stages, possible euphoria, or more severe changes of dementia.

Evaluation of the total clinical picture of multiple sclerosis:
Widespread symptomatology.
Repeated exacerbations and remissions, which may last for years.
Varied and unpredictable clinical course.

Management of multiple sclerosis:
Symptomatic and supportive.
ACTH or corticoids, which may be given at the start of an attack, not for long-term therapy.

Other Demyelinating Disorders

Mention the most frequent congenital diseases with demyelination:

- Tay-Sachs.
- Gaucher.
- Niemann-Pick.
- Hurler.
- Krabbe.

Evaluate the symptoms of *postinfectious encephalitis,* or *acute disseminated encephalomyelitis:*

- Usually follows an acute viral infection; also, a vaccination.
- Symptoms are evaluated under "Encephalitis," in this chapter.

Discuss the symptoms and management of the *Guillain-Barré syndrome:*

- It is supposed to be an immunologic disease of peripheral nerves.
- It may appear 1 or 2 weeks after any common infective disorder, or vaccination.
- It may start with weakness of the lower limbs that in a few days extends to the upper limbs and face.
- Also, symptoms may start peripherally and extend centrally.
- Muscle weakness may be accompanied by tenderness and diminished reflexes.
- Paresthesias may also be felt.
- In severe cases paralysis may become intense and affect the respiratory muscles (death may be due to this paralysis).
- Other symptoms may be edema, hyperhidrosis, livid skin, and postural hypotension.
- Gradual recovery may take weeks, following a course of 1 or more weeks.
- Corticoids are suggested for treatment, but there are doubts about their efficiency.

Discuss the symptoms and management of *optic neuromyelitis:*

- There is acute visual loss, or central scotoma.
- Other symptoms occur similarly to those of multiple sclerosis (q.v.).
- Also, corticoids are suggested for treatment.

Evaluate the symptoms of *Schilder's disease:*

- Optic neuritis, and blindness.
- Muscle spasticity.
- Dementia.
- Fatal outcome in less than two years.

Syringomyelia

Evaluate the characteristic clinical findings for the diagnosis of syringomyelia:

- Loss of sensations for pain and temperature.
- Preservation of deep and tactile sensations.

Evaluate the other findings for syringomyelia:

- Weakness and wasting of muscles, principally of the upper limbs and hands.
- Hypo- or areflexia of the corresponding segments.
- Hyperreflexia and spasticity of the lower limbs.
- Horner's syndrome, nystagmus, Charcot joints in affected limbs.
- Vasomotor and trophic changes, and absence of deep reflexes in the upper limbs.
- Ataxia of the lower limbs, and neurogenic bladder.
- A capelike sensory defect extending over the shoulders and back, not rarely.

Evaluate symptoms when the lesions (syrinx cavity) set at upper levels, thus constituting *syringobulbia:*

- Loss of pain and temperature with preservation of deep and tactile sensations on the face, uni- or bilateral.
- Atrophy and fibrillation of the tongue, with dysarthria.
- Nystagmus, and vertigo.
- Respiratory stridor; dysphonia; dysphagia.
- Symptoms may extend as in pure syringomyelia.

Management of syringomyelia:

- The disease is very slow in its progress, but laminectomy and decompression are usually recommended, with needle aspiration or myelotomy.

Friedreich's Ataxia

Evaluate the symptoms of this, the most common of the hereditary ataxias:

- Onset at puberty.
- Ataxia, with wide-based gait and poor equilibrium (drunkard gait).
- Asynergia of upper limbs, which show incoordination and dysmetria.
- Intense positivity of Romberg's sign, even when sitting.
- Dysarthria, and nystagmus.
- Muscles hypotonic, atrophic, without tendinous reflexes.
- Pes cavus, with hyperextension of the toes; scoliosis.
- Note that some patients may present preferentially the ataxic symptom, others, the pes cavus; others may be oligosymptomatic.
- Electrocardiographically, some of these patients may show anginal changes.

Management of this form of hereditary ataxia:

- Only symptomatic and supportive.

Peroneal Muscular Atrophy (Charcot-Marie-Tooth Disease)

Evaluate the symptoms of this muscular atrophy:

- Onset is insidious, before 30 years of age, with slow progress.
- There is a steppage gait, with a dropping foot with the toes pointing to the ground, the leg lifted high.
- Patient has weakness and atrophy of the muscles of the anterior part of the leg.
- Weakness and atrophy will spread to the posterior muscles of the leg, and to the small muscles of the hand.

Pain and paresthesis will also be noted in the legs.
Sensitivity for pain, temperature, and vibrations is decreased in hands and feet.
Absence of myotatic or stretch reflexes is noted.
There is optic involvement; possibly retinitis pigmentosa.
Physical activity and life span are not affected.

Management of this type of muscular atrophy:
Symptomatic and supportive.

Olivopontocerebellar Atrophy

Evaluate the symptoms of this hereditary ataxia:
The disease begins in adulthood.
The gaze is impaired.
There is palatal myoclonus.
Cerebellar and extrapyramidal signs may be present.
Little or no sensory change takes place.

Management of this condition:
Symptomatic and supportive.

Hypertrophic Interstitial Neuropathy (Dejerine-Sottas Disease)

Evaluate the symptoms of Dejerine-Sottas disease:
Insidious onset, before 30 years of age, and slow progress.
Symptoms similar to peroneal muscular atrophy, q.v., above.
But no eye involvement.
Also, peripheral nerves hypertrophied.

Management of hypertrophic interstitial neuropathy:
Symptomatic and supportive.

Refsum's Syndrome

Evaluate the symptoms of Refsum's syndrome:
There may be cerebellar and sensory changes.
Peripheral and optic nerves may be impaired; there is the possibility of retinitis pigmentosa.
There is impaired hearing.
Electrocardiographic changes are noted.
There is icthyosis.

Management of Refsum's syndrome:
Symptomatic and supportive.

Muscular Dystrophies

Discuss symptoms and management of Duchenne's *pseudohypertrophic muscular dystrophy:*
It starts in boys from 3 to 7 years of age.
A waddling, toe-walking gait is observed.
There is difficulty in climbing stairs and in standing up from the floor (the patient "climbs" with his hands up through the legs).
There is proximal muscle weakness, which shows fatty and fibrous infiltration (pseudohypertrophy).
The pelvic girdle is affected first, followed by the shoulders.
There is a steady progression, disabling the patient at about 12 years of age, or before.
Half the patients have a relatively low I.Q.
Handling is just symptomatic and supportive.

Discuss symptoms and management of *limb-girdle muscular dystrophy:*
It usually begins after 7 years of age.
Symptomatology is as above.
Treatment is symptomatic and supportive.

Discuss symptoms and management of *pelvi-femoral muscular dystrophy* (Leyden-Moebious):
It begins with dystrophy of the pelvic muscles.
Progress is unpredictable.
Outcome is similar to that of pseudohypertrophic muscular dystrophy, q.v., above.
Management is only symptomatic and supportive.

Discuss symptoms and management of Erb's *scapulohumeral muscular dystrophy:*
It is entirely similar to pseudohypertrophic muscular dystrophy, but starts with muscles of the shoulder; the face is not affected.
Outcome and treatment are the same.

Discuss symptoms and management of Landouzy-Dejerine's *fascioscapulohumeral muscular dystrophy:*
It starts during adolescence, affecting both sexes equally.
Affected muscles are those of the face, the shoulder, and the upper arms, bilaterally; there are winging scapulae.
At a later stage pelvic muscles may also be involved.
There is muscle pseudohypertrophy (fat and fibrous tissue).
There is dropping of the eyelids (myopathic facies), and of the upper lip (tapir lip).
The forearms are larger than the upper arms.
Progress is variable, there may be prolonged periods of arrest, and the patients remain active to a normal life span.
As in other instances, treatment is only symptomatic and supportive.

Acute Transverse Myelitis

Evaluate symptoms of this form of cord inflammation:
Usually, it follows a known infectious or parasitic disease.
Frequently, no cause is known.
Onset may occur with sudden back pain.
In a few hours signs of cord transverse lesion occur (see paragraph on "Injury to the Spinal Cord" for information, in this chapter).
The deficit symptoms are usually severe.
Abdominal paralysis will be present in most cases.
The prognosis is bad; it is only relatively good in cases due to edema or to viral encephalomyelitis.

Management of acute transverse myelitis:
Corticoids may be of some help.
Surgical decompression will be discussed.

Posterolateral Sclerosis (Combined System Disease)

Evaluate symptoms of the posterior and lateral degeneration of the cord:

It start after middle age is reached.

The most common association is with pernicious anemia, even antedating it.

First symptoms consist of paresthesias, such as numbness, tingling, and the sensation of pins and needles starting in toes and feet, and later noted in the fingers.

Other sensations may also occur, such as wetness, swelling, and coldness noted in the feet. Mental symptoms may be present.

Weakness of legs, heaviness of feet, unsteady gait may occur.

Secondary symptoms of anemia may be found.

Evaluate symptoms occurring in the *flaccid type* of posterolateral sclerosis:

There is weakness of the distal portions of the lower extremities, and ataxia.

There is tenderness of the soles, and of the calf muscles.

The distal portion of the leg, below the knee, will show decreased sensation to touch and vibrations.

The Romberg sign will be positive.

Diminished reflexes will be noted.

Evaluate symptoms occurring in the *spastic type:*

There are increased deep tendon reflexes.

Clonus, hypertonicity, flexor spasms, and progressive weakness of the legs are noted.

There is loss of sphincter control.

With impaired sensation, decubitus ulcers may occur.

Final stage may occur with paraplegia in flexion.

Management of posterolateral sclerosis:

As for pernicious anemia, q.v.

Aran-Duchenne Atrophy (Myelopathic Muscular Atrophy)

Evaluate the symptoms of Aran-Duchenne atrophy:

It starts in adult life.

Atrophy and fibrillation of the muscles occur, with gradual loss of power.

The small muscles of the hands are involved first.

There is slow progression to muscles of the forearm, the arm, the shoulder, and finally the muscles of the trunk.

Management of Aran-Duchenne atrophy:

Only symptomatic and supportive.

Werdnig-Hoffmann Paralysis

Evaluate symptoms of Werdnig-Hoffmann paralysis:

Beginning of disease in infants, during the first year of life.

Hypotonia and flaccid paralysis, usually starting in the pelvic girdle and the thighs; thereafter symptoms spreading to the limbs and other sites as well.

Absent myotatic or stretch reflexes.

Fasciculations of the tongue, and of other muscles.

Dysphagia.

Delayed neuromuscular development.

Disease usually fatal before age 2; respiratory complications.

A few cases will survive with static weakness.

Management of Werdnig-Hoffmann paralysis or disease:

Only symptomatic and supportive.

Bulbar Palsy (Labioglossolaryngeal Paralysis)

Evaluate symptoms of bulbar paralysis:

There is atrophy with paralysis of muscles of the:

Lips.

Mouth.

Tongue.

Pharynx.

Larynx.

There are difficult chewing, swallowing, and talking; also, drooling, and dysarthria.

There is poor control of emotions.

Cases with dysphagia, that is, difficult swallowing, are of poor prognosis.

The disease affects adults after 40 years of age.

Death may occur in less than 3 years (respiratory paralysis).

Management of this progressive bulbar palsy or Duchenne's paralysis:

Only symptomatic and supportive.

Amyotrophic Lateral Sclerosis

Evaluate the initial stage of the disease:

The usual onset is between 40 and 60 years of age.

It begins with wasting and weakness, generally of the upper extremities, the hands preferentially.

Spasticity, and increased tendon and extensor plantar reflexes may antedate wasting.

Other symptoms of the disease are:

Spastic weakness of the trunk.

Spastic weakness of not only the upper but also the lower limbs.

Muscle fasciculations visible.

Course of the disease:

Fatal within 3 years of the initiation.

Progressively downhill, without remissions.

Management of amyotrophic lateral sclerosis is:

Only symptomatic and supportive.

Juvenile Spinal Muscular Atrophy (Wohlfart-Kugelberg-Welander Disease)

Evaluation of the clinical picture and course of juvenile spinal muscular atrophy:

The clinical picture is similar to that of infantile spinal muscular atrophy, or Werdnig-Hoffmann paralysis, q.v., above.

The differences are:
- The disease starts in late childhood or adolescence, instead of the first years of age.
- The evolution is slower.
- The prognosis is better, for a longer life expectancy.

Management of juvenile spinal muscular atrophy:
- Only symptomatic and supportive.

Amyotonia Congenita (Oppenheim's Disease)

General traits of this congenital atonic pseudoparalysis, or myatonia congenita:
- The infant is born with such a marked hypotonia that it may simulate a true paralysis.
- The infant cannot support limbs, much less the head.
- Tendinous reflexes are diminished.
- No reaction of degeneration is present.
- It may be associated with other anomalies, such as hyperextensive joints, hyperelasticity of the skin, mongolism, etc.

Agreement of authors with respect to amyotonia congenita:
- There are many who protest its legitimacy and would prefer that it be discarded.

Management of this condition:
- Symptomatic and supportive.

Myotonia Congenita (Thomsen's Disease)

Explain onset of the disease, also called ataxia muscularis:
- The disease is noted from birth in the typical case; it is hereditary.
- There is a form called *myotonia acquisita,* which is practically the same, excepting that it starts late in life.

Evaluate symptoms of myotonia congenita:
- There are stiffness and difficulty in relaxation of the entire voluntary musculature because muscles are hypertonic and hypertrophic.
- Physical activity is difficult.
- Periodic attacks of generalized muscle spasm may occur.
- Stiffness is accentuated by cold, and relieved by exercise.

Management of myotonia congenita:
- Quinine.

Myotonia Atrophica (Dystrophia Myotonica, Myotonic Dystrophy)

Explain onset of Steinert's disease:
- It may start at any age.
- The overall symptomatology may be either severe or milder.

Evaluate symptoms of the disease:
- Hypertonus appears together with atrophy and weakness of muscles.
- Muscles mainly affected are those of the face, the hand, the tongue, the jaw, the peroneal, and others.
- Patients cannot release the grip immediately after taking an object.

Other symptoms found in the disease are:
- Atrophy of the face and neck muscles.
- Cataracts.
- Early baldness.
- Testicular atrophy, and other endocrinopathies.
- Mental retardation, or dementia.

Evaluate the symptoms of *paramyotonia congenita:*
- Myotonia that increases with coldness.
- Intermittent flaccid paralysis.
- Possible relationship with hyperkalemic periodic paralysis.

Management of myotonia atrophica:
- Only symptomatic and supportive.

Stiff-Man Syndrome

This syndrome of unknown origin may start as follows:
- There is episodic aching and tightness of the muscles, generally those of the trunk.
- In a few weeks or months the tightness becomes constant, and spreads to the limbs.
- The disease is established as a boardlike hardness and tightness of almost all the muscles of the body.

Other accompanying symptoms of the stiff-man syndrome are:
- Skeletal abnormalities.
- Subluxations and spontaneous fractures.
- Painful paroxysms of muscle spasms lasting for several minutes provoked by sudden stimuli.

Management of the stiff-man syndrome:
- Myoneural blocking agents; diazepam.

Myasthenia Gravis

The initial clinical picture of myasthenia gravis shows:
- Occurrence at birth; among 20% born to mothers with the disease there will be transient symptoms; in a few of them the disease will persist.
- Occurrence in adolescents and young adults, more frequently among females. Onset may be insidious or sudden.
- Occurrence in adults over 40 years of age, usually those who have a thymoma.

Characteristic symptoms of the disease:
- The initial symptom usually is palpebral ptosis.
- Diplopia may also appear early.
- Strabismus may also occur.
- Other muscles may also show severe weakness, such as limb muscles and those used in speech and swallowing.
- There is a high-pitched nasal voice.
- There is a myasthenic smile.
- Reflexes repeatedly obtained, decrease in power; after a short rest they may regain normal power.
- All symptoms are increased with repetitive use of the corresponding muscles.

The outcome of the disease:
- Respiratory muscle weakness is very dangerous.
- The intensity of symptoms may vary, even from day to day.

Remission of symptoms will occur in about 25% of the patients.
Management of myasthenia gravis:
Neostigmine, pyridostigmine, ambenonium, and others may be noted.
Corticoid therapy has been recommended.

Neuromuscular Junction Block

Evaluate drug-induced neuromuscular junction block:
The clinical syndrome is entirely similar to myasthenia gravis, q.v.
Be careful with drugs used to treat myasthenia gravis.
Be careful also with organophosphate insecticides and nerve gases.
Warning symptoms will be miosis, bronchial secretions with tightness of the chest, hyperactivity of the gastrointestinal tract.
The symptoms of myasthenia gravis are prolonged.
Management of this reaction:
Atropine.

Familial Periodic Paralysis

Symptoms common to all forms of familial periodic paralysis:
Periodic attacks of flaccid paralysis, with dropping of objects or falls.
No loss of consciousness.
Variable duration of the attacks.
Normalcy between the attacks.
Characteristics of the *hypokalemic form:*
Attacks last from 1 hour to several days.
At times the patient awakes paralyzed.
Too severe attacks may cause death from respiratory paralysis.
Attacks may be induced by hypertonic glucose, insulin, epinephrine, desoxycorticosterone, etc.
Attacks are relieved or prevented with the administration of potassium.
Characteristics of the *hyperkalemic form (adynamia episodica hereditaria):*
This disease usually appears during childhood.
Attacks are usually shorter and milder.
In this form attacks are more easily provoked by rest after exertion.
Some patients may present symptoms of myotonia.
Paresthesias of the limbs may precede the attakc.
If exercise starts at the beginning of paresthesias, the paralytic attack may be aborted.
Attacks are provoked by potassium administration.
Acetazolamide may prevent attacks.
Characteristics of the *normokalemic form:*
It is not yet well characterized.
It is similar to the hyperkalemic form.
It may respond to acetazolamide.

For more details on "Hyperpotassemia" and "Hypopotassemia" see the corresponding paragraphs in the chapter devoted to metabolism and nutrition.

Cervical Rib (Scalenus Anticus Syndrome)

What may cause, in the thoracic outlet syndrome, the compression of the brachial plexus and the subclavian artery?
Not only a rudimentary cervical rib, but also the following.
First thoracic rib.
Tight scalene muscle.
Fibrous bands.
Evaluate the symptoms corresponding to this syndrome:
Local pain in the base of the neck.
Pain referred to the ulnar side of the forearm and hand.
Paresthesias also noted in the same sites.
Possible impaired perception of pain and light touch on this side.
Muscular weakness of the hand.
Hand that may appear cold and blue.
Diminished pulsations (radial and ulnar arteries).
Occassionally, the Horner's syndrome has been reported.
Explain the Adson's test to check scalenus anticus syndrome:
Patient sits, with hands on thighs.
A rapid deep respiration is taken, and the breath held.
Then, the neck is hyperextended.
In that position, the head is turned as far as possible to the right (check pulse on right wrist), and then to the left (check pulse on left wrist).
Obliteration of the pulse in the affected side is positive.
Handling of the scalenus anticus syndrome:
Surgery gives permanent relief.
Symptomatic and supportive help can also be given.
For additional information, see "Thoracic Syndrome" in the chapter devoted to musculoskeletal diseases.

Acute Brachial Neuritis

Most frequent causes of acute brachial neuritis are:
Damage done by traction to the newborn.
Breast or lung carcinoma, in the adult.
An acute brachial neuritis of unknown origin affecting young adults.
Evaluate symptoms of brachial plexus disorders:
There is shoulder disability if the rostral brachial plexus is involved.
There is hand disability if the caudal brachial plexus is involved.
In the acute disease of young men there may also be supraclavicular pain, weakness, sensory abnormalities, and diminished reflexes, mostly noted in the shoulder area; weakness becomes intense in a few days, and regresses in a few months.

Management of brachial plexus disorders:
- Proceed according to the cause.
- The acute brachial neuritis of young adults may respond to corticoids.

Occipital Neuritis (Occiptal Neuralgia)

Most frequent causes of occipital neuritis are:
- Changes noted in muscles of the occipital area.
- Arthritis changes of the upper spine.
- Other changes, such as those in fascial tissues, etc.
- Very rarely inflammatory or toxic lesions to the nerves.

Most important symptoms of occipital neuritis:
- Severe pain in the back of the neck, and in the head.
- Pain more often unilateral.
- Not rarely history of a previous injury to the area.

Management of occipital neuritis:
- Local infiltration of procaine.
- Manual measures, such as a halter.
- Surgery to be considered in some instances.

Sciatica

Discuss initiation of pain to the sciatic nerve:
- It may be caused by any of the basic motivation also common with low back pain.
- Infections, intoxications, tumors, injuries, etc., are frequently found.
- There are cases not attributable to any cause.
- Most patients are over 60 years of age.

Evaluation of sciatic pain:
- It may be moderate, but in most instances is extremely severe.
- It may be permanent or paroxysmal.
- It starts at the area of the ischium and spreads through the posterior aspect of the lower extremity.
- It may increase on pressure over Valleix's points, close to the ischium in the greater sciatic notch, in the inferior border of the gluteus maximus, in the popliteal area, and at other lower sites.

Evaluation of accompanying symptoms of sciatica:
- There is a flexed leg, with external rotation.
- A limping gait is noted.
- There is muscular hypotonia (poorly marked gluteal crease and muscles of the leg), with a tendency to flat foot; later there will be atrophy.
- Other minor symptoms might be scoliosis, coldness with cyanosis, sweating, ulcers, hypertrichosis, etc.

Evaluation of tests to confirm sciatica:
- The extended leg flexed over the abdomen will exacerbate pain (Lasègue); pain disappears or is attenuated if the lower leg is flexed against the thigh.
- If the patient lying on the bed is suddenly incorporated, the pain is increased, and the leg flexes rapidly to attenuate it.
- Forced abduction of the leg is painful (Bonnet).
- Pain may be induced or increased by flexing the foot, or merely the great toe.

Management of sciatica:
- It depends on the causative factor.
- Give symptomatic and supportive care.

Peripheral Neuropathy (Polyneuritis)

Evaluate the origin of peripheral neuritis:
- Most cases occur in young or middle-aged men.
- There is a slow onset, taking a few weeks for completion of the clinical picture.
- The only rapid onset will occur in alcoholics with an infection.
- Causative factors are manifold (intoxications, infections, mechanical, vascular, nutritional, tumoral, etc.).

Evaluate the symptoms of *mononeuritis:*
- There is pain along the distribution of the nerve.
- Paresthesias also occur on the path of the pain.
- There is weakness of the corresponding muscles.

Evaluate the symptoms of *radial nerve palsy:*
- There is paralysis of the extensor muscles of the hand.
- The thumb is flexed against the hand.
- The hand appears flexed and dropping.

Evaluate the symptoms of *median nerve damage,* or *carpal tunnel syndrome:*
- There is the classical monkey paw, that is, the thumb is in adduction and extension, and cannot be opposed to touch the other fingers.
- The hand in supination, with the palm upward, cannot be easily pronated.
- On intended flexion of the hand, the index and middle fingers will not flex.
- There is muscle atrophy, particularly of the thenar eminence.
- There is anesthesia of the first three fingers and the radial aspect of the fourth; also of the dorsal aspect of the index, middle, and ring fingers.

Evaluate the symptoms of *cubital palsy (ulnar palsy):*
- The classical claw hand, with flexion and atrophy of the hands and fingers.
- Anesthesia of the ulnar border of the hand.
- Decreased transversal diameter of the hand.
- Marked intermetacarpian spaces and eminences.

Evaluate the symptoms of *musculocutaneous nerve palsy:*
- Weak and difficult flexion of the forearm against the upper arm.
- The biceps (and the anterior brachial) paralyzed; no contraction noted.
- Hypo- or anesthesia of the posteroexternal aspect of the arm.

Evaluate symptoms of the *axillary nerve palsy:*
- The arm cannot be elevated above the shoulder.
- The scapulohumeral joint easily shows all the bones.
- There is anesthesia of the deltoid area.

Evaluate the symptoms of *mononeuritis multiplex:*
- More than one nerve is affected.
- It is usually asymmetric.
- The nerves involved may be damaged simultaneously or by steps.
- Each nerve will present its own clinical picture.

Evaluate the symptoms of *polyneuritis* or *multiple neuritis:*
- It is usually symmetric.
- There is slow progression of symptoms.
- Distal extremities are mostly affected.
- There are pain and tenderness, worse at night, aggavated by stimulation.
- Paresthesias are often prominent, sometimes as the initial symptom.
- There is progressive muscular weakness, followed by wasting.
- Hypo- or areflexia is noted.
- There is impaired vibratory sense.
- Trophic changes of the skin occur.

Evaluate *Tinel's sign,* commonly used to check these cases:
- There is percussion over the nerve, usually on the divided part of it, or the adjacent area.
- A tingling sensation in the distal end of the affected limb indicates it is only a partial lesion, or there is a regeneration in the beginning.
- Wait until the acute phase of the problem is over.
- This test is also called distal tingling on percussion (D.T.P.) or formication sign.

Management of peripheral neuropathy:
- Treat each basic condition.
- Avoid toxic agents, and repeated trauma.
- Give physical therapy and symptomatic care.
- A diet with the entire B complex plus thiamine may help.
- Neurosurgery may be indicated.
- During recovery faithfully maintain all possible help.

12. Psychiatry

Schizophrenia (Dementia Praecox)

Evaluate antecedents in cases of schizophrenia:

- Many may belong to the asthenic type; they may show a genetic disposition.
- Many may belong to the schizoid personality, q.v., below; they are autistic.
- They belong to families with high (10%) incidence of the disease or its possible diagnosis.
- Many belong to lower socioeconomic classes, either initially or because they fall thereafter.
- Onset occurs in late adolescence or early adulthood; paranoid psychosis occurs later in life.
- Schizophrenic deterioration may be rapidly established, or may run unrecognized for years.

Evaluate characteristic symptoms of schizophrenia:

- Progressive social withdrawal occurs.
- There is progressive loss of personal care.
- There is awareness of deterioration of psychological traits, in the early stages of the disease; fear of becoming insane, loss of concentration.
- Ego boundaries become loose, and are finally lost; the patient perceives him- or herself as a separate entity.
- There is strong adherence to inner thoughts and beliefs, thus interfering with patient's being on good terms with the outside world.
- Association of thoughts becomes very weak; transit from thought to thought may proceed slowly, or it may shift rapidly.
- There are sexual or religious preoccupations.
- There are delusions, either persecutory or grandiose; visual hallucinations.

Evaluate additional symptoms of schizophrenia:

- There is incongruency of mood and behavior with external circumstances.
- Affections are dull and obtuse.
- There are rapidly alternating mood shifts, unrelated to the surroundings; same happens with behavior.
- Hypersensitivity to stimuli is noted.
- Ability for abstractions (concrete thinking) is lost.
- Depersonalization occurs, as if patient is a mere observer of own actions.

Evaluate delusions in schizophrenia:

- Most frequent are delusions of persecution.
- Also there are frequent delusions about sex, religion, hypochondria, etc.
- Delusions of grandeur are frequent, but they also appear in other psychiatric problems.
- There is delusional interpretation of common facts, or those related to normal life, thus creating personal delusional systems.

Evaluate disorders of thought in schizophrenia:

- Thought is neither clear nor directed to its goal; thus it is diffuse.
- Rapid shifting of thoughts causes incongruency of speech.
- Incongruency of speech is also due to distraction by fringe associations.
- Personal delusion systems make incomprehensible the exposition of thoughts.
- Some patients will complain of thought block.

Evaluate the affective state in schizophrenia:

- It is blunt, inappropriate, and incongruent.
- Patients easily present excitement, depression, anxiety, etc.

Evaluate violent behavior among schizophrenics:

- Beware of even minor agressive bursts.
- Beware of possible violence because of heard voices.
- Beware of the possibility of petty crimes.
- Beware of the risk of suicide.

Evaluate hallucinations among schizophrenics:

- Most common are auditory hallucinations.
- Not rare are hallucinations of sight, smell, touch, etc.

Evaluate catatonia in schizophrenia:

- The former catatonic schizophrenia is becoming exceedingly rare.
- Bizarre positions are maintained for long periods.
- Mannerisms of different types are relatively frequent.

Evaluate acute episodes of schizophrenia:

- Reactive schizophrenia may follow a previous good adjustment.
- In these cases, remission is easily obtained.
- They may or may not be repeated.

Evaluate schizo-affective schizophrenia:

- The prevalent symptomatology includes mood disturbances.

Do not confuse schizophrenia with:

- Primary affective disorders (mania, depression, hysteria, partial seizures).

Organic brain syndromes.
Endocrinological problems (thyroid, adrenal, pituitary).
Drug-induced psychoses (amphetamines, corticosteroids).

Management of schizophrenia:
Antipsychotics are the drugs of choice.
Adjuvant medications are frequently needed.
Discuss hospitalization.
Use a psychological approach.

Paranoia

The basic traits of paranoia are:
A mental disorder built in an apparently logical form.
Ambitions and suspicions as the basic elements.

Evaluate symptoms of paranoid schizophrenia:
There are delusions of persecution.
There are delusions of grandeur.
Hallucinations occur, related to the type of delusion.
The rest of the psychological mechanism may be in good condition, and even work at a very high level.
The disease starts in young adulthood.

Evaluate symptoms of brief paranoid states:
Reactive paranoia among those who are hypersensitive, insecure, suspicious, and have an inferiority complex.
Possibly due to exacerbating problems such as deafness, alcoholism, sexual conflicts (homosexuality), etc.

Evaluate the symptoms of true paranoid psychoses:
Delusions are elaborated in highly apparent logical systems.
Disorganized thinking may progress to frank schizophrenia.
It is relatively frequent that the delusional system centers on some physical defect, either existent or imagined.
Consider also systems built on imagined injustices, religious fanaticism, sexual jealousy (Othello syndrome), and the like.
Beware of the consequences possibly leading to physical assault.

Do not confuse paranoia with:
Mania (less sustained, and with more vacillations).

Management of paranoia:
Hospitalization to be discussed.
Psychotherapy.
Phenothiazines.

Manic-Depressive Psychosis

Evaluate factors favoring the development of manic-depressive psychosis:
It occurs twice as frequently in women as in men.
The disease may start at any age, but more frequently in the thirties, or in the fifties.
Families will present 10 to 15% of close relatives with similar problems.
Genetically, there are the unipolar type (recurrent depression), with later onset of the disease and fewer relatives with symptoms; and the bipolar type (cycles of mania and depression), of younger patients with more relatives similarly affected.
It is more frequent among the higher socioeconomic groups.
Influences of a cultural or family type may also predispose to any of the unipolar or bipolar types.
Most patients are short of stature and of relatively stocky build, that is, belong to the pyknic type, and to the cyclothymic personality type.

Evaluate symptoms of depression, that is, of the depressive phase of the disease:
Rapid onset, with swift progress.
Loss of self-esteem.
Loss of courage, confidence, and hope; different from unhappiness.
Milder symptoms as of apathy, emotional emptiness, or inertia.
Worse feelings during morning; some improvement as the day advances.
Little interest in the outside world.
Lack of response to company or surrounding changes.
Withdrawal from society.
Lack of power of concentration.
Lack of emotional response to others.
Decreased work drive and productivity.
Ideas of guilt and self-reproach, even for minor causes either present or past.
More severe symptoms of delusions of unpleasant or guilt type.
Great risk of suicide (early stages, or during recovery).
Also, risk of murdering close relatives.
Early waking.
Loss of weight.
Lack of appetite, constipation.
Decreased sexual drive.
Psychomotor retardation (speech, movement).
It is important to note that depression may mix with anxiety.

Evaluate the symptoms of involutional melancholia:
It occurs in the elderly patient.
Patient presents an unhappy and depressed emotional state.
There is an abnormal inhibition of mental and bodily activities.
The hypochondriacal reactions are associated with anxiety and other evidence of depression.

Evaluate the symptoms of mania, that is, of the manic phase of the disease:
In about 50% of the patients, occurrence of a previous brief (for only a few days) episode of depression.
Apparent sense of well being, energy, and overactivity.
Great self-confidence and disinhibition.
Excessive gaiety and garrulity, with tactless remarks and advances.

Hostility and resentment when the patient's points of view are questioned.
Delusions of grandeur and decreased sense of judgment, which may cause embarrassing situations.
Diminished sleep span during the disease.
Neglected food intake or other needs that may cause severe inconvenience.
A final stage of the disease that may lead to paranoid psychosis.
The duration of the manic stage is variable; 60% of these cases show a following phase of depression (with a not too great risk of suicide).

Evaluate the symptoms of hypomania:
This may be considered an intermediate state between the cyclothymic personality and the full form of manic-depressive psychosis.
It is more frequent than the disease itself.
Symptoms are almost the same, but considerably milder.
There are mood elevation, overactivity, and heightened energy.
Irritability is frequent; so is distractability.
There is a complete lack of severe symptoms, particularly delusional ones.

The evolution of the disease is characterized as follows:
Depressive phases may last up to 9 months.
Manic phases may last up to 6 months.
Recurrences of the phases are relatively common (80%), particularly with elderly patients, who present longer attacks.
Between attacks the patient is completely well.

Management of manic-depressive psychosis:
Hospitalization is needed in the great majority of cases.
For depression, give imipramine; if there is agitation, give amitriptyline.
Use electroconvulsive therapy for severe cases.
For mania, give chlorpromazine or haloperidol (beware of parkinsonism).
Give lithium for maintenance therapy.

Schizoid Personality

Describe the schizoid personality and its management:
Introverted.
Withdrawn and solitary; always distant from others.
Emotionally cold.
Daydreaming; patients given to theoretical speculations.
Poor practical actions and activity.
Patients reticent, lacking capacity for intimacy with others.
About 40% of schizophrenics found in this personality type.
Psychotherapy (tedious, poor results).

Cyclothymic Personality

Describe the cyclothymic personality and its management:
Patients are extroverted.
These patients like the company of others.
Their mood varies between phases of mirth and gaiety, and phases of pessimistic sadness.
Each of these phases may last for weeks or even months.
In some of the patients the phase of buoyancy predominates; in the rest of them, that of gloom.
Phase changes occur periodically and predictably.
Many accept that this type of personality leads the way to manic-depressive psychosis.
Treatment is psychotherapy.

Hysterical Personality

Describe the hysterical personality:
Egocentric and histrionic.
Emotional immaturity; childish behavior.
A trend to be dependant; a need for protection and affection.
Loose relationship with others.
Poor emotional involvement with others.
Easy forgetfulness of unpleasant or discreditable experiences.

Antisocial Personality

Describe the antisocial personality:
Patient is amoral, impulsive, and irresponsible.
Patient is hostile, and aggressive; does not tolerate frustration or opposition.
Charm and plausibility are used to gain the adherence of others, but the patient will not establish affectionate relationships with them.
Most of these patients will always try to establish rules of social order.
They exhibit poor or no feelings of remorse or guilt for their antisocial behavior.
They will blame on others their antisocial failures, or even crimes.
There is frequent association with alcoholism, addiction.
These patients will not change their points of view, by failure or by punishment.
Some may commit suicide (inward aggression); some are promiscuous or present sexual deviations.
They experience social failure (work, etc.).
They have a diminished life expectancy.
Those who pass 40 years of age may stabilize.

Paranoid Personality

Describe the paranoid personality:
The hostilities they feel, they project as others being hostile toward them.
Excessively sensitive, they interpret as hostile trivial circumstances or actions.
Supposed rejection by others may lead to aggressive feelings or even aggressive behavior.

Envy and inflexibility are common.
Patients are litigious.
Their personality development is helped by personal defects (deafness, lameness, body defects, etc.).

Obsessive-Compulsive Personality

Describe the obsessive-compulsive personality:
Perfectionist, but inflexible.
Methodical, orderly, dependable.
Cautious, resistant to making own decisions and to change according to changing circumstances.
Anxiety feelings because of responsibilities.
Difficult interpersonal relationships.

Obsessional States

Evaluate antecedents in obsessional neuroses:
There is mostly an intensification of a previous obsessive-compulsive personality trait.
They are more common in girls, at about 20 years of age, more or less.
The patients know the acts are absurd and irrational, but anxiety of unfulfilled accomplishment forces them to obey.
Symptoms may be secondary to other psychiatric problems, if these occur in this type of personality.
Evaluate symptoms of obsessional states:
The traits of the obsessive-compulsive personality (q.v., above), notably exaggerated.
Characteristic establishment of obsessive rituals, namely, hand washing, fear of contamination forcing cleansing procedures, continuous checking of possible hazards (cigarettes, kitchen fires, doors and windows well closed, etc.), fear of violence against the family, etc.
Disgusting thoughts.
Disturbed sleep due to fulfillment of obsessions.
Further course of the disease may be:
Mild symptoms may fade in less than 2 years.
In more severe cases a relatively favorable control of symptoms may be achieved in less than 8 years.
Progression of symptoms may lead to some sort of incapacitation.
Management of obsessional states:
Advise psychotherapy (but not analytical!).
Try imipramine.

Alcoholism

Alcoholics will be recognized because of:
Daily ingestion of alcohol, either at social parties or as a routine before having meals; these patients may maintain some control of drinking, and it does not interfere with life.
Intoxications, frequent and destructive, interfering with work and social activities; most of them will end as employed alcoholics, or as indigent alcoholics.
Evaluate symptoms of acute alcoholic intoxication:
Drowsiness, with ataxia and nystagmus.
Disinhibition and errors of commission.
In severe cases, respiratory depression and stupor, leading to shock and final coma, from which death may ensue.
Check for the concomitant use of sedative or addictive drugs.
Organ damage seen in alcoholics:
Cirrhosis of the liver.
Peripheral neuropathy.
Gastritis and pancreatitis.
Hypoglycemia.
Nutritional deficiencies, particularly thiamine.
Cardiomyopathy.
Damage to the brain.
Evaluate alcoholic cerebral hallucinations:
They are terrifying, mostly auditory or also visual hallucinations.
They may simulate paranoid schizophrenia, q.v.
Consciousness may remain relatively clear.
They may respond to chlorpromazine or thioridazine.
Evaluate *delirium tremens,* or alcohol withdrawal syndrome:
It may occur during periods of high alcohol intake, or after a period of abstinence.
In the mild syndrome there will be only tremor, sweating, weakness, hyperreflexia, and gastrointestinal symptoms.
In true delirium tremens there are an initial anxiety attack, confusion, deep depression, sweating, and insomnia.
There are delirium, disorientation, cognitive disruption, profuse diaphoresis, fever or only febricula, restlessness, and tachycardia.
There are hallucinations (often related to terrifying animals), illusions (of performing usual tasks), vestibular disturbances of equilibrium, seizures ("rum fits"), marked ataxia, etc.
The course may last for a few days to 2 or more weeks, after an initial clearance occurring in less than 24 hours.
From 4 to 15% of the patients may die.
Describe *Wernicke's encephalopathy:*
Ataxia.
Ocular palsy.
Polyneuritis.
Describe *Korsakoff's psychosis:*
See below, in this chapter.
Management of alcoholism:
Disulfiram (not in pregnant patient or cardiac patient in decompensation).
Symptomatic treatment.
Psychological treatment.

Opiate Addiction

Evaluate symptoms of acute opiate intoxication:
Flushing and itching of the skin, and other signs of peripheral vasodilation.

Respiratory depression, even leading to massive pulmonary edema or to respiratory arrest; usually, decreased depth and rate.
Drowsiness, deep sleep, even leading to coma.
Gastrointestinal symptoms, mainly nausea and vomiting.
Pinpoint miotic pupils, hypothermia, hypotension, and bradycardia.
Those taking meperidine will not show miosis but mydriasis, and also muscular twitching, confusion, and seizures.

Evaluate the symptoms of mild opiate intoxication:
There is the so-called high, namely, euphoria, relaxation, mental cloudiness, drowsiness, and mood changes.
Dysphoria with anxiety may occur occasionally.
Nausea is relatively common, with occasional vomiting; there may be mild constipation.
Miosis may be noted.

Evaluate symptoms of opiate withdrawal:
Grade 0, after 4 hours of expected administration of the drug, shows anxiety and craving.
Grade I, after 8 hours, adds yawning, rhinorrhea, lacrimation, and perspiration.
Grade II, after 12 hours, adds mydriasis, tremors, piloerection, flashes (cold and hot), generalized aches, and anorexia.
Grade III, after 18 or 24 hours, shows the intensity of the above symptoms increased, and adds fever, tachycardia, hypertension, increased respiratory rate and depth, restlessness, insomnia, and nausea.
Grade IV, after 24 or 36 hours, shows further increase of the above symptoms, plus fetal position, vomiting, and diarrhea with a weight loss of about 2.3 kg a day (5 lb), spontaneous orgasm or simply ejaculation, etc.
In the case of methadone, the course is slower, lasts for a longer time, and may be more severe.

Evaluate complications due to opiate addiction:
Pulmonary edema, in 50% of the patients.
Infections due to contamination.
In heroin addiction, the "stiff-lung syndrome," with hypoxia and aspiration of gastric contents, possible; also, viral hepatitis.
Myositis ossificans due to unskillful manipulations.
Osteomyelitis, also due to infections from injections.
Neurologic disorders, and other disorders as well.

Management of opiate addiction:
Overdosage treated with naloxone.
Methadone substitution; and then, methadone withdrawal.
Symptomatic treatment of incidences.

Marihuana, Mariguana, or Marijuana Addiction

Evaluate symptoms provoked by smoking marijuana:
A mild intoxication will cause mild euphoria followed by sleep.
Ideation becomes disconnected, incontrollable, and flows freely.
Emotions, also, flow freely.
Memory (for recent events) and time perception are impaired.
There is conjunctival congestion.
Also impaired are color, spatial, and other perceptions.
When exaltation, joyfulness, and well-being predominate, it is called a "high."
If there are depression, fear, image distortion, hallucinations, and other panic-causing perceptions, it will be called a "bad trip."
Other symptoms may be due to other drugs used at the same time.
Contrary to popular belief, creative faculties and performing abilities are drastically diminished.

Management of marijuana effects:
No treatment is needed, in most cases.
Treat "bad trips" with haloperidol; trifluoperazine may follow.

Lysergic Acid Diethylamide and Other Hallucinogens

Evaluate the symptoms caused by the use of hallucinogens:
For 1 or 2 hours there is an initial tension, which is followed by a release, with crying or laughing.
For the next 2 or 3 hours, there are visual hallucinations with distortion of perceptions; some may feel that the ego is disintegrating.
During the next 3 or 4 hours, there are major changes in the perception of time, and in mood.
Finally, there are a feeling of detachment and a sense of destiny and control that will occur.
As in the case of marijuana, there may be "bad trips."
Effects vary somewhat according to the type of psychedelic agent.

Management of hallucinogen symptoms:
Protect the patient from injuries.
Give haloperidol; it may be followed by trifluoperazine.

Barbiturate Addiction

Evaluate the symptoms caused by barbiturates:
Drowsiness and sleepiness.
Respiratory depression, ataxia, dysarthria, and nystagmus.
Errors of commission that may result in accidents.
Difficult thinking, slow speech, diminished attention, impaired memory, and freedom from inhibitions.

Evaluate the symptoms due to overdosage:
Marked increase of the above symptoms.
Hypotension, and decreased gastrointestinal activity.
Neurological symptoms, namely, positive Babinski, miosis followed by mydriasis, stupor, shock, and coma that may lead to death.

Evaluate symptoms due to barbiturate withdrawal:
- Restlessness and anxiety.
- Nausea, vomiting, abdominal cramps, anorexia.
- Myoclonic or spasmodic contractions of the limbs, tremors, increasing irritability, seizures, delirium, and hallucinations.
- Paranoid reactions, q.v., above.
- Orthostatic hypotension, muscular weakness.

Management of barbiturate intoxication:
- Symptomatic care for mild cases.
- Maintenance of respiration, gastric lavage in the case of ingestion, parenteral fluids.
- Hemodialysis or peritoneal dialysis.

Cocaine Addiction

Evaluate symptoms of cocaine use:
- Because of the short effects of the drug, repeated intravenous injections the usual form of administration.
- Violent behavior (the patient may be dangerous).
- Hallucinations and delusion of a paranoid type (q.v., above).
- Extreme nervousness, sleeplessness, and miniaturized hallucinations.
- Mydriasis, tachycardia, and hypertension; also, rapid respirations.
- Muscle twitching, and formication ("cocaine bugs").

Evaluate the symptoms due to an overdose of cocaine:
- Tremors and convulsions, of a temporal lobe pattern.
- Delirium.
- Cardiovascular collapse or respiratory failure, which may cause death.
- Restlessness, and irregular respirations.

Management of cocaine intoxication:
- Use washing and lavage to remove the drug; may try emesis.
- Apply tourniquet or ice pack to delay absorption.
- Give symptomatic care.
- May discontinue the addictive substance abruptly.

Insomnia

Evaluate induction and symptoms of this frequent condition:
- Insomnia consists of obtaining an insufficient amount of sleep.
- Very rarely there will be total insomnia.
- There may be initial insomnia, when the patient delays falling sleep.
- There may be late insomnia, when the patient wakes up earlier than usual.
- Schizophrenia and manic-depressive psychosis may cause any form of insomnia, even total insomnia.
- Medical situations that cause pain will cause insomnia at the peak of pain, particularly frequent micturition due to prostatic enlargement, leg cramps, etc.
- Emotional problems of any kind mainly provoke initial insomnia.
- A depressive situation will mainly cause late insomnia.

Management of insomnia:
- Treat the causative factor.
- Beware of suicide attempts indicated by the patient seeking sedatives.

Depressive Neurosis (Reactive Depression)

Reactive depression consists of:
- A neurotic reaction in response to adverse external circumstances.
- The adverse circumstance may be a sudden one or a long-acting depressive situation.
- The reaction is unduly prolonged.

Evaluate symptoms of depressive neurosis:
- Depression is a feeling of dejection, a lowered mood with mild sadness or intense guilt and hopelessness.
- Thinking becomes difficult; patient shows poor concentration, lack of decisiveness.
- There is loss of interest in the surroundings; constant unhappiness.
- Patient has diminished capacity for work and for recreation.
- Fatigue, diminished appetite may occur.
- There may be diminished sexual drive.
- There is some sort of irritability and anxiety.

Patients do not usually recognize depressive neurosis as a disease, but believe it to be a normal psychological reaction; actual differences are:
- Normal depression can be counteracted by rationalizing the situation.
- In depressive neurosis the reaction is usually disproportionate in relation to its cause.
- Depressive symptoms cannot be shaken off easily, as a normal psychological reaction.
- Depressive neurosis may be somewhat long-lasting; but in constrast to depressive psychosis, the mood may improve with congenial company or improved circumstances.

Management of depressive neurosis:
- Psychotherapy; amitriptyline.

Anxiety Neurosis

How anxiety neurosis may be classified:
- Simple anxiety.
- Hyperventilation syndrome.
- Phobias.
- Obsessions and compulsions.
- Dissociative states.
- Conversion reactions.

Simple anxiety is characterized by:
- Sudden onset of fear, and a sense of impending doom, apprehension, uncertainty.

Tension, breathlessness, and restlessness; initial insomnia.
Hyperventilation.
Fatigue, and chronic irritability; lack of concentration.
Hypertension, tachycardia, palpitations, sweating.
Feeling of anger, and dislike of social gatherings.
Secondary depression may occur.

Hyperventilation syndrome consists of:
Attacks of deep tachypnea.
Numbness, and tingling of the skin.
Dizziness, and trembling.
Cramps, which may increase to tetanic spasms.
Vertigo, faintness, and even syncope.

Phobic states may be described as follows:
There is anxiety or fear aroused by a situation or an object to which the true sensation has been transferred or displaced.
Usually, phobic states show an increase in scope, intensity, and number.
Nevertheless, there are monosymptomatic phobias, such as those referring to animals, numbers, and the like.
The extremely large number of words ending with "-phobia" clearly express the variety of these situations.

Obsessions and *compulsions* are characterized as follows:
Repetitive thoughts of a fearful or other irrational content constitute an obsession.
The need to perform a needless or an irrational act constitutes a compulsion.
Usually, the patient recognizes the absurdity of the obsession or the compulsion, and may try to resist it.
If resisted, they create an intense feeling of anxiety, which only can be relieved by the performance of the act.

Dissociative states are characterized as follows:
A form of isolation and repression may help to keep the patient away from any unpleasant situation.
Fugue is a simple dissociative state.
Also, there are amnesia, somnambulism, and multiple personalities.
Symptoms may resemble those of temporal lobe dysfunction.
The condition may last for hours or days.

Conversion reactions are described as follows:
Psychic problems are converted into physical symptoms.
Hysteria is the main source of conversion reactions.

Management of these disorders:
Psychotherapy, and the use of sedatives and minor tranquilizers.

Situational Disorders

Evaluate the stress response syndrome:
The stress response more dependent on the stability of the subject than on the nature of the stress.
Anxiety and/or depression, even with agitation.
Fear, or a sensation of anger or guilt.
Urinary frequency, even with incontinence.
Diarrhea.
Hyperventilation, tachycardia, hypertension.
Restlessness, anxious appearance, tremors, dry mouth.
Mydriasis.

Management of situational disorders consists of:
Psychotherapy; use of mild sedation.

Hysteria

This abused term today refers mainly to:
Conversion and dissociative reactions.

Symptoms of hysteria:
Most cases are women in their middle adult life.
Case usually present a past history of numerous medical and surgical complaints, and present the hysterical personality (q.v., above).
There is also a history of nightmares, enuresis, sleepwalking, phobias, etc., during childhood and early youth.
Conversion symptoms may be of different types, such as blindness, deafness, aphonia, paralysis of a limb, paresthesias, etc.
The classical globus hystericus consists of a subjective sensation of a lump in the throat, sometimes accompanied with a feeling of choking.
A fugue is characterized by amnesia and denial of personal identity.
Symptoms of multiple personalities may also be presented.
Complaints of multiple symptoms may lead to a lifestyle of medical and surgical modalities even reaching the Briquet's syndrome; this syndrome is characterized by shortness of breath and aphonia, due to hysterical paralysis of the diaphragm.

Management of hysteria:
It depends largely on the previous training of the physician, since different modalities of treatment have been advocated.

Sexual Dysfunctions

The different dysfunctions are characterized by:
Decreased sexual drive.
Increased sexual drive.
Homosexuality, and transsexualism.
Pedophilia.
Bestiality.
Necrophilia.
Varied sexual practices.

Evaluate reasons for *decreased* or even *absent sexual drive:*
Genetic or endocrinological diseases, particulary hypogonadism.
Aging.

Abuse of depressant drugs.
Psychological or psychiatric problems.
Diseases that may debilitate, that impair local organs, or are painful.
Deviated preoccupations, or diminished stimulation.
Problems leading to frigidity and impotence.

Evaluate reasons for abnormally *increased sexual drive:*
Abuse of disinhibiting drugs, or androgens.
Hypergonadism.
Central nervous system diseases (hypothalamic or other lesions of the frontal or temporal regions).
Psychiatric problems.

Evaluate *homosexuality:*
Concepts have been changing drastically in recent years; it may not be a criminal offense, but it is not normal.
Bisexuals who have relations with either sex are considered homosexuals who have not "come out"; later on they may set a preference.

Evaluate *transsexualism:*
There is the desire to deny and reverse one's actual sex.
Symptoms may start early in childhood, and may become obsessive in later years, even to consummation of surgical procedures.

Pedophilia is characterized as follows:
There is sexual preference for children, usually experienced by men.
In most instances it is a homosexual manifestation because mostly male children are preferred.

Evaluate manifestations of *bestiality:*
Copulation with animals may mark a severe psychic disturbance.
It will not be so severely evaluated when it happens sporadically in early youth (experimentation) or during drastic deprivation of other sex object.

Evaluate manifestations of *necrophilia:*
Copulation with a dead body usually reveals a severe psychic aberration.

Evaluate *other varied* sexual practices:
Incestuous relations may reveal culturally or socially aberrant situations.
Voyeurism, viewing sex acts or nude bodies, also represents a failure of adequate sexual development.
Sadism (to inflict pain) or masochism (to suffer pain) taken to an excess reveals a dangerous psychiatric problem.
Exhibitionism, exposing the body or the genitals, also reveals a deviation of sexual development.

Management of these problems:
If there is a cause, treat it directly.
Sedatives or tranquilizers may be used at times.
Psychological and behavioral approach may also be used.

Hypochondria

The main characterization of hypochondria is:
Patient irrationally believes self to be sick or to present any other body dysfunction.

The usual symptoms of hypochondria:
Evidence of anxiety neurosis is found in a large number of patients.
History of the obsessive-compulsive personality may be present.
Symptoms of any known disease may be shown, mostly cardiac, venereal, tumoral, cerebral, intestinal, and the like; of course, there is no physical basis for patients' allegations.
Hypochondriacs may also take excessive care of their bodies, with gymnastic rituals, dietary fads, cleansing purgations, and the like.

Management of hypochondria:
Psychotherapy; and also treat anxiety.

Psychosomatic Problems

How psychosomatic problems become apparent:
Directly or indirectly, psychological factors may contribute to the etiology of physical disorders.
Physical disorders may also contribute to the appearance of psychological symptoms.
A practical approach is to consider psychological factors when they do present some etiological influence on physical problems.

Evaluate clinical possibilities of psychosomatic problems:
Symptoms may involve one or more than one organ system.
These symptoms must correlate with psychological stress.
Usually, subjective complaints largely exceed objective findings.
Not rarely, similar problems will be presented by other members of the family.

Evaluate psychological factors as etiological agents:
They are mostly indirect factors.
Any disease, either acute or chronic, may react to psychological factors imposed by the same disease; consider diabetes.
Psychological factors may contribute indirectly to the development of true diseases; consider smoking.

Evaluate the physical reflection of psychological factors:
Symptoms are truly felt, but usually atypically distributed or of a bizarre expression.
Psychogenic pain is among the most frequent symptoms; it may also be due to depression.
Beware of masked anxiety or depression.

Evaluate the psychological reaction to disease:
Depression may aggravate a chronic or acute disease, thus creating a vicious circle.
Given an antidepressive drug, in such cases.

Munchausen's Syndrome

Evaluate this exaggerated, dramatic, and seemingly convincing trend to repeated fabrication of illnesses:
It is not a simply dishonest simulation that must be implicated in most of these patients.

They are quite intelligent, may show histrionic features of their personality, and are resourceful in their simulations.

They can produce the clinical picture of almost any disease.

Management of Munchausen's syndrome:

Psychotherapy.

Organic Brain Syndrome (OBS)

The usual symptoms of organic brain syndrome are:

Cognitive impairment, mostly including the following.

Attention span that is short or may fluctuate.

Disorientation, in both time and space.

Loss of recent memory; impaired capacity for recall.

Thinking, reasoning, judgment that are also impaired.

Defective sensation and perception; also defective and labile temperament, mood, and emotion.

Visual hallucinations, and delusions.

Confabulation, mainly (but not only) noted in alcoholism.

Depression, better noted in less than moderate types.

Defective initiative, drive, and insight.

Possible accompanying symptoms of the causative factor.

Also neurotic or psychotic syndromes may occur.

The usual causes of organic brain syndrome are:

Infections, either acute or chronic.

Intoxications, mostly of any kind, but particularly alcohol, addictive drugs, tranquilizers and antidepressants, etc.

Drug withdrawal.

Trauma, mainly injuries to the head.

Cardiovascular disorders, mainly those involving the central nervous system.

Metabolic disturbances, involving a large number.

Degenerative diseases, such as parkinsonism, multiple sclerosis, and others.

Tumors (neoplastic) of the central nervous system.

Others, such as collagen diseases, immunologic diseases, etc.

Management of organic brain syndrome:

Consider the acute initial onset reversible.

Consider all long-lasting situations irreversible.

Treat reversible problems according to the cause.

Always give overall good care to these patients.

Dementia

This progressive and irreversible cerebral insufficiency shows the following characteristics:

An organic factor is mostly found as the cause of the problem.

The evaluation is in most instances a matter of clinical judgment.

Earlier symptoms may vary and depend on the affected brain area.

There is a slow deterioration of all intellectual functions, including personality, emotions, behavior, etc., that is, all cognitive functions become impaired.

Organic nervous functions may also be impaired, such as speech, motor activity, perceptions, etc.

Symptoms usually start mild, and at times difficult to evaluate, but they progress to be unbearable with time.

Relations with family and peers change, affects become superficial, irritability increases, activities are contrary to common sense, etc.

Some form of depression is a common finding.

Neurologic symptoms will occur in accordance with the site of the basic lesion.

Evaluate symptoms of some the causes of dementia:

In *Huntington's chorea* symptoms may start at any age, but mostly between 35 and 50 years.

Choreoathetoid movements may initiate the clinical picture.

Also, initial symptoms may be personality and behavioral changes.

Gait may become wide-based, and prancing.

Paranoic symptoms are common; also euphoria or violence.

With progress of the disease, the patient becomes disabled.

Children of one affected parent are at 50% risk, the fate unknown until later in life.

In *normal* or *low pressure hydrocephalus* symptoms start at middle age.

There may be history of a previous meningitis, encephalitis, or head injury; a few cases may be due to tumors.

Average symptomatology of dementia is found, plus shuffling gait.

It may improve with a shunt.

In *chronic progressive traumatic encephalopathy* there is a history of repetitive cranial injury.

Symptoms of dementia occur; boxers may show the syndrome, which is progressive, even when they abandon boxing.

Other causes may also account for dementia, such as hypovitaminoses of the B complex, multiple sclerosis, myxedema, alcoholism, intracranial hemorrhages, poisoning (particularly lead or carbon monoxide), and also other possibilities.

Alzheimer's Disease (Presenile Dementia)

Clinical evaluation of Alzheimer's disease, or presenile dementia, shows:

It usually begins close to 50 years of age.

Symptoms are those quoted for dementia, q.v., above.

The clinical picture resembles that of senile dementia, profound and rapid.

The outstanding fact is the earlier onset of the disease.

Memory shows a rapid and deep deterioration.

There is excessive talking, without any sense.
Excessive dirtiness is noted.
Management of presenile dementia:
Supportive and symptomatic.

Pick's Disease (Lobar Atrophy)

Clinical evaluation of Pick's disease:
Essentially, the same as Alzheimer's disease.
Pathology makes the principal difference between both diseases.
Specialists may find small differences, enough for a clinical differentiation.
Management of Pick's disease:
Supportive and symptomatic.

Senile Dementia

Evaluate symptoms due to the loss of cells from the cerebral cortex and other areas of the brain:
Onset is mostly in the late seventies, and more frequent among women.
There is a steady, inexorable progress of symptoms, to be completed and maximal in about 2 or 3 years.
There is mostly some evidence of organic brain syndrome, q.v., above.
Common symptoms are irritability, depression, and paranoid ideation.
It may start with loss of recent memory, while remote memory is better preserved, at least for a while.
There is spasmodic laughter or crying.
There are egotism, fear (of death), greediness, suspiciousness.
Finally total deterioration occurs.
Management of senile dementia:
Supportive, and symptomatic.

Transient Global Amnesia

Evaluation of transient global amnesia:
There is severe loss of recent memory.
Confusion, and disorientation in time and space are noted.
Attacks last for minutes or hours.
Attacks may recur.
There may be previous episodes of mild cloudiness of consciousness.
Most attacks will occur in elderly men.
Management of transient global amnesia:
Try to improve causative cerebral ischemia due to vertebro-basilar involvement.

Sclerotic Dementia

Evaluate the symptoms of arteriosclerotic dementia:
Most patients are men in their late sixties or early seventies.
There is evidence of arteriosclerosis of the cerebral vessels.
The vessels of the neck may show greater evidence of sclerosis.
Evidence of cerebral infarctation may also be shown.
Hypertension is a frequent finding.
Intellectual, personality, and emotional changes are less marked than in senile dementia, and other forms of dementia, at least at onset.
Symptoms progress in a steplike manner.
Depression is common; beware of suicide.
Organic symptoms may also appear, such as hemiplegia, parkinsonism, etc.
Management of sclerotic dementia:
Prophylactically, treat hypertension and hypercholesterolemia.
Try to improve circulation, whenever possible, by surgical means.
Otherwise, give supportive and symptomatic care.

Creutzfeldt-Jakob Disease (Subacute Spongiform Encephalopathy)

Evaluate the clinical aspects of this disease:
It is caused by a slow viral infection.
The disease runs a subacute course.
Myotonic attacks are frequent.
There are also ataxia, visual symptoms, and pyramidal or extrapyramidal features.
Symptoms of dementia are progressive.
Management of this disease:
Symptomatic and supportive.

Korsakoff's Psychosis (Dysmnesic Syndrome)

Situations that usually precede Korsakoff's psychosis are:
Chronic alcoholism.
Head injury, including neurosurgery procedures.
Cerebral tumors of the invasive type.
Bilateral infarction.
Acute necrotic encephalitis from herpes simplex.
Subarachnoid hemorrhage.
Consider the central feature of the disease:
There is total loss of recent memory; incapacity to learn the easiest skill.
Guidance by remote memory may give the idea that there is not any intellectual loss.
Other symptoms of Korsakoff's psychosis are:
Confabulation, that is, the ready answer regardless of truth, which may even appear convincing.
Disorientation, particularly in time.
Little response to events, even those eliciting responsibility or causing fear.
No feelings of distress because of the sickness.
Prognosis dependent on the cause: good in head injury and subarachnoid hemorrhage; bad in alcoholism and other forms of irreversible lesion.

Possibly also hallucinations, falsification of memory, and some evidence of polyneuritis, such as wrist-drop, etc.

Management of Korsakoff's psychosis:

Treat the causative factor.

Give symptomatic and supportive care.

Frontal Lobe Syndrome

Evaluate the core of the clinical picture of frontal lobe syndrome:

Emotions and inhibition are markedly decreased.

There is impairment or loss of foresight.

Patient becomes an extroverted version of himself.

Other symptoms of the disease are:

The patient becomes unreliable, either among the family or at work.

The patient becomes careless, and habits deteriorate.

There is lack of concentration and of continuity in any task.

Inopportune euphoria or persistent indifference is noted.

Insight is lost.

The patient deteriorates, though he will not complain (but the family will complain a lot).

There may be an ulterior course to dementia.

What are the most common causes of frontal lobe lesions?

Degenerative diseases.

Cerebral tumors.

Head injuries.

General paresis.

Management of frontal lobe syndrome:

Treat the causative condition.

Give symptomatic and supportive care.

13. Mental Retardation

Mental Retardation

Mental retardation is characterized as follows:
- Intelligence is below accepted averages.
- Social competence is also below average.
- There is a gradation for both defects.
- Borderline retardation is encountered in 14% of the population.
- Frank mental retardation is found in 3% of the population, only fewer than 1.5% of the cases are identified.
- I.Q. under 50 is present in 36 children out of 10,000.

Usual causes of mental retardation:
- In the great majority of patients (80%) the cause is unknown.
- Prenatal conditions include chromosomal defects, hereditary disorders, infections, or accidents before birth.
- Perinatal complications may also cause retardation.
- Postnatal diseases may cause retardation when they affect the normal physiology of the brain; malnutrition is an important factor.

Evaluation of the grade of retardation:
- Borderline retardation shows an I.Q. between 84 and 71; these persons are slow learners and make up about one seventh of the total population.
- Mild retardation shows an I.Q. between 70 and 50; these persons are educable, and even may learn to read.
- Moderately retarded persons, with an I.Q. between 49 and 35, may speak, are trainable, but cannot live independently.
- The severely retarded, I.Q. between 34 and 20, are only minimally trainable.
- Finally, the profoundly retarded, I.Q. below 19, will not even be able to walk, and at most will learn only a few words, if we do not want to call them merely sounds.

Mongolism (Down's Syndrome, Trisomy 21)

Evaluate the incidence of mongolism:
- There is one mongoloid born in each 700 births (close to 300,000 in the United States).
- Younger mothers will give birth to one in each 2,000 live births.
- Older mothers will have more children with the defect; mothers over 35 years of age will have about 50% of all mongoloids.

Evaluate symptoms of mongolism:
- There is mild or moderate retardation.
- Mongoloids have brachycephaly, flat bridge of the nose, and slanted eyes with epicanthal fold (which is different from that of Orientals).
- There is an open mouth, usually with a protruding tongue; the tongue is large.
- The tongue is furrowed; it lacks the central fissure.
- Hands and feet are short and broad.
- Hands have only one palmar crease (simian crease); fingers are short, and the 5th presents clinodactyly, or with internal incurvation.
- Feet present a wide gap between the great and 2nd toes; and a plantar furrow extending backward.
- Mongoloids are of short stature.
- They are usually friendly, and love rhythm and music.
- When born, they appear hypotonic and placid, rarely cry, and will present Brushfield's spots like salt grains in the periphery of the iris; these spots may persist almost through life, or may disappear at about 1 year of age.
- There are characteristic dermatoglyphics (dermal prints).
- Hip bones show decreased acetabular and iliac angles.
- Congenital heart diseases are prone to occur among mongoloids.
- Watch for acute leukemia.

Management of mongoloids:
- Special education and care.

Klinefelter's Syndrome (XXXY Syndrome)

Evalute the incidence of Klinefelter's syndrome:
- One in 700 live male births will be affected.
- One out of 50 institutionalized patients will present the syndrome.

Evaluate symptoms of Klinefelter's syndrome:
- Clinical diagnosis is made after puberty is reached.
- Patients are of tall stature, with eunuchoid proportions.
- Testes are small and firm.
- Gynecomastia is frequent.

Retardation is usually mild to borderline; some patients may be of almost normal intelligence.
There is a Barr body, as if the person were a female.
Patient is infertile.

Turner's Syndrome (Agenesia Ovarica, XO Syndrome)

Evaluate the incidence of this gonadal dysgenesis:
There will be one in 3,000 live female births.
Evaluate symptoms corresponding to Turner's syndrome:
At birth, most infants will show a marked lymphedema of hands and feet.
If there is also, at this time, a loose fold of skin on each side of the neck, the diagnosis is almost sure.
The webbing of the neck is more evident with most adult patients.
Patient has a wide, shield-like chest, with broadly spaced nipples.
Patient is of short stature, usually below 5 feet.
Not all cases present mental retardation; but retardation may be of the mild to moderate type.
Other symptoms that may also be presented by these patients:
Multiple pigmented nevi.
Hypoplastic nails, and short 4th metacarpals.
Organic malformations, such as coarctation of the aorta, renal anomalies, etc.
Evaluate the usual symptoms of ovarian infantilism occuring in the disease:
Infantile external genitalia.
Infantile internal genitals, and lack of ovaries.
No breast development, nor development of sex hair.
Amenorrhea, and infertility.
Management of cases with Turner's syndrome:
Use of estrogens.
Removal of streaks or abnormal forms of ovarian residues, which may undergo neoplastic transformation.

Klinefelter-Mongolism Polysyndrome

Evaluate this possible combination:
It has been found to be more frequent than is indicated by figures obtained by estimation from incidence of both diseases.
Symptoms of both diseases mix in each particular patient.
Mental retardation exists in all cases.
Treat as for mongolism.

Turner-Mongolism Polysyndrome

Evaluate this possible combination:
Symptoms of both diseases mix in each particular case.
The diagnosis can be made from clinical evidence.
Mental retardation has been noted in all cases reported.
Treat as for Turner and mongolism.

The XXX Syndrome

Evaluate this possible situation:
The patient will present two Barr bodies.
There is mental retardation in an apparently normally developed woman.
It may appear in 12 or 13 out of 10,000 normal females, in routine surveys of newborns.
A few patients will present absence of secondary sex characters.
Also, some may present menstrual disturbances.

The XXXX Syndrome

Evaluate this possible situation:
Patient will present three Barr bodies.
Patient will be an apparently normal female, with mental retardation.

The XXXXX Syndrome

Evaluate this possible situation:
Patient will present four Barr bodies.
Mental retardation is present.
There will be mongoloid features, mainly noted in the face and the simian crease.
There may be skeletal defects.

The XXXY Syndrome

Evaluate this possible combination:
An apparent male will present two Barr bodies.
The clinical syndrome will be that of Kilnefelter's.
Mental retardation will be more marked.
There will be testicular atrophy.

The XXXXY Syndrome

Evaluate this possible situation:
An apparent male will present three Barr bodies.
Mental retardation will be marked.
The face will present some traits similar to mongolism.
There will be external hypoplastic genitals.
There will also be skeletal defects.

The XYY Syndrome

Evaluate this possible situation:
Mental retardation possible, but of the mild or moderate type.
Large stature, above 6 feet.
Cryptorchidia.
Irregular teeth.
Radioulnar synostosis.

The XYYY Syndrome

Evaluate this possible situation:
Mental retardation, together with motor retardation, both of the mild to moderate type.

Cryptorchidia.
Simian crease on hands.
Dental dysplasia.
Pulmonary stenosis, and inguinal hernia.

Deletion Syndromes

Evaluate the clinical features of these deletions of autosomal chromosomes:

4p–, constituting Wolf's syndrome, shows severe retardation, markedly delayed growth, seizures, midline scalp defects, abnormal facies, and hypospadias.

5p–, the cri-du-chat syndrome, is characterized by a high-pitched catlike cry, this only present during a brief time after birth, a grotesque appearance of the face with wide-set, antimongoloid slanting eyes and a broad-based nose, microcephalia, micrognathia, short neck, syndactyly, etc. Retardation is very severe.

8q– shows mental retardation, anomalies of the ribs and the vertebrae, and limited joint mobility.

13q– presents both mental and physical retardation, microcephaly, broad base of the nose, hypertelorism, eye defects, webbing of the neck which is short, hypoplastic or absent thumbs, and other defects.

21q– also presents mental and growth retardation, skeletal defects that include microcephaly, abnormal facies that include antimongoloid slant, palebral fissures, hypotonia.

22q– is characterized by mental retardation, microcephaly, abnormal facies, syndactyly, and hypotonia.

Trisomy 8

Evaluate the clinical features of trisomy 8:
Mental retardation, mild to moderate.
Speech delayed and badly articulated.
Unusually deep palmar and plantar creases characteristic.
Stature normal; pateints are slender.
Skeletal abnormalities, mainly of ribs, vertebrae, and patellae.
Large and asymmetric head.
Strabismus, and low-set, dysplastic ears.
Contractures, and limitations of movement.

Management of trisomy 8:
Symptomatic, and supportive.

Trisomy 9

Evaluate the clinical features of trisomy 9:
Mental retardation, worse than moderate.
Microcephaly and abnormal facies.
Small palpebral fissures, low-set ears, prominent nose.
Cryptorchidia, and small penis.
Long flexed fingers.
Congenital heart disease, of a severe type.
Dislocation of hips.

Trisomy 13 (Patau's Syndrome)

Evaluate the clinical features of Patau's syndrome:
There is mental retardation, worse than severe.
It occurs once in 5,000 births.
There is a low birth weight.
Most (70%) die before 6 months of age; few (less than 20%) survive 1 year.
During the first months there are apneic spells.
There are skull and cerebral malformations, such as microcephaly, sloping forehead, wide sutures and fontanels, forebrain not divided (holoprosencephaly), abnormal olfactory bulbs, etc.; also cleft lip or palate.
Half of the cases will present myelomeningocele.
There is frequent deafness; ears are ill-shaped and low-set.
Patients have abnormal facies, with microphthalmia, colobomas, retinal dysplasia, shallow supraorbital ridges, slanted eyes.
There are congenital heart defects, such as interventricular opening, patent ductus arteriosus, anomalous heart valves, and others; these defects will be present in about 80% of the cases.
Hands will show flexed fingers, hyperconvex and narrow fingernails, frequent polydactyly, and simian crease.
Feet show rocker-bottom shape and posterior prominence of heels.
There are cryptorchidism and abnormal scrotum.
Bicornuate uterus is found.
Other middle-line defects may include hemangiomas, dermal sinuses, webbing of the neck, etc.

Trisomy 18 (Edward's Syndrome)

Evaluate the clinical features of Edward's syndrome:
Mental retardation, worse than severe.
One in 3,000 live births; three times more females affected.
Low birth weight; during gestation very little activity.
Skeletal muscles and subcutaneous fat hypoplastic.
General hypotonia, and weak cry.
Microcephaly, prominent occiput, narrow bifrontal diameter, hypoplasia of the orbital ridges, micrognathia.
Small palpebral fissures, epicanthus, low-set abnormal ears, small mouth, cleft lip or palate.
Overall aspect of the face as if it were pinched with large tongs or pliers.
Characteristic clenched fist with the thumb overlapping 3rd and 4th fingers; but the thumb may be absent.
Distal crease of 5th finger absent.
Hypoplastic nails, syndactyly, and other foot abnormalties.
Congenital heart disease, such as ventricular or atrial defects, valvular abnormalities; also congenital defects of the lungs, the diaphragm, or the urinary tract.

Cryptorchidia, and hernias; webbing of the neck is not rare.
Survival for more than a few months is rare.

Trisomy 21 (Mongolism or Down's Syndrome)

For information, see above in this chapter.

Trisomy 22

Evaluate symptoms of partial trisomy 22, or cat-eye syndrome:
- Characteristic coloboma of the iris.
- More than severe mental and motor retardation.
- Other eye defects, such as hypertelorism, antimongoloid slanting.
- Abnormal ears, with preauricular tags or fistulas.
- Congenital heart disease.
- Anal atresia.

Evaluate symptoms of full trisomy 22:
- Mental retardation.
- Retarded growth.
- Microcephaly with micrognathia.
- Abnormal facies.
- Abnormal thumbs.
- General hypotonia.

Other Autosomal Disorders

Evaluate other autosomal disorders not yet mentioned, which are also accompanied by mental retardation:
- *1q+,* with micrognathia and peaked nose, long and tapering fingers, small, enlarged or absent thymus, and congenital heart disease.
- *4p+,* with growth retardation, microcephaly, abnormal facies, and abnormal vertebrae and pelvis.
- *4q+,* with low birth weight, hypotonia, and early closure of fontanels.
- *7q+,* with low birth weight, abnormal facies, wide fontanels, fuzzy hair, kyphoscoliosis, dislocated hips, or other skeletal anomalies.
- *9p+,* with microcephaly, brachycephaly, abnormal facies, and hypoplastic phalanges.
- *10q+,* with severe motor and growth retardation, abnormal facies, and abnormal digits with webbing and wide spacing.
- *11p+,* with abnormal facies, strabismus, and generalized hypotonia.
- *11q+,* with low birth weight, abnormal facies, and congenital heart and kidney disease.
- *14q+,* with microcephaly, abnormal facies, seizures, and failure to thrive.
- *15q+,* with severe motor retardation, abnormal facies, strabismus, seizures, and general hypotonia; growth is normal.

Cretinism

For information, see the chapter devoted to endocrinology.

Phenylketonuria

Hartnup Disease

Maple Syrup Urine Disease

Homocystinuria

Hydroxykynurinemia

Histidinemia

Hypermethininemia

Carnosinemia

Hyperammoniemia

Isovaleric Acidemia

Argininosuccinic Acidemia

Hypervalinemia

Citrulinemia

Hyperglycinemia

Hypersarcosinemia

Hyperprolinemia

Lysine Intolerance

Hyperlysinemia

For information on the above diseases, see the chapter devoted to metabolism and nutrition.

Methylmalonic Acidemia

Evaluate clinical features of methylmalonic acidemia:
- Mental retardation.
- Physical retardation.
- Evidence of acidosis.
- Lethargy that may lead to coma.

Management of methylmalonic acidemia:
- A diet low in protein, particularly including restriction for isoleucine, valine, and threonine.
- Large doses of vitamin B_{12} (cyanocobalamine).

Propionicacidemia

Evaluate clinical features of propionicacidemia:
- Mental retardation.
- Physical retardation.
- Evidence of acidosis.
- Lethargy that may lead to coma.

Management of propionicacidemia:
Diet low in protein, with restriction of threonine, isoleucine, and methionine.
Large doses of biotin.

Tyrosinemia

Evaluate the clinical features of tyrosinemia:
Mental retardation.
A defective tyrosine aminotransferase.
Management of tyrosinemia:
Decreased intake of tyrosine and phenylalanine.

Hydroxyisovaleric Aciduria

Evaluate clinical features of hydroxyisovaleric aciduria:
Mental retardation.
Muscle atrophy.
Unpleasant odor of the urine.
Management of hydroxyisovaleric aciduria:
Decreased intake of leucine.

Methylacetoacetate Accumulation

Evaluate clinical features of methylacetoacetate accumulation:
Mental retardation.
Episodic attacks of acidosis, which may lead to coma.
Management of this situation:
Decrease protein and isoleucine in diet.

Saccharopinuria

Evaluate clinical features of saccharopinuria:
Mental retardation.
Defective aminoadipic semialdehyde-glutamate reductase.
Management of saccharopinuria:
Decrease lysine intake.

Pipecolicacidemia

Evaluate clinical features of pipecolicacidemia:
Mental retardation.
Defective pipecolate oxidase.
Management of pipecolicacidemia:
Decrease lysine intake.

Arginemia

Evaluate clinical features of arginemia:
Mental retardation.
Spasticity of muscles.
Seizures.
Defective arginase.
Management of arginemia:
Diet low in protein.

Pyroglutamic Acidemia

Evaluate clinical features of pyroglutamic acidemia:
Mental retardation.
Episodic attacks of vomiting.

Glutamicacidemia

Evaluate clinical features of glutamicacidemia:
Mental retardation.
Physical retardation.
Trichorrhexis nodosa, a condition in which the hairs show white nodes (fractured cortex) through which they may break.
Seizures.

Lesch-Nyhan Syndrome

Characteristic symptoms of Lesch-Nyhan syndrome are:
Mental retardation.
Choreathetosis, and cannibalism.
Spasticity.
Hyperuricemia.
Management of Lesch-Nyhan syndrome:
Reduce hyperuricemia.

Abetalipoproteinemia

Niemann-Pick Disease

Tay-Sachs Disease

For information on the above diseases, see the chapter devoted to metabolism and nutrition.

Gaucher's Disease

Fabry's Disease

The above diseases do not always present any evidence of mental retardation, but some of the patients may present it. For information see the chapter devoted to metabolism and nutrition.

Metachromatic Leukodystrophy

Evaluate clinical features of metachromatic leukodystrophy:
There is mental retardation, with symptoms corresponding to dementia.
There is a progressive paralysis of muscles.
Metachromatic lipids accumulate in the nervous system, but also in the spleen and kidneys.
Symptoms usually begin before 2 years of age.
Practically all patients die by age 10.
No treatment is known.

Krabbe's Disease (Globoid Leukodystrophy)

Characteristics of Krabbe's disease:
- A familial disease with progressive mental retardation.
- Blindness and deafness.
- Paralysis and pseudobulbar palsy.
- No known treatment.

Galactosemia

Evaluate symptoms of galactosemia:
- There is a normal appearance at birth.
- After a few days or weeks of milk feeding patients begin to show gastrointestinal symptoms, such as vomiting, anorexia, and then hepatomegaly, with jaundice.
- There is growth failure.
- Proteinuria and aminoaciduria are noted.
- Finally, there are edema and ascites.
- Survivors will show mental retardation and cataracts.
- Mild cases may occur, almost without symptoms.
- There is an urgent need for an early diagnosis, to avoid ulterior damage.

Management of galactosemia:
- Complete avoidance of milk, even to a trait carrier mother during pregnancy.
- Maintenance of the diet no less than 2 years; better, 6 years.

Hunter's Syndrome

Evaluate symptoms of Hunter's disease, one of the mucopolysaccharidoses:
- Mild or at most moderate mental retardation.
- Apparently normal at birth.
- Coarse facies, with thick lips and open mouth, flat nose.
- Short stature, and bone dysplasia.
- Hirsutism.
- Enlarged liver and spleen.
- No treatment; attempts have been done with skin implants and plasma infusions.

Morquio's Syndrome

Evaluate symptoms of Morquio's syndrome:
- Most cases will not present mental retardation, but it may occur at times.
- There are severe bone deformities, better noted when the child begins to walk.
- There is muscular and ligamentous hyperextensibility.
- The cornea becomes cloudy; the sclerae may be bluish.
- There is aortic regurgitation.

Management of Morquio's syndrome, or disease:
- Symptomatic and supportive.

Sanfilippo's Syndrome

Give the clinical evaluation of both Sanfilippo's syndromes, A and B:
- Both show identical clinical appearance.
- There are somatic defects, not too marked.
- Neurological defects are found, usually of a severe type.

Hurler's Disease (Gargoylism)

For information see the chapter devoted to metabolism and nutrition.

Malnutrition

How malnutrition may provoke mental retardation:
- If the nutritional deficiency occurs before birth.
- If the nutritional deficiency occurs shortly after birth.
- If malnutrition occurs together with environmental deprivation.

Causes of malnutrition are:
- Inadequate amounts of food to meet individual needs.
- Inadequate absorption of foods because of disease.
- Impaired metabolism.
- Errors from cultural or education habits.
- Influence of drugs.

Management of malnutrition:
- Urgent diagnosis, to help correction, as in phenylketonuria and other similar diseases.
- Evaluation of the correct diet needed.
- Avoidance of causative factors.

Kernicterus

When hyperbilirubinemia will cause kernicterus:
- When large amounts of bilirubin are deposited in the brain.

What is the symptomatology of kernicterus?
- Evidence of jaundice.
- Anorexia and vomiting.
- Lethargy.
- Upward deviation of the eyes, and opisthotonos.
- Seizures.
- Death, not a rare final outcome.

What is the clinical symptomatology in most survivors of kernicterus?
- Mild mental retardation.
- Choreoathetosis and other evidence of cerebral palsy.
- Hearing loss.
- Loss of upward gaze.

What are the common causes of kernicterus, because of symptomatic jaundice?
- Excessive production of bilirubin caused by fetal-maternal blood incompatibility, other forms of hemolytic anemias, intestinal atresia, meconium ileus, Hirschprung's disease, etc.

Diminished excretion of bilirubin caused by some nonhemolytic type of jaundice, metabolic diseases, diabetic mother, effects of some drugs, etc.
Mixed types due to intrauterine infections, etc.
Management of kernicterus:
Exchange transfusion.
Phototherapy, if feasible.

Lowe's Disease

For information, see the chapter devoted to metabolism and nutrition.

Craniofacial Abnormalities

What are the most common craniofacial abnormalities accompanied by mental retardation?
Treacher Collins syndrome, with a small mandible due to mandibulofacial dysostosis; may also present respiratory obstruction, and mental retardation.
Pierre Robin syndrome, which may also present small mandible and respiratory problems; may also present mental retardation.
Hypertelorism, with widely spaced eyes, but only rarely accompanied by mental retardation.
Microcephaly, almost always accompanied by mental retardation, and very frequently a joyous character.
Management of craniofacial abnormalities:
Symptomatic, supportive, and surgery whenever feasible.

Arthrogryposis

Evaluate clinical manifestations of arthrogryposis:
Joints appear fixed in flexion (less frequently in extension), the abnormality noted at birth.
There is secondary underdevelopment of skeletal muscle mass.
Most patients, but not all, will also show mental retardation.
Management of arthrogryposis:
Orthopedic reeducation.
Symptomatic and supportive.

Crigler-Najjar Syndrome

How this type of hyperbilirubinemia will cause mental retardation:
This nonhereditary jaundice of neonates, when severe and belonging to type I cases, will show central nervous system damage due to kernicterus, q.v., above.
Mild cases belonging to type II may survive, and may respond to therapy with phenobarbital.

Cystic Fibrosis

For information see the chapter devoted to metabolism and nutrition.

Tuberous Sclerosis

Evaluate clinical manifestations of tuberous sclerosis:
Most cases will show profound mental retardation.
There will be seizures, or decerebration spasticity.
Some cases may show rarefaction of the phalanges.
The presence of sebaceous adenomatosis may be characteristic of the disease in numerous instances.
Management of tuberous sclerosis:
Symptomatic and supportive.

Myotonia Atrophica (Dystrophia Myotonica, Steinert's Disease)

Evaluate the clinical features of Steinert's disease:
There may be mental retardation, but it will not affect all the patients; mental symptoms may also be demential.
The disease may start symptomatologically at any age.
There is hypertonicity of some of the muscles (fist, tongue).
There are atrophy and weakness of muscles of the face, jaw, peronei, etc.
After grasping an object the patient is unable to release the grip immediately.
There may be early baldness.
Cataracts are found.
There is evidence of glandular dysfunction, particularly testicular atrophy.
Management of Steinert's disease:
Symptomatic and supportive; physiotherapy may help.
For more information see the chapter on neurology.

Cerebral Palsy

For information, see the chapter devoted to neurology.

Perinatal Complications

Evaluate perinatal complications that may lead to mental retardation:
Improper feeding may lead to malnutrition, q.v., above.
Asphyxia neonatorum may induce severe cerebral damage if it is sufficently prolonged; *blood loss* may act the same way.
Hyaline membrane disease or respiratory distress syndrome will also result in cerebral damage in cases not adequately controlled.
In *meconium aspiration* mental problems may result if the secondary asphyxiation lasts for a prolonged time.
Injuries to the central nervous system, particularly those accompanied by hemorrhage, show a very poor prognosis because a large number of the survivors will present more or less marked nervous damage.

Hypoglycemia, notably that occurring among infants from diabetic mothers but in other instances as well, has to be efficiently and rapidly treated if we want to avoid severe brain damage.

Infections, inborn errors of metabolism, blood incompatibility, some forms of *anemia,* hyperbilirubinemia *(kernicterus),* or any other disease that may damage the central nervous system must be seriously considered as a possible cause of mental retardation.

14. Infectious Diseases

Influenza (Flu)

How does the usual onset of influenza occur?
Rapidly.
With fever, generally accompanied by chills, malaise, and generalized aches, notably of muscles and joints.
With catarrhal symptoms of the type of coryza with cough, and headache.

Evaluate the clinical symptomatology of influenza:
There is a worsening course of the foregoing symptoms.
Fever, aches, and prostration are worse than those symptoms corresponding to a catarrhal syndrome.
Headache increases, accompanied by photophobia and retrobulbar ache.
Cough becomes severe and productive, and appears as a dominant symptom.
Symptoms of pharyngitis also appear, together with mild conjunctivitis, lacrimation, etc.
There is also a flushed face.
Weakness is another dominant symptom.

Further course of influenza will show:
There is a rapid subsidence of symptoms in less than 5 days, in uncomplicated cases.
Complications appear in severe cases.
Beware of severe viral pneumonia if fulminant dyspnea, cyanosis, hemoptysis, and pulmonary edema develop.
Watch also, particularly in the elderly, for any form of pneumonia, hemorrhagic bronchitis, myocarditis, encephalitis, Reye's syndrome, etc.

Positive diagnosis of influenza depends on:
Serologic tests or virus isolation.

Management of influenza:
Prophylactic vaccination; amantadine recommended for virus A.
Symptomatic and supportive.

Parainfluenza

What are the viruses that may cause the parainfluenza type of disease?
Type 1, common in early childhood, occurs mainly in the fall, may show cyclic forms of epidemics; incubation lasts longer (4 to 5 days); the disease is mild and may recur once or twice.
Type 2 is more sporadic in occurrence; the main clinical syndrome is in the form of acute laryngotracheobronchitis in infants.
Type 3, also frequent in childhood, occurs in summer, causes explosive epidemics, lasts longer (7 to 8 days), shows a short incubation period, and may recur.
Type 4, rarely, is the cause of mild respiratory syndromes.

Evaluate the clinical symptomatology of parainfluenza:
It is essentially the same as for influenza; type 3 being the most severe and type 4 the mildest.
Symptoms of other respiratory diseases may also occur, the more severe being those of acute laryngotracheobronchitis in type 2 or so-called walking pneumonia in type 3.

Clinically, a positive diagnosis of parainfluenza cannot be made; it requires:
Virus isolation, tissue culture inoculation, serologic tests.

Management of parainfluenza:
Symptomatologic, and supportive.

Common Cold

For information, see the chapter devoted to respiratory diseases.

Respiratory Syncytial Virus

The usual symptoms of the disease are as follows:
There is cough, with dyspnea and wheezing.
There is fever.
Crepitants are heard on auscultation; signs of bronchopneumonia are seen on X-ray films.
The clinical picture presents a resemblance to influenza and parainfluenza, and bronchiolitis.
Care will be taken for complications, such as pneumonia.
Occurrence is more frequent in late fall and winter.

Positive diagnosis of the disease depends on:
Virus isolation (difficult) or serology.

Management of respiratory syncytial virus disease:
Symptomatic, and supportive (particularly respiratory support).

Acute Febrile Respiratory Disease

Evaluate clinical features of this adenoviral disease:
It is more frequent among children.
Usually it is due to viruses 1, 2, 3, 5, and 6 (there may be others).
Transmission is air- or waterborne; also by direct contact.
Incubation is from 2 to 5 days.
Fever may be the only symptom.
Also, there may be fever and pharyngitis; or fever with pharyngitis plus other respiratory symptoms (those corresponding to tracheitis, bronchitis, or even pneumonia); coughing is important.
Complications may include otitis media, or lymphadenitis.
Diagnosis of acute febrile respiratory disease depends on:
Virus isolation, serologic tests.
Management of the disease:
Symptomatic and supportive.

Acute Respiratory Disease

Evaluate clinical features of the disease:
It is almost exclusively seen among the military; it is sporadic among civilians.
Usually it is due to viruses 4 and 7; there may also be 14 and 21.
The disease starts with fever, chills, malaise, and headache.
There are cough, nasopharyngitis, and hoarseness; exudate is found on the pharynx.
There is lymphadenitis, but nodes are not too tender.
Macular rash may appear on the body; also, conjunctivitis.
Very few patients (10%) will present rales and X-ray changes.
The complete course of the disease will take 2 to 4 days; convalescence requires about 10 to 14 days.
Positive diagnosis depends on:
Virus identification, serological tests.
Management of the disease:
Symptomatic and supportive.

Epidemic Keratonconjunctivitis

Evaluate the clinical features of this—like the former one—adenoviral disease:
It is called "shipyard eye" because it most frequently affects shipyard workers.
Usually it is due to virus 8, or type 19; there is a mild form due to types 3 and 7.
There is a sudden onset.
There is unilateral conjunctivitis, with pain and tearing, chemosis, and swelling.
Keratitis may lead to corneal ulcerations with subepithelial opacities.
Preauricular lymph node, frequently of a large size, is noted.
The second eye may be involved in one week.
Course lasts for 3 or 4 weeks.
Opacities persist for a long time, and may become permanent.
The milder infections cause very little impairment.
Management of keratoconjunctivitis of the adenoviral type:
Positive diagnosis with virus isolation or serology.
Use of topical corticoids, better in hospital and by an ophthalmologist.

Viral Pneumonia of Infants

Evaluate clinical features of this adenoviral infection due to a virus of type 7, more rarely due to types 1 or 3:
Infants are affected during the first weeks of life.
There is a sudden onset, involving upper and lower respiratory tract.
There is elevated fever.
Evidence of lobar pneumonia is found (for information see under respiratory diseases).
There is a maculopapular rash, or encephalitis (for information see under nervous diseases), mostly seen in severe cases; also focal necrosis of brain, lungs, or skin.
Diagnosis is made by identification of the virus, or serology.
Management of viral penumonia of infants:
Close supervision in hospital; supportive, and symptomatic.

Acute Follicular Conjunctivitis

Evaluate clinical manifestations of this adenoviral infection:
It is due to a virus of type 3 or 7; rarely to other types, such as 2, 6, 9, 10, and 21.
Adults are mostly affected; children will also show systemic and respiratory involvement.
There is a rapid onset.
One eye is involved; half the patients will show less acute involvement of the second eye after a few days.
Inflamed conjunctivae are observed, both palpebral and bulbar, with redness and lacrimation; there is a sensation as of a foreign body.
There is follicular enlargement of submucoid tissue (may resemble trachoma).
Enlarged lymph nodes, preauricular and postcervical, are found.
There may also be a sore throat, conjunctival hemorrhages, and periorbital edema.
Diagnosis is to be made as usual (viral identification and serology).
Management of acute follicular conjunctivitis:
Symptomatic and supportive.

Acute Pharyngoconjunctivitis

Evaluate clinical features of acute pharyngoconjunctival fever:
- It is due to virus types 3 and 7; less commonly to types 1, 2, 5, 6, 14, and 21.
- It is sporadic in adults and epidemic among children; incubation is about 1 week.
- It is more frequent in the summer time, principally among swimmers.
- There will be fever, conjunctivitis, and pharyngitis.
- A few patients will show only one or two elements of the disease.
- Fewer cases will show involvement of the lower respiratory tract.
- Total duration of the disease is about 1 week; the conjunctivitis may last another week.
- Diagnosis is by viral identification or serology.

Management of acute pharyngoconjunctival fever:
- Symptomatic and supportive.

Encephalitis

Meningitis

For information on both subjects, see the chapter devoted to nervous diseases.

Aseptic Meningitis

This enteroviral disease is caused by:
- Poliovirus 1, or 3; less frequent after introduction of vaccination.
- Coxsackieviruses of Group A (2, 4, 7, 9, 23, and others), or Group B (1, 2, 3, 4, 5, or 6).
- Echoviruses 4, 6, or others less commonly found.

Evaluate the clinical manifestations of the disease:
- It affects preferentially infants and children; older persons may also be affected, in these cases because of other viruses.
- There is a prodromal stage at times with fever, malaise, and vomiting.
- Onset is usually sudden, with headache, pain and stiffness of the back, other muscular pains, positive Kernig and similar signs.
- There may be occasional encephalitic symptoms.
- The whole course may last about 1 week.
- Residual weakness and irritability may persist for months.
- Diagnosis is made by virus isolation or serology.

Management of aseptic meningitis:
- Treat as for poliomyelitis, q.v.

Measles

This paramyxovirus infection is characterized as follows:
- Incubation lasts from 1 to 2 weeks; communicability from 2 to 4 days before rash, to 2 to 5 days after onset.
- Prodromic symptoms are fever, and a coryza-like syndrome with cough, conjunctivitis, and photophobia.
- Koplik's spots are almost pathognomonic (like grains of salt surrounded by erythema, in front of 2nd and 3rd upper molars).
- At the same time, there may also appear symptoms of pharyngitis, laryngitis, or tracheobronchitis.
- As a last stage of the disease there will be worsening of the prodromal symptoms, with added periorbital edema, and itching; and the classic rash.

Evaluate the characteristics of the morbilliform rash:
- It follows after 1 or 2 days of Koplik's spots and 3 to 5 days from the onset of symptoms.
- It will start behind the ears and on the face; the following day it will begin to coalesce on the face and will appear on the trunk; the third day it will be confluent on the trunk and will appear on the extremities, while it will be fading on the face.
- Fading of the eruption will follow the same pattern as its appearance.
- Slight desquamation will follow; some fair-skinned persons may remain hyperpigmented, at least for a time.
- The rash consists of very small papules that coalesce forming brick-red, irregular maculopapular lesions; in severe cases it may reach the aspect of a uniform erythema, or even be petechial.
- A generalized enlargement of lymph nodes is frequent.

Evaluate diagnostic procedures:
- Clinical diagnosis.
- Viral identification and serology.

Management of measles:
- Symptomatic and supportive.
- Isolation.

Rubella (German Measles)

This infection, probably due to a togavirus, is characterized as follows:
- Incubation lasts 2 or 3 weeks; communicability from a very few days before appearance of the rash to its end (infected newborns may be infective for months).
- There is a sudden, but mild, onset of symptoms with fever and the eruption.
- Systemic symptoms, besides fever, are malaise, headache, rhinitis and other coryza-like symptoms, enlarged and tender nodes behind the ears and on the postcervical area, and arthralgia, particularly present among young women.

Evaluate the characteristics of the rubella rash:
- There is a fine maculopapular rash, with pinkish elements that may become confluent or scarlatiniform.
- There is rapid progression from face, trunk, to extremities.
- Rapid extinction occurs in the same order.
- There may be cases of rubella without the rash.

Total duration of the rash is about 3 days, or less.
Erythema of palate and throat may be present.

Evaluate the implications of rubella during pregnancy:
Expectant mothers will be carefully examined for contagion by serologic followup whenever necessary.
There is a high risk during the first 2 months of pregnancy.
Infection acquired in utero is prone to cause different sorts of abnormalities.

Management of rubella:
Symptomatic and supportive.
Abortion to be considered in cases of pregnancy.

Cytomegalovirus Infection

This cytomegalic inclusion disease is characterized by:
Sudden onset.
Fever and malaise.
Pains of muscles and joints.
Generalized enlargement of lymph nodes.
Hepatomegaly, most often with tenderness; occasional jaundice.
A rash, in some cases.
There are asymptomatic patients.

What may be the relation of cytomegalovirus disease to transfusions?
It may be due to transfusion.
Symptoms will appear after 2 to 4 weeks.

How the immunosuppressed host may react to the disease:
May present a severe pneumonia, or other gastrointestinal or renal involvement.

Manifestations of the congenital form of the disease are:
Soon after birth there is jaundice with hepato- and splenomegaly; fever.
There are signs of encephalitis, with purpura and hematuria.
There is a low birth weight.
These infants may develop microcephaly, intracranial calcifications, optic atrophy, deafness, seizures, paralyses, and mental retardation.
Some will present asymptomatic disease.

Frequency of the disease shows the following characteristics:
The virus is present in about 1% of all newborns.
The virus is in the cervix of about 10% of healthy women.
The virus is in the salivary glands of 10 to 25% of all healthy persons.
The frequency of the infection increases with age; from 60 to 90% of adults have been infected.
The positivity of the infection can be assured by viral identification or serology.

Management of the disease:
Symptomatic and supportive.

Roseola Infantum (Exanthema Subitum)

Evaluate the symptomatology of exanthema subitum:
There is high fever of unknown cause, lasting 3 or 4 days, and of sudden onset.
There may be convulsions during the febrile stage; at least, there will be irritability.
Enlarged lymph nodes will be noted behind the ears and on the postcervical area; splenomegaly is observed.
The fourth day fever falls by crisis, coinciding characteristically with the appearance of the rash.
There is a maculopapular rash; transient; abundant on the chest, and less marked on face and extremities.
In some instances the rash may be unnoticed.

Management of this benign disease:
Symptomatic and supportive.

Erythema Infectiosum (Fifth Disease, Exanthema Infectiosum)

Evaluate the clinical appearance of "slapped cheek" disease:
There are sporadic outbreaks, affecting children.
Mild generalized symptoms are noted; fatigue or malaise, at most.
There is a fiery red maculopapular rash that becomes confluent and edematous; mainly noted on the face, but also on other body areas.
For about 7 to 9 days, the rash comes and goes.
No treatment is needed.

Chickenpox (Varicella)

What are the characteristics of the chickenpox-zoster virus?
The same virus causes varicella and herpes zoster.
Varicella seems to be the acute invasive phase of the disease.
Herpes zoster seems to be a reactivation of the latent phase.
The incubation may last from 2 to 3 weeks; contagiousness lasts from a few days before onset of symptoms to the end of the crusting stage.

Evaluate the clinical symptomatology of varicella:
Moderate fever and malaise, milder in children than in adults.
Headache, and sore throat.
Characteristic itchy eruption.

Evaluate the characteristics of the varicella rash:
It starts shortly after onset of symptoms.
It appears first on the trunk, and then spreads to the neck, face, and extremities.
Palms and soles are rarely affected.
The initial lesion is a macule, which progresses to form a papule, which vesiculates and then breaks, forming a crust.
Lesions appear as successive crops.
There will be lesions of different ages at each given time.
New lesions are formed during the first 5 days of the disease.
The changes of lesions may occur in a matter of hours, at most from one day to the next.
Final sloughing of the crusts will take 1 or 2 weeks.

Precautions to be taken with varicella patients:
In immunosuppressed patients it may disseminate and be fatal.
Zoster immune globulin (ZIG) is effective in preventing the disease when given to susceptible patients (there is a small supply).
Management of varicella:
Care is symptomatic and supportive.
Treat susceptible patients, as early as possible, with adenine arabinoside.
Antibiotics and corticoids will help in some instances.

Smallpox (Variola)

This viral disease—which is said to be practically conquered all over the world—presents the following epidemiologic facts:
Incubation lasts from 1 to 3 weeks (average, 12 days).
Contagiousness extends 1 or 2 days before onset of symptoms until disappearance of all crusts.
It is very easily transmitted, either directly or indirectly, including the air route for dried droplets.
All ages and races are susceptible.
The starting symptoms of the disease are:
There is a sudden onset of elevated fever, usually with chills, and tachycardia.
There is pain, severe in most cases, along the spine and in muscles; there is also intense headache.
Most patients will also present nausea, vomiting, and prostration.
Also, there may be dizziness, constipation, tachypnea, and convulsions in the case of small children.
There is the possibility of eruption of an unspecific rash (morbilliform, scarlatiniform, petechial), of no help for diagnosis.
The elevated temperature abates after 2 to 4 days, the characteristic rash appears, and the temperature rises again.
Evaluate the characteristics of the variola rash:
There is only one crop of lesions, all of the same age.
Lesions begin for 2 or 3 days and change from macules to papules and then vesicles at the third day; at about the sixth day of the eruption all lesions pustulate, and after less than 1 week all become crusts.
The fever increases again at the pustulation stage.
Pink macules appear first on face and scalp (forehead, temples, mouth, ears), rapidly invading neck, extremities, and trunk; palms and soles may also be affected, particularly in severe cases.
Macules rapidly turn into papules deeply set in the skin, feeling shotty on palpation.
Vesicles present a characteristic umbilication; are multilocular, filled with clear serum, and surrounded by a pinkish areola.
In about 2 days the vesicles pustulate, then they shrink or break, and soon the skin is covered with crusts and other purulent material.
In most instances the lesions appear confluent.
Hemorrhagic lesions are almost always fatal.
Lesions with the characteristic umbilication may be seen in mucous membranes (mouth, pharynx, vagina, urethra, and rectum).
The final stage may show extensive desquamation, with loss of hair or nails, or other serious lesions.
Evaluate diagnostic possibilities:
Clinical diagnosis.
Virus isolation, serology, and other laboratory procedures.
Prophylaxis of smallpox:
Vaccinate, and revaccinate (3-year term).
Immediately revaccinate on exposure, if vaccination has occurred more than 3 years previously.
Consider contraindications (ill persons, immunosuppressed or immunodeficient patients, those with cancer, extensive skin diseases); use vaccinia immune globulin in case vaccination is essential for such cases.
Revaccinate if results are not satisfactory.
Management of variola:
Only symptomatic and supportive.
Isolation.

Vaccinia

Evaluate reactions of vaccinia:
In nonimmune persons a lesion entirely similar to that of smallpox will appear in 3 to 5 days, with a total evolution of about 12 days.
Fever, malaise, and adenopathy may occur (sixth to eighth days).
A scar will remain, the whole process constituting a major reaction.
In previously vaccinated persons, the reaction will be accelerated, with similar lesions, but of smaller size and less systemic symptoms.
If the subsequent vaccinations give an entirely different reaction, it will be an equivocal reaction requiring revaccination.
What are usual complications of vaccinia?
Secondary bacterial infections.
Generalized vaccinia, including autoinoculation.
Hypersensitive noninfectious rashes.
Severe reactions of the type of eczema vaccinatum, vaccinia necrosum, and central nervous system complications.
Management of vaccinia:
No treatment or dressing usually needed.
Antibiotics for secondary bacterial infections.
Vaccinia immune globulin for severe cases; also methisazone may help in these instances.

Herpes Simplex (Fever or Cold Sore)

What are the accepted viruses for herpes simplex?
Herpesvirus hominis type 1, causative of herpes labialis and keratitis.

Herpesvirus hominis type 2, causative of genital herpes, with a possible oncogenic effect.

Evaluate the general symptomatology of *herpes simplex:*

Neuralgic pain may precede and accompany the attack; itch may occur.

Lesions consist of small tense vesicles on an erythematous base that will occur in small groups elsewhere on the body, particularly lips, mouth, and genitals; also on conjunctiva and cornea.

Those that set on ears, nose, or fingers may be very painful.

Clusters of vesicles may vary in size, up to 1.5 cm; groups may coalesce.

Other local symptoms may be burning and stinging; regional enlarged lymph nodes may be painful.

The total evolution of symptoms may take about 3 weeks; or occur at a slower pace if there is secondary infection or the lesion is moistened.

Evaluate symptoms of primary acute *herpetic gingivostomatitis:*

In the mouth, there will appear multiple shallow ulcers, which are very painful.

There is evidence of gingivitis (inflammation and pain).

Pain will subside in 4 or 5 days, and the total disease in 3 to 5 more days.

There may be enlarged lymph nodes, also fever and malaise.

Fatal viremia may occur among infants; rarely among older children.

Evaluate symptoms of recurrent *herpes labialis:*

There is a previous sensation of fullness and burning itch at the junction of mucosa and skin around the lips on the site of the eruption.

A small crop of vesicles will develop, most of it on the skin side.

At a later stage, the vesicles become yellowish and crusted.

The whole disease will last for about 10 days.

Evaluate the symptoms of *herpes simplex keratitis:*

In *dendritic keratitis* there are lesions resembling the veins of a leaf with knoblike terminations; there are photophobia, lacrimation, and a red conjunctiva; there is almost characteristic corneal hypo- or anesthesia; watch for corneal ulceration, which may lead to a permanent scarring.

In *disciforme keratitis* the cornea will react with a deep disc-shaped inflammation, usually with iritis.

Evaluate the symptoms of *genital herpes:*

It starts with soreness and itching.

Then, there appears a small area of erythema on skin or mucosae.

Next stage shows a small crop of vesicles that ulcerate rapidly; round ulcers with a red areola; they are painful.

The total evolution of the disease takes about 10 days.

Any part of the genital area may be involved; scarring is left.

Regional lymph nodes are mildly enlarged, and tender.

Evaluate diagnostic procedures for herpes simplex:

Virus isolation, serology, and positive Tzenck test (vesicle scrapings stained with Giemsa).

Management of herpes simplex:

Avoid corticoids, particularly for herpes simplex keratitis.

Symptomatic and supportive; local care, including ethyl ether.

Idoxuridine solution is helpful for both herpes labialis and herpes simplex keratitis.

Herpes Zoster

Evaluate the symptoms of this varicella-zoster virus infection:

There is prodromal pain along the path of a nerve; it may persist even for years.

There may be systemic manifestations, such as fever (may be with chills), malaise, and gastrointestinal discomfort.

In 2 to 5 days crops of tense deep-seated vesicles appear along the path of the affected nerve; the base is erythematous.

After about 5 days of eruption, vesicles dry and scab.

Local enlargement of lymph nodes may occur at times.

Usually, lesions are unilateral, but in rare instances zoster may become generalized.

Evaluate the symptoms of thoracic zoster:

It is one of the most frequent forms.

It follows the path of one of the intercostal nerves.

All symptoms are as above.

Evaluate the symptoms of ophthalmic herpes zoster:

It is also a frequent form.

Lesions appear around the eyes, from the forehead to the nose, on one side of the face.

There will also be edema, inflammation of tissues (conjunctiva, ciliary body); general symptoms, as above.

Beware of corneal ulcerations, which may lead to opacities.

Occasionally, there may be paralysis of the 3rd cranial nerve (oculomotor).

Evaluate symptoms of otic herpes zoster:

Lesions will appear around the auricles and the aural canal.

Other lesions may be noted on the soft palate and the pharynx.

There will be severe ear pain, loss of hearing, tinnitus, and possibly vertigo.

Other cranial nerves may be involved, manifested by facial paralysis, nystagmus, and perhaps other symptoms.

Mild symptoms from the central nervous system (encephalic, meningeal) may also be noted in some cases.

General symptoms are as stated above.

Management of herpes zoster:
- Care is symptomatic and supportive.
- Corticoids should be given as soon as possible (do not give in herpes simplex!).
- Use adenine arabinoside, or zoster immune globulin whenever needed, particularly for immunosuppressed patients.

Poliomyelitis (Infantile Paralysis)

Evaluate characteristics of poliovirus infections:
- This variety of enterovirus (of the picornavirus group) presents three types; type I is the most important one.
- Incubation may last 1 or 2 weeks; but incubation may last 35 days.
- Contagiousness is maximal during the first week, but may last several weeks.
- There may be transient carriers, from contacts.
- An average 21,000 cases a year were active before vaccination; presently there are almost no cases (7 in 1974).
- The overall mortality is about 5 to 10%; bulbar polio, the most severe form of the disease, occurs in 10 to 20% of cases.
- Less than 1% of all infected cases will show symptoms of the disease.

Evaluate symptoms of the minor illness or abortive poliomyelitis:
- Incubation may be shorter, only 3 to 5 days.
- About 90% of all the cases will present the minor illness.
- Symptoms are unspecific, and of almost no help for diagnosis.
- There are mild fever, headache, sore throat, and gastrointestinal disturbances.
- There is no evidence of central nervous system involvement.
- Recovery takes place in 1 to 3 days; there may be recurrence in a few cases.

Evaluate symptoms of nonparalytic poliomyelitis:
- Symptoms as for abortive poliomyelitis, but worse; plus the following.
- Pain in the neck, back, and extremities; also, abdominal pain.
- Irritability, and lethargy.
- Muscle spasm noted in all these patients (extensors of the neck and back, flexors of the leg); resistance to flexion of the neck or straightening of the leg.
- Muscles tender to palpation.

Evaluate the symptoms of the major illness or paralytic polio:
- Symptoms are as above, plus the following.
- Tremors and muscle weakness will be added.
- Paresthesias, retention, constipation, or ileus may occur.
- Paralysis will occur at any time of the disease.
- Paralytic symptoms may belong to the spinal or the bulbar type.
- Symptoms of spinal polio are those of paralysis of one or more limbs.
- The type is that of flaccid paralysis; this is the classic form of poliomyelitis.
- Symptoms of bulbar poliomyelitis are those involving dysfunction of the swallowing mechanism, respiratory distress (respiratory paralysis is the most dangerous result of the disease), etc.
- Other symptoms of bulbar polio are those evidencing central nervous system impairment (encephalitis), diplopia, facial weakness, dysphonia with nasal voice, neck drop, etc.
- In all forms deep tendon reflexes are diminished or lost.
- Some patients may show tachycardia, rarely convulsions, and changes of blood pressure, either high or low.

Evaluate diagnosis of poliomyelitis:
- Virus isolation (throat washings at the beginning, stools also at the beginning or late), serology after the first or second week.

Management of poliomyelitis:
- Vaccination for prevention.
- Symptomatic and supportive; reeducation when needed.

Rabies (Hydrophobia)

Evaluate characteristics of the rabies virus:
- Contamination from rabid dogs, cats, or wild animals.
- Incubation period usually is from 3 to 7 weeks, but may vary from 10 days to 2 years.
- Incubation may be shorter with large wounds or wounds close to the head.
- Dogs are infective only 5 to 7 days before death.
- The disease is almost uniformly fatal.

Evaluate symptoms of rabies:
- There is history of a bite.
- Prodromal symptoms are fever, depression, restlessness, and pain followed by tingling at the site of the bite.
- There are intense irritability and excitement, profuse salivation (thick and tenacious), and extremely painful laryngeal spasms (hydrophobia).
- The skin is very sensitive; convulsions may be present.
- Laryngospasm is easily precipitated even by mild stimulation.
- Exhaustion, general paralysis, or asphyxia will cause death in about 3 to 10 days.

Management of rabies:
- Aggressive and vigorous supportive treatment may help some cases.
- Prevention is the best resource, with serum or antirabies immune globulin, or with vaccine.

Herpangina

Evaluate clinical features of herpangina:

It is caused by any of the coxsackieviruses, and at times by some of the enteroviruses.

Most commonly it affects infants and children.

There is a sudden onset with fever, sore throat, pain (neck, limbs, abdomen), and headache.

Characteristically, there will be some small grayish papulovesicular lesions on an erythematous base on the pharyngeal area, including palate and tongue.

In about 1 day the lesions will uclerate; they will heal in 1 to 5 days.

Fever may be high, and then accompanied by convulsions.

Diagnosis is helped by viral and serologic studies.

Management is only symptomatic and supportive.

Hand, Foot, and Mouth Disease

Evaluate clinical features of the disease:

Most are due to coxsackievirus type 16; but other viruses may also be incriminated.

Epidemics may occur; particularly affecting young children.

Symptoms resemble those of herpangina, q.v., above.

The vesicular rash will be extended to hands and feet; also on the diaper area, with infants.

Usual viral or serological studies are made.

Treatment is only symptomatic and supportive.

Epidemic Pleurodynia (Bornholm Disease)

Evaluate clinical features of Bornholm disease:

It is caused by any of the six viruses of coxsackievirus Group B.

It may occur at any age, but most frequently among children.

A sudden onset of recurrent diaphragmatic pain is felt in the lower chest or epigastric area.

Fever may present during the attacks of pain.

There are also headache, sore throat, nausea, and malaise.

Other symptoms may be tenderness, hyperesthesia, muscle swelling, myalgia, which are not present in all instances.

As complications, there may be orchitis, pleurisy, and more rarely aseptic meningitis or pericarditis.

Relapses may occur.

Diagnosis is helped by the occurrence of epidemics; will rely on viral or serologic studies.

Treatment is only symptomatic and supportive.

Summer Grippe

Evaluate the clinical features of summer grippe:

It is caused by coxsackieviruses A and D.

It affects mostly children.

There are mild general symptoms.

There is some evidence of respiratory involvement.

It lasts for only 1 to 4 days.

Diagnosis is proved by viral or serologic studies.

Treatment is symptomatic and supportive.

Dengue (Breakbone or Dandy Fever)

Evaluate the characteristics of the causative agent:

Any of the four subgroups of the Group B arbovirus may be involved.

It is transmitted by the bite of a mosquito (*Aëdes*).

It is prevalent in the tropics and subtropical areas.

Incubation lasts from 3 to 15 days, average 5 to 8.

Immunity lasts for 1 year, sometimes more.

Evaluate the clinical findings in dengue during the initial phase:

There is a sudden onset, with high fever, chills, severe "breakbone" pains in the head, back, and extremities, together with sore throat, depression, and prostration.

There are relative bradycardia and hypotension.

Red conjunctivae and flushed skin of a macular aspect are noted.

There is a mildly enlarged, soft spleen.

There are enlarged lymph nodes.

After 2 to 4 days the fever decreases rapidly, with profuse sweating.

The remission of fever may not occur; when present, it may last for only a few hours or up to 2 days.

Evaluate the clinical findings in dengue during the second phase:

The second phase usually follows the defervescence period, but it may take place without a noticeable afebrile period (with a feeling of well-being).

The dengue triad will be present with fever, pains, and rash.

The rash may last only a couple of hours, but may extend to 2 days; appears in about 80% of the cases; may be scarlatiniform, morbilliform, maculopapular, or petechial; spreading from limbs to trunk (except face), with bright red and edematous palms and soles.

Convalescence is prolonged, but mortality is nil.

Evaluate diagnostic help:

Viral studies, and serology.

Management of dengue:

Symptomatic and supportive care.

Eradication of the vector; keep patients under mosquito netting during the entire febrile process.

Colorado Tick Fever

Evaluate characteristics of the causative agent:

It is a Diplornavirus (reovirus-like) transmitted by bites of the *Dermacentor andersoni* tick.

Disease is mainly confined to the western part of the United States.

It is mostly transmitted during the tick season, from March to August.

Incubation lasts 3 to 6 days; disease will start that length of time after the tick bite.

Evaluate the clinical course of Colorado tick fever:

Sudden onset, with elevated temperature that may be accompanied by chills.

Severe pains affecting muscles and head.

Photophobia, generalized weakness, anorexia, nausea, and vomiting.

A faint rash possible.

Remission of fever after 3 days; it may last for 2 or 3 days.

Then, a recrudescence of fever, lasting 3 or 4 days.

A third bout of fever possible.

Check viremia by fluorescent antibody stain of the patient's red cells with adsorbed virus, or inoculate mice; serology is performed after 3 weeks.

Management of Colorado tick fever:

Symptomatic and supportive.

Saint Louis Encephalitis

Evaluate the clinical features related to St. Louis encephalitis:

It occurs in the western and central parts of the United States, and Florida.

It is transmitted by mosquitoes and birds.

Older people present the greatest morbidity and mortality.

An arbovirus of Group B causes the disease.

The clinical picture shows fever and central nervous system symptoms.

Treatment is symptomatic and supportive.

California Encephalitis

Evaluate the clinical features related to California encephalitis:

It occurs all over the United States.

It is transmitted by mosquitoes and small mammals.

It is caused by a virus of the California Group.

Children are mainly affected.

The clinical picture shows fever and central nervous system symptoms.

Treatment is symptomatic and supportive.

Eastern Equine Encephalitis

Evaluate the clinical features related to eastern equine encephalitis:

It occurs mainly in the eastern part of the United States and South America; also in eastern Canada.

It is transmitted by mosquitoes, birds, and small rodents.

It occurs in horses of the area, and may affect young children or elderly adults.

It is caused by a Group A arbovirus.

Mortality is relatively elevated.

Treatment is symptomatic and supportive.

Western Equine Encephalitis

Evaluate the clinical features related to western equine encephalitis:

It extends over the western hemisphere, to Brazil and Argentina.

It is transmitted by mosquitoes and birds.

It is caused by a Group A arbovirus.

It may occur at all ages, but principally under 1 year.

Mortality is not too high.

The clinical picture shows fever and central nervous system symptoms.

Treatment is symptomatic and supportive.

Lymphocytic Choriomeningitis

Evaluate characteristics of the causative agent:

It is caused by an arenavirus (RNA virus).

It is endemic in rodents; also transmitted by domestic animals; not transmitted by man.

Incubation period may last from 8 to 13 days.

The disease only appears east of the Rocky Mountains.

The disease may be more frequent among adults during the winter.

Fatalities are rare.

Evaluate clinical features of lymphocytic choriomeningitis:

It may begin as an influenzalike syndrome.

Less frequently, it may begin as a case of aseptic meningitis, q.v.

Occasionally, it may start as an influenzalike syndrome with a remission and then the meningitic syndrome.

The virus may be identified.

Serology will not be informative before the second week.

Management of the disease:

Symptomatic and supportive, as for encephalitis.

Yellow Fever (Black Vomit)

Evaluate characteristics of the causative virus:

It is caused by a Group B arbovirus.

It is endemic in South America and Africa.

It is transmitted by mosquitoes of the *Aëdes aegypti* type, in towns; the jungle or sylvatic yellow fever is transmitted by *Haemagogus* and similar types of mosquitoes.

Incubation lasts from 3 to 6 days.

Evaluate symptoms of the mild form of yellow fever:

There is fever, with headache and malaise.

Bradycardia may occur.

There are photophobia and retro-orbital pain.

Nausea and vomiting occur; jaundice may be present.

This syndrome strongly resembles a case of hepatitis.
Mortality is very low in this form of yellow fever.

Evaluate symptoms of the severe form of yellow fever:
- During the phase of invasion there are:
  - Sudden onset with elevated temperature.
  - Severe pains all over the body; headache.
  - Flushed face and injected eyes.
  - Red margins and furred center of the tongue.
  - Epigastric distress, nausea, vomiting, and constipation.
  - Initial tachycardia followed by relative bradycardia the second day (Faget's sign).
  - Prostration, irritability, and restlessness.
- During the phase of calm or remission:
  - After 2 to 5 days of invasion, fever falls by crisis.
  - Temperature remains normal or about normal.
  - This period lasts for hours or days.
- During the phase of intoxication there are:
  - Again, rise of temperature, with bradycardia and hypotension.
  - Fever, jaundice, and albuminuria (the essential clues in the past).
  - Bleeding in the skin and mucosae (black vomit).
  - Worsening of same symptoms of invasion.
  - Oliguria or anuria.
  - Dullness, confusion, delirium.
- Final stage may be that of a short convalescence, after about 1 week, or death in a high number of cases at about 6 to 9 days (more than 10%).

Evaluate positive diagnosis, at the present time:
- Viral studies and serology may be used.
- Clinically, the triad fever, jaundice, and albuminaria or the Faget's sign is highly suggestive.

Management of yellow fever:
- Symptomatic and supportive.

Infectious Mononucleosis

Evaluate characteristics of the infective virus:
- It is the Epstein-Barr herpes virus.
- Incubation period is about 5 to 15 days; also said to be 4 to 7 weeks.
- Disease may occur at any age, but mostly among younger persons.
- Fever will subside in about 10 days, enlarged lymph tissue (nodes and spleen) in a month; rare cases will show some problems even after 2 or 3 months.
- Usually, there are no sequelae or deaths.

Evaluate symptoms of infectious mononucleosis:
- There is fever, with sore throat and malaise.
- There is lymphadenopathy, moderately enlarged and painful, particularly noted in the posterior cervical chain.
- Splenomegaly will present in about 50% of the cases; beware of ruptures!
- A rash (macular, papular, petechial) will be noted in about 50% of the cases.
- Some patients may show symptoms of hepatitis, q.v.
- Some patients may show symptoms of encephalitis or meningitis, or of the Guillain-Barré syndrome, q.v.
- Some patients may present pulmonary or myocardial involvement.
- About 10% of the cases will present a typhoidal form of the disease.
- Symptomatology may be extremely varied.

Diagnostic procedures for infectious mononucleosis:
- Paul-Bunnel test (also Paul-Bunnel-Davidsohn test, or heterophil antibody test) is positive, but may be delayed until the fourth week.
- Specific serodiagnostic tests are also available.
- Blood smears are also informative, with atypical lymphocytes.

Management of infectious mononucleosis:
- Symptomatic and supportive.

Mumps (Parotitis, either Endemic or Epidemic)

Evaluate characteristics of the infective virus:
- It is a paramyxovirus.
- The disease may occur at any age, but usually among children.
- Incubation lasts from 2 to 3 weeks, averaging 18 days.
- Contagiousness precedes 1 day and is maximal 3 days after the onset, but will be present until swelling of the gland disappears.
- The disease occurs more frequently in late winter and early spring.
- Very rarely a relapse of the disease may occur after 2 weeks.

Clinical symptoms and course are as follows:
- There is a gradual onset of fever (minimal in very young children; maximal with orchitis or miningoencephalitis), with chilly sensations, malaise, headache, and anorexia.
- After 12 to 24 hours the parotid glands enlarge and become tender (also other salivary glands); both glands are affected in 75% of the cases; enlargement of glands may occur in succession 1 to 3 days apart.
- There are difficulties in chewing, swallowing, or tasting acids.
- The orifice of the gland (Stensen's duct) may be swollen and red.
- There is sensitivity to pressure over the angle of the jaw.
- There may be edema on the surroundings of the enlarged gland; the skin may be tense and shiny.
- Orchitis will occur in 25% of adults; testicles are painful and swollen; fever will be high.
- In females, oophoritis will cause low abdominal pain and enlarged ovaries.
- Increased headache and lethargy and elevated temperature will suggest meningoencephalitis; there will also be neck stiffness.

Pancreatitis will be suggested by epigastric tenderness.
There may also be symptoms of nephritis, mastitis, myocarditis, inflammation of other glands, etc.
Evaluation of diagnostic procedures:
Isolation of virus; serology.
Management of mumps:
Symptomatic and supportive.

Typhus (Classic or Epidemic)

Characteristics of the *Rickettsia prowazekii* causative factor:
It is louse-borne; not transmitted by humans.
Incubation lasts from 10 to 14 days.
Evaluation of clinical findings and course of the disease:
There is a prodromal stage with headache, malaise, chest pain, and cough.
There is a sudden increase of symptoms, with fever slowly rising to 40°C (104°F), chills, and prostration, in an influenzalike syndrome.
Headache increases to intolerable proportions.
There are flushed face, conjunctivitis, some auscultatory signs in the base of the lungs, and not rarely splenomegaly.
There may be hypotension; vascular collapse may occur; also renal insufficiency; and stupor and delirium.
Close to the end of the first week of disease, a rash will appear on the upper trunk and axillae, rapidly spreading to the extremities.
The rash is maculopapular, soon becomes papular, starts pinkish and thereafter darkens, and in severe cases becomes petechial or hemorrhagic.
The rash will spare the face, the palms, and the soles.
Recovery will occur 13 to 16 days after the onset, with a rapid fall of fever; but over 50 years of age mortality rises to 60%, even though among youngsters it may not exceed 10%, and is nil among children under 10 years of age.
Evaluation of diagnostic procedures:
Isolation of the causative germ from blood.
Agglutination tests for proteus OX19.
Management of epidemic typhus:
Give tetracyclines and chloramphenicol.
Treat symptoms, and support the patient.

Endemic Typhus (Murine Typhus)

Characteristics of the *Rickettsia typhi (mooseri)* causative factor:
It is transmitted by rat fleas.
Incubation lasts from 6 to 14 days.
Evaluate clinical features of endemic typhus:
There is a gradual onset of fever.
The rash is maculopapular, only present on the trunk for a short time.
The total duration of the disease is 6 to 13 days.
Other secondary symptomatology involving organs or systems is very rare.
Fatalities are very rare, limited to older people.
Evaluate diagnostic procedures:
Serology for *R. typhi* antigens.
Agglutination tests for proteus OX19.
Management of endemic typhus:
Tetracycline, or even nothing.

Brill's Disease (Brill-Zinsser's Disease)

Evaluate symptoms and course of this type of recrudescence of epidemic typhus:
There is a history of a previous attack of epidemic typhus, or the abode of the patient at infected areas.
Symptoms are the same (q.v.) but milder and of shorter duration.
The fever is not as elevated and steady, but fluctuates.
The rash is evanescent, or may even be absent.
Total duration of the disease will be from 7 to 11 days.
Mortality is practically absent.
Serology is positive, but the Weil-Felix reaction may be negative.
Management of this form of typhus:
Prefer tetracycline; but chloramphenicol may be needed.

Rocky Mountain Spotted Fever (Tick Fever)

Evaluate characteristics of the *Rickettsia ricketsii* causative factor:
It is limited to the western hemisphere, North and South America.
It is transmitted by ticks (harbored by generations in the same tick family).
Incubation lasts from 3 to 10 days; average 1 week.
Late spring and summer will show the most cases, in areas infested by ticks and open for recreation or work.
Evaluate symptoms and course of the disease:
There is a possible history of exposure.
There is a sudden onset of an influenzalike syndrome with fever, muscle and joint pains, headache, sore throat, gastrointestinal symptoms such as anorexia, nausea, and vomiting, and abdominal pain.
There may be chills, malaise, restlessness, insomnia, irritability, and final lethargy, stupor, delirium, or even coma.
There are flushed face and conjunctivitis.
Some patients may show spleno- or hepatomegaly, jaundice, myocarditis, gangrene, or uremia.
A characteristic rash will appear between the second and sixth day of fever, on wrists and ankles; it will spread through extremities and then the trunk.
There will be small and red macules, which then turn petechial and grow larger, the total spreading time being 2 to 3 days; they may ulcerate.

Total duration of the disease will be up to 10 or even 15 to 20 days.

Evaluate the diagnostic procedure for spotted fever:

Isolate the germ from blood during the first week.

Check for antibodies after the second week.

The Weil-Felix reaction will be positive during convalescence.

Management of spotted fever:

Use tetracycline or chloramphenicol early in the disease, since otherwise it may be deadly to 70% of adults and 20% of children.

Fièvre Boutonneuse (Eastern Hemisphere Rickettsioses)

Evaluate characteristics of the infective agent:

It may vary according to the country (*R. sibirica, R. australis,* and *R. conorii*).

It is transmitted by ticks; incubation is 5 to 7 days.

Evaluate symptoms and course of the disease:

Onset occurs with fever, headache, conjunctivitis, and malaise.

At the site of the bite, a 2- to 5-mm ulcer will develop, which will present a black center (eschar or tache noire).

The fourth day a rash will appear on forearms and will spread to the rest of the body, even covering palms and soles.

Lymphadenopathy will be noted.

Total duration will be about 2 weeks.

There will be almost no complications or mortality (except for the aged).

Evaluate diagnostic procedures:

Check for antibodies; the proteus OX2 gives higher agglutinations.

Cross-immunity tests in guinea pigs, and other reactions may be used.

Management of this form of typhus:

Early treatment with tetracycline.

Scrub Typhus (Tsutsugamushi Disease, Tropical Typhus, Mite-Borne Typhus)

Evaluate characteristics of the *R. tsutsugamushi:*

It is transmitted by mites (also kept in mite families for generations), usually in the form of a larva (chigger).

Incubation lasts for 1 to 3 weeks; average 10 to 12 days.

It occurs in the Pacific islands and India.

Evaluate symptoms and course of scrub typhus:

There are nonspecific prodromal symptoms, such as fever, headache, backache, chilliness, and lymphadenopathy.

More or less simultaneously with fever there will be a papule at the site of the bite, not always seen in infected Asians.

The papule vesiculates, ruptures, and will show a black scab.

There will also be conjunctivitis and splenomegaly, and some patients will appear confused and obtunded.

At the end of the first week of fever a rash will be noted on the trunk, which may extend to the extremities.

The rash will start with macules, and may be fleeting, or may be changed to intensely colored maculopapules.

Cough may be present during the first week; pneumonitis may develop during the second week.

Also, during the second week there may appear complications such as encephalitis, and cardiac problems (tachycardia, hypotension, etc.).

Evaluate diagnostic procedures for scrub typhus:

Isolate organism from blood or tissues.

Check agglutinins against Proteus mirabilis OXK (second week).

Management of scrub typhus:

Tetracycline or chloramphincol (defervescence usually in 36 hours).

Repeat treatment the seventh and the fourteenth days after end of therapy.

Rickettsialpox (Vesicular Rickettsiosis)

Evaluate characteristics of the disease:

It is transmitted by mites.

It is caused by *R. akari.*

Incubation lasts from 7 to 12 days.

Sudden onset occurs, with fever, chills, headache, body pains, and photophobia.

An initial lesion antedates the aforementioned onset for 1 week, that is, a small papule which ulcerates and presents a dark crust.

There will also be lymphadenopathy, profuse sweating, and a rash.

The rash starts 2 to 4 days after fever; it is papular, vesiculates, is widespread, and spares palms and soles; the crusts shed in about 10 days.

The Weil-Felix test is negative; check for antibodies.

No treatment is usually needed; but tetracycline may be given for rapid improvement.

Q Fever

Evaluate characteristics of the infective factor, *Rickettsia burnetti:*

It is also called *Coxiella burnetti,* and is present all over the world.

It is transmitted by inhalation from infective animals or humans.

Incubation lasts 1 to 3 weeks, averaging about 20 days.

It may also be transmitted by infected milk.

Evaluate symptoms and course of Q fever:

Onset may be either sudden or slow.

Main symptoms are fever with prostration, headache, and cough with evidence of pneumonitis, particularly from X-ray films.

There are also abdominal pains, muscle pains, and possibly jaundice.
The disease usually lasts for 2 or more weeks.
Cardiovascular symptoms may be present; endocarditis is rare, but mostly fatal.
Mortality is far below 1% if treated properly; only pneumonia or cardiac complications will cause death to the aged or debilitated.

Diagnostic procedures for Q fever are:
Isolate the germ from blood.
Check for complement-fixing antibodies (Weil-Felix test is negative).

Management of Q fever:
Tetracycline will control fever within 48 hours, but will not always eradicate the infection.

Trench Fever (Wolhynian Fever)

Evaluate characteristics of the infective factor, *Rickettsia quintana,* also called *Rochalimaea quintana:*
It is transmitted by lice, now probably found in Mexico and Central America.
Incubation may last from 2 weeks to 1 month.

Symptoms and course for trench fever are:
Sudden onset occurs, with fever, weakness, severe pain behind the eyes, and pains also in back and legs; dizziness.
Lymphadenopathy and splenomegaly are noted; also hepatomegaly.
There is a maculopapular rash, which will be only transient.
Fever will persist for 3 to 5 or 6 days; there will be a pause of about the same length, and a relapse will occur.
Relapses may occur up to eight times.
The total disease may last for 1 or 2 months.
Subclinical infection and carrier state are not too rare.
The infective organism can be recovered from blood cultures.
No treatment is always needed, but tetracyclines and chloramphenicol may help.

Cat's Scratch Disease (or Fever)

Clinical considerations in cat's scratch disease:
The causative factor is unknown, but Chlamydiae have been incriminated.
Frequently (30% of the cases) a papule or pustule will develop at the site of the scratch.
One to three weeks after the vesicle or pustule appears there will occur an infective syndrome.
Fever, malaise, headache, and regional lymphadenopathy occur.
There is enlargement of lymph glands, with no evidence of lymphangitis; nodes appear tender and fixed, with overlying inflammation, or merely enlarged.
Eventually, the nodes become fluctuant and may discharge sterile pus; there may be fistula formation.
Complications (encephalitis, erythema nodosum, osteolytic lesions, purpura) may occur, but are rare.

Diagnostic criteria are:
Clinical evaluation.
Intradermal (tuberculinlike) test.

Management of cat's scratch fever:
Symptoms may last 5 to 14 days; the disease is benign.
Tetracycline may help; surgery is often needed.

Tuberculosis

For more information, please refer to other sections of the book (on respiratory, gastrointestinal diseases).

Evaluate clinical features of *tuberculous pyelonephritis:*
It responds to hematogenous spread from other sites.
Prodromal stage may be asymptomatic, or may only show fever and loss of weight.
Symptoms of pyelonephritis will eventually evolve; thereafter, cystitis or other evidence of lower urinary teact infection will be noted.
Also, fistulas of perineal masses may be noted.
X-ray films will give good information; also, laboratory procedures.
Multiple antituberculous drug therapy will be given.

Evaluate clinical features of *tuberculous peritonitis:*
There is a chronic syndrome, with evidence of a systemic infection, abdominal tenderness, and under palpation a doughy-feeling sensation.
There are symptoms of acute peritonitis, q.v.
Usually, there is a rapid response to antituberculous therapy, even with only one drug (INH).

Evaluate clinical features of *tuberculosis of the pleura:*
There is evidence of pleurisy with effusion, q.v.
Systemic manifestations may be either intense or mild.
Mycobacteria may be recovered from fluid (33% of cases); tuberculin reactions are intensely positive.
Symptoms of empyema are only progressive, following a previous usually known pulmonary infection.
Give the usual treatment for tuberculosis.

Evaluate clinical features of *tuberculous meningitis:*
It may follow a focus in the subarachnoid space, or miliary tuberculosis.
Symptoms may be either intense or mild (see section on meningitis).
Complications may occur (hydrocephalus, focal symtoms, convulsions).
Diagnostic procedures will be carried out as usual; check spinal fluid.
Treatment is as for active tuberculosis, q.v.

Evaluate clinical features of *miliary tuberculosis:*
In early septicemia, or hyperacute miliary tuberculosis, there are very high fever and symptoms of intense toxicity.

In this instance the presence of choroidal tubercles and cultures of sputum or gastric contents are almost essential for diagnosis.

In late dissemination multiple and spaced episodes of bacteremia will be noted; there will be fever, weight loss, anorexia, etc.

In this instance the diagnosis will depend on cultures from fluids and good results from antituberculous therapy (only INH may be needed).

Evaluate clinical features of other possible tuberculous infections:

Pericarditis	Either acute or gradual onset; signs of constrictive pericarditis; pericardial biopsy; intense therapy.
Adrenal tuberculosis	Addison's disease, q.v.
Spondylitis (Pott's disease)	Back pain, evidence of spinal abscess, and symptoms of compression.
Tuberculosis of joints	Usually monoarticular; cultures from affected site.
Scrofula (lymphadenitis)	Enlarged lymph nodes, mainly of the neck; excisional biopsy.

Leprosy (Hansen's Disease)

Clinical facts regarding leprosy are as follows:

It is endemic in some regions of the world (America, Asia, Africa, the Pacific islands, etc.).

There is an extremely slow onset.

Initial lesions occur in the cooler areas of the skin, superficial nerves, eyes, mucosae, testicles.

Lesions will show as lepromatous and tuberculoid.

In lepromatous leprosy the lesions are small and very numerous, with diffuse margins, mostly nodular, involving almost the whole body; symmetric nerve involvement occurs slowly; the resistance of the patient is low, and the course progressive.

In tuberculoid leprosy there are macular lesions, large, asymmetric, anesthetic, and few in number; also there is asymmetric nerve involvement.

Nerve involvement in leprosy is noted by thickening of the trunk, anesthesia, signs of neuritis, and resultant ulcers and bone resorption, with shortening of digits, and extreme disfigurement of face and other traits.

Other symptoms may be of the type of keratitis, iridocyclitis, corneal ulceration, conjunctivitis, etc.; nasal ulcers that provoke deformity of the organ; loss of the eyebrows and enlargement of the lobes of the ear, which are very suggestive warnings; orchitis and gynecomastia; anemia, lymphadenopathy, etc.

Diagnostis of leprosy is by:

Biopsy.

Lepromin test.

Culture of bacilli in animals.

Management of leprosy:

Dapsone.

Diphenylthiourea, thalidomide, rifampin.

Watch for reactions (use corticoids).

Rheumatic Fever

Syndenhan's Chorea

Hutchinson's Chorea

For information, see other sections of this book, i.e., those devoted to musculoskeletal and nervous diseases.

Pertussis (Whooping Cough)

Evaluate characteristics of the causative *Bordetella pertussis:*

There is worldwide distribution.

Epidemics occur every 2 to 4 years.

Transmission is by inhalation.

Incubation lasts 7 to 17 days (rarely 21 days); contagiousness may extend up to 8 weeks.

A *B. parapertussis* may cause parapertussis, a similar but milder disease.

Symptoms and course of pertussis are as follows:

There is a prodromal or catarrhal stage or phase, similar to a common cold, only with the nocturnal coughing becoming diurnal.

The paroxysmal stage will occur 10 to 14 days after the start, characterized by very intense coughing (rapid consecutive coughs ending in a deep hurried inspiration called the whoop), repeated up to 50 times every day.

The paroxysmal coughing produces large amounts of viscid mucus, which may be expelled or swallowed.

Vomiting is not rare, occuring during the paroxysmal attacks of cough.

About 1 month after the initiation of paroxysms the convalescent stage begins, with a decrease in frequency and intensity of the attacks.

The total duration of the disease may be 6 weeks.

Final diagnosis depends on:

Causing a paroxysmal attack of cough by irritation of the pharynx.

Positive cultures from nasopharyngeal secretion, which may be positive in 80 to 90% of the cases in early stages.

Specific fluorescent antibodies tests.

Management of pertussis:

Use active prophylactic immunization.

Hyperimmune globulin and antibiotics are of dubious help.

Give symptomatic and supportive help.

Typhoid Fever

Characteristics of the causative *Salmonella typhi* are:
- Most infections may come from carriers.
- Entrance is via the gastrointestinal tract.
- Incubations last from 5 to 14 days, rarely 25 days.

Clinical symptoms and course are as follows:
- Usually, an insidious onset (rarely sudden, as with children) characterizes the prodromal stage.
- They will be a gradually increasing sensation of bad health, fever with chills or chilly sensations, headache, epistaxis (at times considered a warning sign), body aches, anorexia, and constipation.
- At about the second week of disease, symptoms reach their peak; that is, fever will be high, abdominal discomfort ends in distention, the constipation may appear worse or turn into pea-soup diarrhea, and the patient will feel very bad and probably will develop the typhoid state.
- In the typhoid state the patient is obtunded, stays motionless and almost unresponsive, or at most responds to carry out very simple orders.
- During this fastigium the temperature is sustained high, and the pulse appears bradycardic and dicrotic; the almost characteristic rose spots will emerge at about the seventh to tenth day on the chest and abdomen, but only in some 10% of the cases, and will fade in no more than 5 days; the spleen will enlarge; and occasionally there will be meningismus or heart arrhythmia.
- At about the third week of the disease symptoms will start to decrease, if the patient does not die; in 7 to 10 days patient will appear almost normal.
- Relapse may occur after 1 or 2 weeks of apparent normalcy.

Complications that may occur with typhoid patients are:
- A consequence of no treatment or insufficient treatment.
- Intestinal hemorrhage, during the third week, q.v.
- Intestinal perforation, also during the third week, and mainly with males, q.v.
- Also to be considered, pneumonia (pneumo-typhus), myocarditis, cholecystitis, spondylitis (typhoid spine), urinary retention, etc.

Laboratory findings for typhoid fever are the following:
- Blood culture, the first week.
- Stool culture, the second week.
- Urine culture that may be positive at any time.
- Widal test, the second week, and after that time.

Management of typhoid fever:
- Preventive vaccination.
- Ampicillin or chloramphenicol.
- Supportive and symptomatic care.

Paratyphoid Fever

Evaluate clinical features of paratyphoid fever:
- It is due to infections with other type of salmonellas, namely, *S. typhimurium, S. derby, S. heidelberg, S. infantis,* etc.
- Clinical symptoms simulate gastroenteritis, q.v.
- The causative organisms can be recovered from the stools.
- Treat symptomatically; only in special cases give ampicillin or chloramphenicol.

Shigellosis (Bacillary Dysentery)

Characteristics of the causative factor for bacillary dysentery:
- *Shigella dysenteriae* is the most virulent.
- *S. sonnei* is the most frequently found in the United States.
- Other forms are *S. flexneri* and *S. boydii.*
- Infection is carried by contaminated foods.
- Incubation lasts from 1 to 4 days.
- Most cases resolve in 2, 3, or 6 weeks; very mild ones in about 1 week.

Clinical characteristics of shigellosis are as follows:
- Sudden onset is usual.
- There are lower abdominal cramps with diarrhea and tenesmus.
- Diarrhea may be bloody, and tenesmus may end in rectal prolapsus.
- There may be fever (elevated among children, even absent among adults), with or without chills, headache, lethargy.
- Severe cases will add meningismus, seizures, and coma.
- Stool culture will be positive for *Shigella.*

Management of shigellosis:
- Symptomatic and supportive.
- Ampicillin or trimethoprim with sulfamethoxazole (spare antibiotics!).

Cholera

Characteristics of the causative *Vibrio cholerae:*
- It is mostly found in Asia; also in Africa, Japan, Australia, etc.
- It is transmitted by ingestion of contaminated water or food.
- Incubation lasts from 1 to 3 days; it may be 5 days.
- Recovery will occur in 3 to 6 days; 50% of those untreated will die.

Clinical symptoms and course for cholera will be:
- There is a fulminant onset of diarrhea (cases may be very mild or fulminantly lethal).
- Diarrhea is watery; stools are gray, turbid, but rarely with pus.
- Losses may amount to 7 liters in 24 hours; to this, some patients may add losses from vomiting.
- Consequent dehydration and acidosis will be evident, q.v.

Diagnosis of cholera:
- Isolate the causative organism from stools.
- Agglutination may also be performed.

Management of cholera:
- Preventive vaccination; treat contacts with tetracycline.
- Careful treatment of dehydration and acidosis.
- Early treatment with tetracycline (will reduce mortality to less than 1% and terminate diarrhea in about two days).

Food Poisoning

The clinical picture of food poisoning usually runs as follows:
- Sudden onset.
- Anorexia with nausea and possibly vomiting.
- Diarrhea.
- Lack of fever and other systemic manifestations (with some exceptions).

The infective causes of food poisoning are:
- The milder cases of shigellosis, cholera, and salmonellosis.
- Also, milder cases of botulism; consider *Clostridium perfringens.*
- Staphylococcal infection.
- *Escherichia coli* infections.
- *Vibrio parahemolyticus* infections.

Noninfective causes of food poisoning are:
- Chemical contaminants.
- Fish, shellfish, and mushrooms.
- Ergot, and other nonbacterial causes.

Clinical evaluation of *Clostridium perfringens infections:*
- There is a history of eating rewarmed meats.
- Symptoms are as above.
- *Clostridia* will be found in cultures from food or feces.
- Recovery will occur in less than 4 days, even without treatment.
- For severe cases use penicillin and type-specific antisera.

Clinical evaluation of *staphylococcal infections:*
- The germ grows in meats, dairy products, and bakery foods.
- Symptoms are as above.
- A group of people eating the same food will be affected.
- Recovery is in less than 2 days, even without treatment.
- If needed, restore fluids and electrolytes.

Clinical evaluation of *Escherichia coli infections,* which are also known as *traveler's diarrhea* (also Montezuma's revenge):
- Symptoms are as above, usually with little vomiting.
- Symptoms subside in less than 3 days.
- Laboratory procedures (serotyping, bioassays) will give the diagnosis.
- Serious disease will occur only among neonates or small infants, the elderly, or debilitated patients.
- Treat symptomatically and give good supportive help.
- Diphenoxylate may be given.

Clinical evaluation of *Vibrio parahemolyticus infections:*
- The causative agent grows in seafood.
- Symptoms are as above, but there may be bloody diarrhea.
- It will affect groups of persons eating the same food, particularly crabs and other shellfish.
- Cultures are positive from food and stools.
- Recovery will occur in less than 3 days.
- There is no need for treatment; but check for dehydration and electrolyte defects.

Evaluation of *noninfective causes* of food poisoning:
- *Lead poisoning* may cause, in addition to the above symptoms, headache, ataxia, insomnia, convulsions, etc.; if needed, do chelation therapy.
- *Arsenic poisoning* may also cause throat constriction, dysphagia, and evidence of dehydration, pulmonary edema, and failure of kidneys and liver; if needed do a gastric lavage, chelation therapy, BAL, etc.
- Other causes may be due to *insecticides* (DDT, Parathion, etc.), *cadmium* (cadmium-lined containers), etc.
- *Shellfish poisoning* will add perioral paresthesias, and perhaps serious central nervous symptoms, or disturbed coagulation; treatment will be mainly supportive and symptomatic.
- *Fish poisoning* may also cause circumoral paresthesias, general aches, fever, sweating, etc.; cholinesterase reactivators have been recommended.
- *Mushrooms* may be the cause of severe poisoning, with added symptomatology of nervous involvement and perhaps a lethal outcome; treat with atropine (muscarine poisoning) and combat hypoglycemia (phalloidine poisoning).
- *Ergot poisoning* adds burning feet, hypotension, gangrene of distal sites, etc.; treatment is mainly supportive.

Plague (Bubonic Plague)

Characteristics of the causative *Pasteurella* (or *Yersinia*) *pestis:*
- It is transmitted from rodents to men by means of fleas.
- Human transmission by inhalation may occur with pneumonic plague.
- Incubation lasts from 2 to 10 days; possibly hours to 12 days.

Symptoms and course of the disease are:
- Sudden onset occurs, with elevated fever, malaise, headache, myalgias, and tachycardia.
- The patient rapidly becomes anxious and delirious.
- In *bubonic plague* there will be a pustule or an ulcer at the site of inoculation, enlarged lymph nodes (inguinal, axillary, less frequently the cervical).
- The buboes (lymphadenopathy) are firm, fixed, and tender; the overlying skin is red and smooth; may eventually suppurate and drain.
- In *pneumonic plague* (by inhalation) there will be no lesion of inoculation; cough will develop rapidly, with a sputum that also rapidly will become bloody; there will be dyspnea with tachypnea, and few auscultatory signs; it is lethal if treatment does not start immediately.

In *septicemic plague* the illness is fulminant, with few symptoms; purpuric spots (black plague) will be seen on the skin.
The causative germ will be cultured from blood, buboes, etc.

Management of plague:
With early treatment mortality will be less than 5%.
Give streptomycin, tetracycline.
Order isolation, and supportive care.

Brucellosis (Undulant Fever, Malta Fever)

Considerations about the infective factor:
It is a *Brucella*, either *B. melitensis, B. abortus,* or *B. suis,* etc.
It is distributed all over the world.
Transmission occurs mainly through abraded skin or mucosae, or through the respiratory tract; also from milk.
Incubation varies from a few days to several weeks, or months.

Evaluation of symptoms and course of brucellosis:
There is an insidious onset; it is rarely sudden.
Initially, there will be intermittent fever, with chills and sweating; or merely weakness and exhaustion from minimal activity, lasting for a few weeks.
Relatively characteristic symptoms will include the establishment of a typical undulant fever; during the febrile stage the temperature will drop in the morning with profuse sweating; half of the cases will present splenomegaly and lymphadenopathy, and some will show complications of the type of orchitis, bone lesions, hepatic or nervous symptoms.
There may also be gastrointestinal symptoms (anorexia, pains, and a marked constipation).

Evaluation of diagnostic procedures:
Intradermal test is of little or no value.
Cultures are positive from blood, urine, etc., but bacteriologic identification may be difficult, at least in late stages.
Agglutination tests will help.

Management of Malta fever:
Tetracycline; with streptomycin to the severely ill.

Tularemia (Rabbit Fever)

Considerations regarding *Francisella tularensis,* which causes the disease:
It is an infection of wild rodents.
It is transmitted by contamination, inoculation, or ingestion.
It is most frequent among hunters, butchers, and fur-handlers.
Incubation may last from 1 to 10 days (average 2 to 4 days).

Evaluation of the symptomatology and clinical course of tularemia:
There is a sudden onset with high fever, chills, headache, nausea (possibly with vomiting), and intense prostration.
After 1 or 2 days a papule, which soon ulcerates, appears at the site of inoculation.
The initial lesion will occur on the skin of a finger or an arm in the great majority of cases (87%), characterizing the ulceroglandular type of infection; or around one eye (3%), mostly in the form of multiple ulcers, thus characterizing the oculoglandular type.
There may be also a typhoidal type (8%) and a glandular type (2%), these without inoculating ulceration.
Enlarged regional lymph nodes will be noted.
There may be a pneumonia.
The typhoidal type will resemble typhoid fever, and will be caused by ingestion.

Evaluate diagnostic procedures:
Culture of the *Francisella* (or *Pasteurella*) *tularensis* is made from blood or ulcers or lymph nodes.
Agglutination tests will be informative after the second week.
About 50% of the patients will present a positive skin test.

Management of tularemia:
An early adequate treatment will eliminate mortality (5% in regular instances; 30% in cases with pneumonia).
Give streptomycin; preferably with tetracycline; also, chloramphenicol.

Glanders (Farcy)

Evaluation of clinical features of glanders:
It is caused by *Malleomyces mallei,* also called *Actinobacillus* or *Pseudomonas mallei.*
There is a history of exposure to horses, about 1 week previously.
Sudden onset occurs, with elevated fever, chills, headache, and prostration.
There is a painful ulcer at the site on infection.
Other ulcers may also develop; regional adenopathy will follow.
There may be intense coryza-like symptoms.
The cutaneous form of glanders may present an acute or a chronic syndrome; in the first instance together with symptoms of nasal glanders; in the second, with abscesses around the joints.
The nasal glanders presents a nasal mucosa swollen and ulcerated, a severe rhinitis with bloody secretions, and dyspnea.
Culture of the causative organism will give the diagnosis.
It is treated with the specific antibiotic, or a combination of two, while the patient is hospitalized.

Melioidosis

Evaluation of clinical features of melioidosis:
- It is caused by *Pseudomonas pseudomallei.*
- It is transmitted by contamination, ingestion, or inhalation.
- Latent illness may last for years.
- Acute illness may be in the pulmonary form with cough, rales, and tachypnea; the sputum is tinged with blood, and X-ray findings will reveal consolidation and cavitation.
- It also may be in the septicemic form with confusion, intense dyspnea, colic with diarrhea, and skin pustular lesions.
- Cultures will give the diagnosis; also agglutination tests.
- Treat with tetracycline, or other antibiotics or sulfas.

Diphtheria

Evaluation of the causative *Corynebacterium diphtheriae:*
- There are three different biotypes of the bacillus; only the toxigenic variety produces exotoxin.
- Transmission is direct or by contaminated objects.
- Incubation lasts from 1 to 7 days; average, 2 to 4 days.

Clinical features related to diphtheria:
- There is a short and noncharacteristic prodromal stage.
- There is a noncharacteristic, usually relatively mild, infective syndrome.
- The development of the membrane is almost characteristic of the disease.
- Thereafter, severe evidence of toxemia and possibly complications (heart, nervous system) will develop.

Evaluation of pharyngeal diphtheria:
- The membrane, gray and tenacious, grows on the pharynx and anterior pillars.
- There is a surrounding erythema, and a larger edematous area.
- There are symptoms of sore throat and respiratory difficulties.
- Complicating myocarditis may terminate in decompensation.
- Complicating neuritis may cause weakness (nasal voice, regurgitation, difficult swallowing, diplopia or strabismus, etc.).

Evaluation of laryngeal diphtheria:
- It may follow pharyngeal diphtheria, or be the initial manifestation.
- Obstruction of airway tract is more severe in this condition.
- Evidence of toxicity is worse in this condition.
- When there is a severe local edema, because of diffusion of endotoxin, there will be a bull-necked patient; this may also happen in cases of pharyngeal diphtheria.

Evaluation of nasal diphtheria:
- There is less toxemia than in the pharyngeal and laryngeal forms.
- There is a serosanguinous discharge from the nostrils.
- The membrane will develop in the nasal passages.

Evaluation of cutaneous diphtheria:
- It is found mostly among indigents and those with poor personal hygiene (in the tropics).
- Usually the membrane will grow on wounds or other breaks of the skin.
- Lesions may look like vitiligo.
- Check for nasopharyngeal invasion in all these cases.

Diagnosis of diphtheria:
- Confirmed by bacterial cultures.

Management of diphtheria:
- Active immunization.
- Diphtheria antitoxin to be given to all patients.
- Penicillin, or erythromycin.
- Other symptomatic and supportive measures.

Tetanus

Characteristics of the causative organism, *Clostridium tetani:*
- Distribution is almost universal.
- The germ lives on soil and feces.
- Even a supposedly clean wound may become infected, particularly if it has been in contact with soiled matter.
- Average incubation will last for 5-8 to 10-12 days, but may extend from 2 to even 100 days.
- Neonates may be infected through the umbilical cord.
- Heroin users are at risk (particularly females).

Evaluate clinical features of tetanus:
- There are pain, tingling, and muscle spasticity at the site of inoculation.
- The characteristic symptom is jaw stiffness with trismus because of spams of other jaw muscles.
- There are stiffness of the neck, dysphagia, hyperreflexia.
- There are irritability, and stiffness of other muscles (risus sardonicus).
- There are painful tonic convulsions following minor stimulation; opisthotonus.
- At most, a febricula will be present.
- The patient is alert at all times.
- Spasm of upper respiratory muscles may cause severe obstruction.

Evaluate diagnosis of tetanus:
- Clinical diagnosis (spasms and convulsions), following history of a recent wound (as a better help).

Management of tetanus:
- Active immunization.
- Tetanus immune globulin (human); check convulsions (diazepam, etc.).
- Treatment of other symptoms, and support of the patient.

Histotoxic Clostridial Disease (Gas Gangrene)

Characteristics of the causative clostridia:
- The most frequent is *Clostridium perfringes,* but there may also be *Cl. novyi,* or *Cl. septicum.*
- They grow in anaerobic conditions, usually in penetrating or crushing injuries.
- Also, they may complicate appendicitis, perforating intestinal lesions, or other similar diseases.

Evaluate clinical features of gas gangrene:
- Usual sudden onset, with pain and edema on contaminated area.
- Watery exudate of a brown or bloody color, and foul odor.
- Skin discoloration.
- Tachycardia, and hypotension; mild fever.
- Later development of vesicles, and crepitation noted from gas.
- There may be prostration, stupor, delirium, coma; and complications of the type of jaundice and renal failure.

Evaluate clinical facts of other clostridial infections:
- In clostridial myonecrosis the progress is rapid, a matter of only hours.
- In clostridial uterine infection a previous septic abortion is the cause; the uterus is tender, and the lochia foul smelling.

Diagnostic data to be considered:
- Moderate amounts of gas will arouse suspicion.
- *Clostridia* will be found on cultures or smears of exudate, but this finding will not suffice for diagnosis by itself.

Management of clostridial infections:
- Careful debridement and exposure of the lesion.
- Very high doses of penicillin, and polyvalent gas gangrene antitoxin; the latter questionable, and the former to be changed to tetracycline or cephalothin for allergic patients.

Botulism

The *Clostridium botulinum* that causes this form of food poisoning shows the following characteristics:
- The ingestion of its toxin causes the symptoms.
- It is found in canned food (particularly homemade), and also smoked meats, vacuum-packed fish, etc.
- Incubation lasts 12-18 to 36 hours, but may extend from 4 hours to even 8 days.

Clinical facts about botulism are:
- There is a history of eating suspect food.
- There may be a short prodromal stage with weakness.
- Diplopia is the commonly found first symptom; but there may be other sorts of visual changes (diminished vision, blepharoptosis, involvement of pupillary reflexes).
- There are dysphagia, dysphonia, dryness of mouth.
- Muscle weakness may lead to respiratory paralysis.
- Nausea, vomiting, and diarrhea may occur (particularly with canned fish containing type E of the clostridia).
- Temperature and sensorium remain normal.
- In rare cases it may occur from a wound infection.
- The toxin can be identified from serum or foods.

Management of botulism:
- Urgent administration of trivalent botulinus antitoxin (check for sensitivity to horse serum).
- Symptomatic and supportive care.

Anthrax (Malignant Pustule)

Evaluate clinical findings regarding malignant pustule:
- The causative *Bacillus anthracis* has an incubation period of 3 to 5 days, but it may be as short as 12 hours.
- The disease is almost controlled all over the world.
- Cutaneous anthrax is the most frequent finding; the malignant pustule appears as a papule that vesiculates and enlarges, showing a very dark center (purple or black) surrounded by numerous vesicles on an indurated area.
- There are regional lymphadenopathy, fever (usually with fever symptomatology), and sepsis manifested by sweating, cyanosis, collapse, and final shock.
- Pulmonary anthrax (also called woolsorter's disease) presents a pneumonia picture, with congestion of the nose, throat, and larynx.
- Mortality is elevated, particularly for pulmonary anthrax.
- The causative organism may be isolated from sputum or blood; antibodies can be detected by indirect hemagglutination test.

Management of anthrax:
- Early administration of high doses of penicillin by the intravenous route, in the cases of pulmonary anthrax; lesser amounts in the case of cutaneous anthrax.

Syphilis (Lues)

Evaluate clinical features of *primary syphilis:*
- Inoculation (sex, kiss, or other form of close body contact) occurs 3 to 4 weeks previously, but this lapse may be extended from 1 to 13 weeks.
- At the site of inoculation there appears a chancre (similar origin to that of the word cancer).
- The chancre starts as a red papule or small erosion, rapidly turning into a painless ulcer on an indurated hard basis (rarely more than one chancre present).
- No bleeding will occur; on abrasion a clear serum rich in *Treponema pallidum* is obtained.
- Regional lymph nodes become enlarged, rubbery, nontender, and discrete.
- Most chancres are found in genital areas; some may appear on lips, fingers, etc.
- Diagnosis is made from dark field examinations; serologic tests will be positive only 1 or 2 weeks after the initial clinical finding.
- Treat with penicillin.

Evaluate clinical features of *secondary syphilis:*

Symptoms will appear 2 or more months (up to 6 months) after the chancre.

There may be fever, and generalized lymphadenopathy (about 50% of cases).

Skin or mucosal lesions are the most common findings (80%).

Skin lesions may mimic a large number of dermatologic conditions.

They are usually symmetrical and generalized, involving palms and soles, maculopapular in most instances, pinkish in whites and pigmented in blacks; they are not itchy and take a rounded form, becoming confluent.

Mucous lesions are papules or ulcers noted on mouth, genitalia, and anus.

Both types of lesions, cutaneous and mucous, are highly contagious.

Condylomata lata are fused papules on the moist areas of skin and mucosae, presenting a hypertrophic, flattened, and grayish aspect.

Other symptoms and complications are alopecia, iritis, jaundice, nephrotic syndrome, and meningeal, hepatic, kidney, bone, and similar manifestations.

Lesions are rich in treponemas, and serologic blood tests are positive.

Treat with penicillin; but consider that with inadequate treatment lesions may relapse; they will also relapse if not treated at all.

Evaluate clinical features of *tertiary* (or *late*) *syphilis:*

A latent or hidden stage of syphilis will occur following secondary syphilis; there will be no symptoms, but serology will remain positive.

Appearance of symptoms will occur at any time after secondary syphilis, even several years.

Gummata are lesions in the skin, submucous tissue, long bones, or any organ in the body.

A gumma is a localized lesion with central necrosis surrounded by granulomatous tissue; it is painless, and after healing will leave a scar.

Skin gummata are nodular and ulcerative; in other sites, they will result in punched-out ulcers, or perforation.

More serious tertiary lesions of diffuse inflammatory character will occur in the cardiovascular or neurological systems.

Evaluate symptoms of syphilitic *aortitis:*

About 80% of those untreated or deficiently treated will develop it.

Main symptomatology will be that of obstruction or of aneurysmatic dilatation.

Symptoms of obstruction will lead to Martorell's or Takayase's disease, q.v., in the chapter devoted to cardiovascular diseases.

Aneurysms of the aorta are dealt with in the same chapter.

Evaluate symptoms of *neurosyphilis:*

In *meningovascular involvement* together with usual symptoms there may be poor concentration, neck stiffness, blurred vision, papilledema, nerve deficiencies (aphasia, paralysis, etc.), and the characteristic Argyll Robertson pupil (irregularly shaped and with no reaction to light but reacting well to accommodation).

In *general paresis* change of behavior is the important sign; delusions and other important symptoms will come later.

In *tabes dorsalis* there are stabbing fulgurant pains, mainly felt in the legs, followed by difficult gait, particularly in the dark, and the also characteristic positive Romberg's sign (poor equilibrium with the eyes closed) and visceral crises.

Evaluate other consequences of tertiary syphilis:

Trophic lesions.

Charcot's arthropathy.

Respiratory involvement.

Gastrointestinal involvement.

Evaluate diagnosis and management of tertiary syphilis:

Rely on clinical evidence and serology.

Regular penicillin courses will be given.

More severe neurologic involvement may require larger doses of penicillin and even additional courses; in neurologic cases the spinal fluid will be carefully examined every few months.

Evaluate *congenital syphilis:*

It affects offspring of syphilitic untreated mothers.

In early congenital syphilis skin lesions are present, mainly bullous eruptions, but also other manifestations of syphilis may be noted; the infant will fail to thrive and will show the classic old-man appearance.

In late congenital syphilis (also later in early syphilis) there will be Hutchinson's teeth, and possibly keratitis, deafness, saber shins, parietal bossing, etc.

Treat these cases with penicillin; a good followup is needed.

Treponematoses

Evaluate these diseases, which occur mostly in foreign countries:

Bejel, caused by *Treponema pallidum II,* is a nonvenereal form of infection, with prevalent moist ulcerated lesions appearing on the skin and mucous membranes, and rare visceral involvement.

Pinta, caused by *Treponema carateum,* provokes the appearance of papulo-squamous plaques with a variety of colors, mostly on the limbs; later, there will be atrophy and depigmentation.

Frambesia, or *yaws,* caused by *Treponema pertenue,* begins with a mother yaw in the site of inoculation (usually a limb) accompanied by enlarged lymph nodes, the initial lesion being a papule that eventually ulcerates and is followed later on by similar secondary lesions; those noted on the feet are called crab yaws, on the nose they are gangosa, and if in the lower jaw they constitute goundou.

Evaluate diagnosis and treatment for these treponematoses:
- Serology is employed, as for syphilis.
- Treponemas may be found on lesions.
- Treat with penicillin, as soon as possible to avoid disfigurement.

Chancroid (Soft Chancre)

Evaluate the causative factor, *Haemophilus ducreyi:*
- It is transmitted by venereal contact.
- Incubation lasts 3 to 5 days.

Evaluate clinical features of the soft chancre:
- There is an initial macule or vesicopustule that soon ulcerates.
- The soft, painful ucler is on a necrotic base surrounded by erythema.
- The edge is undetermined, and there is no induration as in the case of syphilitic ulcerative chancre.
- Multiple lesions may occur; and phagedenic erosion may destroy tissues.
- Lymphatic involvement may cause buboes, which may suppurate and form a sinus.
- There may be phimosis, strictures of the urethra, and other forms of tissue destruction.
- Diagnosis depends on clinical evidence, since cultures are difficult to obtain; rule out other venereal diseases.

Management of soft chancre:
- Prefer sulfonamides; tetracycline may also be given.
- Surgical measures may be needed.

Granuloma Inguinale

Evaluate features of the causative factor:
- It is believed that *Calymmatobacterium* (or *Donovania*) *granulomatis* is possibly the causative agent.
- It is believed that sexual contacts may be the spreading route.
- Incubation may last from 1 to 12 weeks.

Clinical features of granuloma inguinale are:
- There is a slow onset.
- Initial lesions are on the genital area, or other areas used for sex.
- Lesions are painless infiltrated nodules of a beef-red color that grow to a rounded, elevated, velvet granulomatous mass.
- Lesions may spread by contiguity, may be very extensive, and will heal slowly, leaving a scar.
- Secondary infections may occur; cachexia may follow neglected cases.
- Diagnosis may depend on the finding of the characteristic Donovan bodies from scrapings of the ulcerative bases.

Management of granuloma inguinalis:
- Give streptomycin or tetracycline.
- Follow the patient for at least 6 months after treatment.
- Carefully rule out other venereal diseases.

Lymphogranuloma Venereum (or Inguinale)

This infection by one of the members of the Chlamydia group presents the following clinical features:
- Incubation may last from 5 to 28 days (7 to 21).
- The initial, at times unnoticed, primary lesion is a vesicle that very rapidly ulcerates and heals.
- First notice is usually given by enlarged groin lymph nodes.
- Lymph nodes are bilateral, fuse, soften, and leak through sinuses, which produce extensive scarring.
- Similar manifestations may occur in the anorectal area, leading to stricture, constipation, and fistula formation.
- Systemic symptoms will be fever, arthralgia, skin rashes, and eye complications; there may be also headache and meningeal irritation.
- Large polypoid masses may lead to elephantiasis.

Diagnosis of lyphogranuloma inguinale may be assesed by:
- Frei test.
- A more sensitive complement fixation test.

Management of the disease:
- Give tetracycline.
- Sulfas may also be given, particularly if syphilis is suspected.
- Elephantiasis will require surgery.

Gonorrhea (Blenorrhagia)

Evaluate characteristics of the causative *Neisseria gonorrhoeae:*
- There is venereal transmission.
- Incubation lasts from 2 to 8 or 10 days.

Symptoms and other clinical findings in gonorrhea affecting women:
- A large number (60%) do not show symptoms.
- Symptoms may be mild; only a moderately increased discharge, or a modest cervicitis.
- In other cases there will be dysuria (with frequency and urgency), a purulent discharge from the urethra (either spontaneously or by expression), and other evidence of vaginitis, cervicitis, and inflammation of the adjacent glands (Bartholin, Skene).
- Infection may progress to the uterus and the adnexa structures.
- Rectal infection (also pharyngeal) may occur.

Symptoms and other clinical findings in gonorrhea affecting men:
- It starts with a tingling sensation of the urethra.
- Rapidly, dysuria and purulent discharge develop.
- There are frequency and urgency of a very painful micturition.

There is a yellowish-green purulent discharge from the urethra.
The lips of the urethral meatus are swollen and red.
Spread of infection may involve prostate, epididymis, and periurethral glands, all becoming painful and inflamed.
Other initial sites of infection may also occur, particularly pharyngeal, and anorectal among homosexuals.

Diagnosis of gonorrhea:
Detection of the gonococcus by smears or cultures.

Consequences of gonococcal bacteremia:
Intermittent fever, with arthralgia and skin lesions.
Gonococcal arthritis.
Iritis and conjunctivitis (may lead to panophthalmitis with destruction of the eye, particularly in neonates).
Rarely, endocarditis or meningitis.

Management of gonorrhea:
Penicillin (never the benzathine form).
If needed, ampicillin or a tetracycline.

Psittacosis

For information, see the chapter devoted to respiratory diseases.

Carrión's Disease (Oroya Fever, or Bartonellosis)

Evaluate clinical features of verruga peruana:
The causative germ is *Bartonella bacilliformis.*
It is endemic in the Andean valleys.
It is transmitted by the bite of a phlebotomus.
Oroya fever is the first stage, which lasts from 2 to 6 weeks and may end in apparent recovery or death.
Verruga peruana is the second stage.

Evaluate clinical features of the first stage of Carrión's disease:
Remittent fever, or it may be intermittent.
Malaise and pains (head, bone, joints).
Hepatomegaly, severe anemia (macrocytic), hemorrhagic lymph nodes; jaundice.
Possibility of thrombosis.
Gradual improvement of symptoms, or deterioration and death.

Evaluate clinical features of the second stage of Carrión's disease:
If Oroya fever was not apparent, this might give the erroneous impression of being the first stage.
Multiple hemangiomas (miliary and nodular) appear in crops.
They mainly set on the face and extremities.
They bleed easily; they may ulcerate.
Cutaneous lesions last from 1 to 12 months.
They heal without a scar.

Evaluate diagnostic procedures:
Blood cultures may be used in early first stage.
Bartonellas are found in endothelial cells (second stage).

Management of Carrión's disease:
Chloramphenicol or tetracycline.
Symptomatic for anemia.

Relapsing Fever (Recurrent Fever)

Evaluate the causative factor of this spirillum fever:
It is caused by a group of almost identical clinical entities.
The causative factor may be one of different spirochetes, but the principal one is *Borrelia recurrentis.*
Borrelias are transmitted by lice or ticks.
Incubation lasts about 1 week.

Evaluate clinical features of the disease:
A sudden onset occurs.
There are fever, chills, tachycardia, severe headache, pain in muscles and joints, nausea and vomiting, and mental changes.
There are hepatomegaly, splenomegaly; on occasion there is bronchitis, and there may be jaundice.
Some cases will present a rash (erythema on trunk and limbs, which later changes to rose spots); petechia may occur.
After 3 to 10 days of symptoms, they improve, and the fever falls by crisis.
For about 1 week (4–5 to 10–14 days) there will be a remission.
Then a relapse of similar symptomatology will occur.
Relapses are less and less severe; but there may be jaundice, cranial nerve lesions, iritis, conjunctivitis, and hemorrhagic phenomena.
Relapses usually occur from 2 to 10 times; then recovery follows.
Mortality may reach 2 to 8%.

Diagnostic procedures:
Check for spirochetes during a paroxysm.
Cultures in rats.
Positive Weil-Felix test.

Management of recurrent fever:
Tetracycline or penicillin (not close to the end of a paroxysmal recurrence); also chloramphenicol.
Resistant cases treated with an arsenical.

Leptospirosis (Weil's Disease, Infectious Jaundice)

The infective leptospiras are characterized as follows:
Leptospira icterohemorrhagiae, L. canicola, L. pomona, or perhaps others as well (about 130 serotypes of the genus) may cause infection.
Infection may occur at any age, from direct or indirect contact with contaminated water or soil; most cases appear from June to September.
Incubation lasts from 2 to 20 days (average 1 or 2 weeks).

Clinical features for leptospirosis in its first stage (leptospiremic):
There is a sudden onset, with high fever, chills, pains (head, abdomen, muscles), and vomiting.

Conjunctivitis is characteristic.
Hepatomegaly and splenomegaly are not too frequent.
Defervescence occurs at about the fourth to ninth day.

Clinical features for leptospirosis in its second (immune) stage:
After 2 or 3 days of defervescence former symptoms reappear.
There may be evidence of meningismus (aseptic meningitis).
There are capillary hemorrhages and purpuric skin lesions.
Jaundice will characterize Weil's disease, usually with azotemia, continued fever, mental changes, perhaps more marked hemorrhagic features, and other renal abnormalities.
Mortality is nil for patients without jaundice, and 15% if jaundice is present (over age 60, it will 30%).

Diagnostic features for leptospirosis:
Identify the *Leptospira* from blood (only during the first 10 days of disease), or from cultures.
Use specific agglutination tests, after 7 days.

Management of leptospirosis:
Start urgent treatment (before the fourth day of disease) with penicillin, tetracycline, or another potent antibiotic.
In severe illness use large intravenous amounts.
Provide symptomatic and supportive treatment when needed.

Rat-Bite Fever (Sodoku)

Clinical features of rat-bite fever are:
It may be caused by either *Streptobacillus moniliformis* (more frequent in the United States) or *Spirillum minus.*
These organisms are transmitted by rat bites.
Symptoms start less than 10 days after the bite (may extend from 1 to 22 days).
In streptobacillary infections there is a flulike initial symptomatology, with a skin rash (morbilliform and petechial) on hands and feet and polyarthralgia of large joints; the germ may be cultured from blood or joint fluid, and serology will help after the second or third week.
In spirillary infections inflammation recurs at the site of the bite with relapsing of fever and adenopathy; there may also be a rash, but it is less prominent; also, the germ will be identified from blood.

Management of rat-bite fever:
Penicillin, or tetracycline.

Erysipeloid

Clinical features of erysipeloid are:
The infection is caused by *Erysipelothrix rhusiopathiae.*
It mostly occurs from handling fish or animal tissues (fishermen or butchers).
Incubation lasts about a week.
In a finger or the back of a hand a lesion appears, red, raised, indurated, itchy, and giving a burning sensation; it gradually extends.
Local swelling occurs, even to inhibit use of hand; but there is no lymph node involvement.
The disease may last for 2 or 3 weeks.
Germs may be obtained for identification from the edge of the lesion.
Penicillin or any broad spectrum antibiotic is curative.

Listeriosis

Clinical features of listeriosis are:
Disease is caused by *Listeria monocytogenes.*
Higher incidence occurs in neonates, adults over 40 years, and during the months of July and August.
Infection is lethal to the fetus.
Postpartum infections cause meningitis.
Adults will also present meningitis; in less frequent instances there will be endocarditis, oculoglandular infection, typhoidal syndrome.
Diagnosis is made by identification of the causal *Listeria.*
Treatment is with penicillin; give tetracycline for meningitis; erythromycin is also active.

Coccidioidomycosis (San Joaquin Fever, Valley Fever)

The causative fungus presents the following characteristics:
It is *Coccidioides immitis.*
It is endemic in the southwestern United States.
Transmission occurs by inhalation, mostly by men between 25 and 55.
Most cases (60%) are subclinical.
Incubation may last from 10 to 30 days.

Essential features of the clinical presentation of primary coccidioidomycosis:
Mild or severe influenzalike syndrome.
Pleural pain, usually severe; same for headache and muscular pains; a skin rash (morbilliform, erythema multiforme or nodosum).
Nasopharyngitis and bronchitis, with coughing.
Arthralgia and periarticular swelling of knees and ankles.
This desert rheumatism includes arthritic symptoms, conjunctivitis, and erythema nodosum.

Essential features of the clinical presentation of progressive coccidioidomycosis:
Symptoms depend on the site of dissemination.
Pulmonary symptoms become more marked; there may be pulmonary abscess.
It may invade the skin, the bones, and peri- or myocardium.
Meningitis will take place in 25% of the cases with disseminated disease.
Other forms of abscess may occur.

Diagnostic procedures for coccidioidomycosis:
- Find the characteristic spherules (better to use well-trained technicians).
- Serology results are a good help, but they appear late in the disease.

Management of the disease:
- Give symptomatic and supportive care.
- Try amphotericin B (may help).
- Surgery is performed whenever needed (using amphotericin B before and after).

Blastomycosis

Characteristics of the occurrence of *North American blastomycosis:*
- The responsible organism is *Blastomyces dermatitidis,* a fungus found in southeastern states and the Mississippi valley.
- Most cases are men 20 to 40 years of age.

Its symptomatology is characterized by:
- An insidious bronchopneumonia with cough, chest pain, dyspnea, together with fever, chills, and drenching sweats.
- Hematogenous spread that will affect skin, prostate and other genital organs, bones, etc.; most lesions being destructive and proliferative.
- Raised, verrucous skin lesions that spread slowly; other forms of skin lesion are not rare.
- Diagnosis dependent on isolation and identification of *B. dermatitidis.*

Occurrence of *South American blastomycosis,* or *paracoccidioiomycosis,* is as follows:
- *Paracoccidioides brasiliensis,* a fungus found in Central and South America, is the causative organism.
- Men between 20 and 50 years of age are mostly affected (coffee-growers in Brazil).

Its symptomatology is characterized by:
- A *cutaneous* typical lesion on the borders of nose and mouth, in the form of an ulcer with granular base and many tiny yellow-whitish areas; there are enlarged lymph nodes that may suppurate.
- A *lymphatic* form, with enlarged lymph nodes in the neck, the supraclavicular area, and the axillae.
- A *visceral* form with enlarged liver, spleen, and lymph nodes, usually with abdominal pain.
- A *mixed* form with several involvements simultaneously.
- Diagnosis dependent on identification of the *P. brasiliensis.*

Management of blastomycosis:
- Amphotericin B may help in these very serious diseases.

Histoplasmosis

This fungal disease is due to:
- *Histoplasma capsulatum,* found in the United States in the Ohio and Mississippi valleys.
- Transmission probably through inhalation.

Essential features of the clinical presentation of histoplasmosis:
- Most cases are asymptomatic.
- Primary acute form cases present an influenzalike syndrome.
- Progressive disseminated form cases present a hematogenous spread from the lungs, with hepatomegaly, splenomegaly, lymphadenopathy, and ulcerations in the mouth or gastrointestinal tract; there is the possibility of developing Addison's disease.
- Chronic cavitary form cases entirely mimic cavitary pulmonary tuberculosis, with cough, dyspnea, and increasing respiratory embarrassment.
- Diagnosis depends on the identification of the fungus by cultures from sputum, lymph nodes, or other tissues.

Management of histoplasmosis:
- Try amphotericin B; it may help in some instances.

Torulosis (Cryptococcosis)

Characteristics of the fungus that causes torulosis:
- It is *Cryptococcus neoformans,* which mainly affects men over age 40.
- It is found all over the world; in the United States mainly in the Southeast.
- Transmission is believed to occur by inhalation.

Symptoms and clinical course of the infection:
- Many patients are almost asymptomatic with pulmonary cryptococcosis.
- Some will present a subacute respiratory syndrome, with febricula, pleural pain, cough, sputum production, and some evidence of bronchitis or pulmonary consolidation.
- Infections of the kidney are also common, with symptoms of pyelonephritis or perhaps papillary necrosis.
- Meningitis is a common form, with headache, blurred vision, behavior changes, disturbances of speech, vertigo, nausea, neck rigidity, positive signs of meningeal irritation, etc.
- Skin lesions of acneiform shape, swollen and painful bone lesions, eye involvement, etc., may also be noted.

Management of torulosis:
- Amphotericin B; flucytosine.

Candidiasis (Moniliasis)

The characteristics of the *Candida* fungi are:
- Normally they are present in about 65% of the population (more in debilitated persons).
- *Candida albicans* is the most frequently found.
- Superficial infections are frequently found, mainly as secondary invaders.

Evaluate clinical features of systemic candidiasis:
- Endocarditis may be related to heart surgery or previous heart damage.

In cases of endocarditis there are fever, heart murmurs, possible emboli, splenomegaly and petechiae, and occasionally renal involvement.

Septicemia usually follows a fulminant course, with fever, oliguria, azotemia, and final renal shutdown with shock.

Meningitis is relatively benign and follows a chronic course.

Pyelonephritis, particularly among elders, presents the fungi in the urine.

All these types of candidiasis usually follow therapy with antibiotics and corticoids for debilitating diseases.

Cultures and serologic tests will help to establish the diagnosis.

Management of candidiasis:

Amphotericin B for serious infections.

Also, flucytosine; and local treatment for superficial infections.

Asperigillosis

Evaluate clinical features of aspergillosis:

Aspergillus fumigatus is the most frequent causative agent of the disease.

After antibiotic or antifungal therapy the aspergillus may invade damaged bronchi (bronchitis, bronchiectasis, tuberculosis, etc.).

The aspergilloma (fungus ball) forms a compact mass, not adherent to the walls of the affected organ.

Aspergillomas produce a dense round mass in X-ray films.

Dissemination to the brain or kidney will cause fever, chills, hypotension, delirium, and other evidence of septicemia.

Smears will help, together with the clinical picture.

Amphotericin B may give some help.

Actinomycosis (Lumpy Jaw)

Characteristics of the causative fungal organism, *Actinomyces israelii:*

In tissues it forms a compact mass called "sulfur granules."

Entry into tissues (usually gums through decayed teeth) allows its pathogeny to become manifest under anaerobic conditions.

It usually associates with other anaerobic germs.

Evaluate clinical symptoms and course of actinomycosis:

Lesions are hard, indurated, granulomatous, suppurative, and most frequently give rise to sinus tracts.

About 60% of the cases will occur in the *cervicofacial area,* following some sort of trauma (extraction, etc.).

There is slow onset and course of an indurated area under reddish or cyanotic skin of irregular surface.

Abscesses eventually suppurate, with the classic sulfur granules in the pus.

Adjacent areas may also be invaded.

Abdominal actinomycosis causes pain, fever, emaciation; a tender ileocecal area; vomiting, and diarrhea or constipation; a mass may be noted; and draining sinuses may develop.

Thoracic actinomycosis gives a picture entirely similar to tuberculosis; perforating sinuses may open on the chest.

Other sites, particularly adjacent areas, may also be invaded, particularly identified by the suppurative sinuses leaking sulfur granules.

Management of actinomycosis:

Give penincillin, in large doses and for a relatively long time.

Tetracycline or other broad spectrum antibiotics may be used instead.

Mucormycosis (Phycomycosis)

Evaluate clinical features of mucormycosis:

It is usually caused by a *Rhizopus* or a *Basidiobolus, Mucor, Absidia,* etc.

In the United States a form complicating diabetic acidosis may set on the nose, the sinuses, or the orbit.

There will be fever, severe local pain, discharge, local destruction of tissues (septum, palate, orbit), and possible invasion of vessels giving rise to central nervous system involvement (convulsions, paralyses, etc.).

Control diabetes carefully; use amphotericin B.

In Asia and Africa there is a subcutaneous form causing grotesque disfiguration of the neck and chest.

Sporotrichosis

Evaluate clinical features of sporotrichosis:

It is caused by *Sprotrichum schenckii,* found in soil, plants, or decaying wood.

It enters through a trauma to the hand, foot, or arm; more rarely will cause pneumonia, if inhaled.

The usual initial lesion is an induration (chancriform) of the skin, which generally spreads along the lymphatic channels (lymphangitis), and stops before the lymph nodes are invaded.

Pneumonic symptoms are usually mild.

Cultures will help diagnosis.

Treat with potassium iodide; give amphotericin B to severe cases.

Mycetoma (Madura Foot, Maduromycosis)

Evaluate clinical features of maduromycosis:

About 50% of the cases are caused by *Nocardia* species; others by *Streptomyces* or any of 20 other different fungi.

Barefoot people, mostly from 20 to 40 years of age and living in the tropics or southern parts of the United States, will present the disease.

It mostly affects the feet, but also other tissues.

Lesions are papulovesicles on an indurated base, which ulcerates and forms a fistula; the entire area ulcerates, becomes granulomatous, progresses slowly, and finally destroys muscles, tendons, bones, etc., discharging an oily serosanguineous fluid and distorting the form of the extremity.

Check for the characteristic invading organism.

Nocardia infections may respond to soluble sulfas.

Other infections are difficult to treat.

Nocardiosis

Evaluate clinical features of nocardiosis:

It is caused by *Nocardia asteroides* (not a fungus!), related to *Actinomyces israelii.*

Most cases occur in patients with neoplastic diseases (leukemia, etc.).

Pulmonary invasion is similar to that of actinomycosis; there is a relatively rapid hematogenous invasion (to the brain in the first place, also to kidneys, etc.).

Treat with sulfa drugs.

Rhinosporidiosis

Evaluate clinical features of rhinosporidiosis:

It is caused by *Rhinosporidium seeberi,* when swimming in stagnant water (India).

Large, friable, sessile polyposis will appear in mucous membranes.

Areas mostly affected are eyes, nose, larynx, vagina; also may set on ears or penis.

Check for the causative organism.

Remove the polyps.

Chromomycosis (Chromoblastomycosis)

Evaluate clinical features of chromomycosis:

It is caused by fungi with a dark mycelium (*Hormodendrum, Phialophora*).

Most cases are men between the ages of 30 and 50; there is worldwide distribution, but particularly in the tropics.

The lesion starts on the foot or leg, or any other exposed part of the body with an abraded surface.

A papule or ulcer slowly expands, becoming verrucous or papillomatous and forming hard, red or gray nodules with the appearance of cauliflowerlike or dry verrucous plaques.

Elephantiasis, secondary infections, and ulceration may occur.

Finding the causative organism will help diagnosis.

Early removal is the best treatment.

Try amphotericin B.

Fever of Unknown (or Undetermined) Origin, FUO

Explain what is considered to be a fever of unknown origin:

Temperature must be over 38°C (100.4°F), though some claim it must be over 38.5°C, particularly with children.

Duration of the fever has to be over 3 weeks (2 weeks for those who require higher fever).

Temperature should be checked daily, but at least on four different occasions during its duration.

Routine procedures will be carried out in all instances, to rule out infections, neoplasm invasion, collagen diseases, milk allergy, thyroiditis, etc.

Clinical evaluation of fever of undetermined origin:

Most cases are not so; they will be ascribed to some of the prevalent diseases in a given area.

Symptoms are those corresponding to the fever syndrome.

If there is evidence of localized symptoms, beware of a fatal outcome.

Skin rashes may also identify a poor prognosis.

Proceed in all instances with a well-planned diagnostic schedule.

Check in the first instance for systemic infections; then, for localized ones.

Check immediately for neoplastic problems, leukemia and lymphoma in the first place.

Check for autoimmune diseases, particularly rehumatoid arthritis, polyarteritis, and the like.

Check for sarcoidosis and other granulomatous conditions.

Check for pulmonary embolism, thyroiditis, or any other condition that may arouse suspicion.

Perform any other procedure suggested by the history, the course of the disease, or any hint that may be obtained.

Sarcoidosis (Boeck's Sarcoid)

Evaluate etiologic conditions for sarcoidosis:

Cause unknown (possibly a virus?).

Preferential occurence in temperature zones, and among blacks (14:1).

Age, between 20 and 40 years.

Evaluate clinical symptomatology and course of sarcoidosis:

It may start with fever, weight loss, and joint pains.

Symptoms depend on the site of involvement.

Pulmonary symptoms occasionally start with cough and dyspnea, but these will be apparent later in the disease.

In spite of the mildness or paucity of pulmonary symptoms, X-ray films may show extensive lesions (fine ground-glass appearance).

End results will be pulmonary fibrosis, cystic changes, or cor pulmonale.

Skin involvement will show nodules, erythema nodosum, plaques, papules, etc., most of them on face, ears, nose, extensor surfaces, and conjunctivas; atrophic scars may follow healing.
Rarely, there will be other organ involvement, such as liver involvement (though hepatic granulomas may be seen in 70% of the cases examined), uveitis (also noted in 15% of those examined), polyarthritis, myocardial lesions, and others.
Diagnosis depends on biopsy.
Management of sarcoidosis:
No treatment is known; try prednisone.

Reye's Syndrome

Elements constituting the syndrome are:
Acute encephalopathy.
Fatty degeneration of viscera.
Unknown etiology; though a number of cases follow acute viral infections.
Characteristic etiological conditions for Reye's syndrome:
More frequent among youngsters under 18 years of age.
More frequent in late fall and winter.
Known cases in association with influenza B virus, varicella, toxins (*Aspergillus*), metabolic defects (urea-cycle enzymes).

Evaluate symptoms and course of Reye's syndrome:
Initial symptomatology is as for a viral infection, mainly of the upper respiratory tract.
There may be an exanthema.
About the sixth day nausea and vomiting appear, and a change in behavior and mental condition (if associated with varicella, mental changes will occur the fourth or fifth day of the rash).
Symptoms may increase to lethargy, disorientation, agitation, and final coma.
During coma other changes may occur, such as progressive deterioration ending in decerebrate and decorticate symptoms.
Evalute diagnostic procedures:
Check carefully an acute encephalopathy not associated with heavy metals or toxins, particularly if there is also evidence of hepatic dysfunction, of the fatty infiltration type.
Also, evalute the history together with the known changes that may occur in the disease, such as increased transaminases, hyperbilirubinemia, and others.
Management of Reye's syndrome:
In fatal cases death occurs relatively early (4 days after hospitalization).
Always try an intensive supportive care, particularly with intravenous fluids and electrolytes.

15. Parasitology

Amebiasis

The characteristics of the causative *Entamoeba histolytica* are:

- Transmission occurs by contaminated water or food.
- The cystic form is the infective organism; it is very resistant.
- In endemic areas with poor sanitation 50% of the population may be carriers.

Evaluate symptoms and course of amebiasis:

- A large number of patients are asymptomatic.
- There is gradual onset of diarrhea with abdominal pain.
- Sudden onset may indicate a complication with *Shigella.*
- Main symptomatology is recurrent bouts of abdominal pain and diarrhea that may alternate with constipation; tenesmus.
- Stools (5 to 10 a day) are semifluid with flecks of mucus tinged with blood; in severe cases stools are more abundant (over 20 a day) and will present copious mucus and blood.
- The clinical course may lead to important weight loss, debility, and prostration.

Evaluate complications of amebiasis:

- Hepatic abscess, most frequently among males, with pain in the liver area, tenderness on palpation, pain referred to the right shoulder, fever, sweats, possible mild jaundice, weight loss; perforation may occur.
- Subacute appendicitis, or perforation of the bowel.
- Infection of the lungs, brain, or skin.

Evaluation of diagnostic procedures:

- Trophozoites identified in fresh stools.
- Cyst identification also.
- Proctoscopic procedures.
- Serologic tests (among carriers, positive in only 10% of cases).

Management of amebiasis:

- Metronidazole.
- Paromomycin, which may be used only for intestinal amebiasis.
- Emetine.
- Also to be considered, diiodohydroxyquine, chloroquine, etc.

Enterobiasis (Oxyuriasis, Pinworm Infestation)

Considerations about the causative organism:

- Present name is *Enterobius vermicularis;* formerly was *Oxyuris vermicularis.*
- Children are principally affected; possible 20% of the general population, and 90% in institutionalized cases.
- Eggs are very resistant; transmission is mostly by ingestion; reinfestation is easily produced.

Evaluation of symptoms and course of pinworm infestation:

- Most cases do not present symptoms.
- Some present perianal itching, particularly nocturnal.
- Some children may present irritability, insomnia, restlessness, and even enuresis.
- Ectopic disease (appendicitis, urethritis, etc.) is rare.
- Outcome is of relatively little importance.
- Identify the parasite for diagnostic purposes (female or ova in perianal area), obtained with adhesive tape.

Management of enterobiasis:

- No treatment may be needed.
- Give pyrvinium pamoate.

Lambliasis (Giardiasis)

Discuss clinical features related to lambliasis:

- It is caused by *Giardia lamblia* (or *Lamblia intestinalis*).
- Transmission is by ingested cysts.
- A large number of patients are asymptomatic.
- Prevalent symptoms may be abdominal pain, mucous diarrhea, and weight loss; also alternating constipation, flatulence, and bulky stools with offensive odor.
- Check for lambliasis in patients with cholecystitis, peptic ulcer, pylorospasm, immunoglobulin defiency, so-called traveler's diarrhea, etc.
- Find the parasite or its cysts in stools.
- Treat with metronidazole or quinacrine; no need of treatment for asymptomatic patients.

Schistosomiasis (Bilharziasis)

Considerations about the infective fluke:

- *Schistosoma mansoni* in South America, the Caribbean, and Africa.
- *S. haematobium* in Africa and the Middle East.

S. japonicum in Asia.

Snails are the intermediate host; they infest water that may come in contact with the skin.

Evaluate clinical features of schistosomiasis:

An itchy erythematous or petechial rash occurs at the site of entry.

Allergic symptoms occur 4 or 5 weeks later, such as urticaria, malaise, and eosinophilia.

Other symptoms may be fever, respiratory involvement, hepatomegaly, and splenomegaly.

After 2 to 8 weeks, the patient becomes asymptomatic again.

Final stage will occur 6 months to several years later.

Symptoms will depend on the number and site of implantation of eggs.

There are diarrhea (dysentery) and abdominal pains.

Hematuria, frequency, and painful dysuria are noted.

There is hepatic fibrosis, with portal hypertension and hepatic insufficiency.

Diagnosis depends in finding the eggs in feces or urine.

Management of bilharziasis:

Give tartar emetic (antimony potassium, or sodium, tartrate), particularly for *S. japonicum* infections.

Niridazole is to be tried first in most infections.

Other drugs to be considered are stibophen, stibocaptate, and perhaps some other brands; consider surgery, also, for some patients.

Fascioliasis (Fasciola Hepatica Infestation)

Evaluation of clinical features of fascioliasis:

Transmission is by ingestion of aquatic vegetables in sheep-raising countries.

Mild infections may be asymptomatic.

Acute fascioliasis will present fever and hepatomegaly; not rarely symptoms of cholecystitis or hepatic colic.

Ova in the feces will give the diagnosis.

Treat with bithionol.

Chlonorchiasis

Evaluation of clinical features of chlonorchiasis:

Transmission of *Chlonorchis sinensis* is by ingestion of infected fish.

It is endemic in Asia; imported cases are seen in the United States.

Hepatalgia, jaundice, and progressive hepatomegaly are found.

There is the possibility of some gastrointestinal symptoms, and even malignant changes.

Eggs are found in stools and in duodenal contents.

Poor therapeutic results have been obtained; try chloroquine phosphate or bithionol.

Fasciolopsiasis and Other Intestinal Flukes

Evaluate clinical features of infections with *Fasciolopsis buski:*

Infection is from contaminated aquatic vegetables.

In the United States it is mostly imported from the Orient.

Incubation lasts several months.

Symptoms occur mostly in severe cases, with gastrointestinal manifestations, crampy pains, diarrhea with intermittent constipation; also, edema of the face, and ascites.

Eggs, and occasionaly flukes, in the stools will give the diagnosis.

Treat with tetrachloroethylene.

Evaluate clinical features regarding infections with *Heterophyes katsuradai* (Japan) or *H. heterophyes* (Egypt):

Transmission from fresh-water fish, via the mouth.

Symptoms of intestinal toxemia; there may be obstruction.

Diagnosis from finding eggs in the stools.

Treatment with tetrachloroethylene.

Evaluate clinical features of infections with *Metagonimus ovatus* or *yokogawai:*

See above entry.

Evaluate clinical features of infections with *Echinostoma ilocanum, E. echinatum,* and perhaps others:

Transmission is by ingestion of material contaminated by snails.

There are symptoms of intestinal toxemia; there may be obstruction.

Check for eggs in the stools.

Treat with aspidium oleoresin or tetrachloroethylene.

Tapeworm Infections

Evaluate clinical features of beef tapeworm or *Taenia saginata:*

Transmission is by ingestion of poorly cooked meats.

There is poor, or no symptomatology.

Active proglottids may be felt crawling through the anus.

Diagnosis depends on finding proglottids (rarely the scolex) in feces.

Treat with niclosamide; otherwise, use aspidium oleoresin, quinacrine hydrochloride, paromomycin.

Evaluate clinical features of pork tapeworm or *Taenia solium:*

Transmission is by ingestion of poorly cooked pork.

Adult worm infection causes mild or no symptomatology.

Larval infection may cause cysticercosis with myalgia, weakness, and possibly central nervous system manifestations (meningoencephalitis, seizures).

Check for proglottids, scolex, or eggs in the stools.

Treat with quinacrine.

Evaluate clinical features of dwarf tapeworm or *Hymenolepsis nana* infection:
- Transmission is by ingestion of eggs.
- There may be abdominal discomfort, with diarrhea and dizziness; it may be symptomless.
- Children may present inanition.
- For diagnosis, find eggs in the stools.
- Treat with quinacrine or niclosamide.

Evaluate clinical features of fish tapeworm or *Diphyllobothrium latum:*
- Transmission is by ingestion of poorly cooked infested fish.
- There is no, or mild, gastrointestinal symptomatology.
- There is anemia, similar to pernicious anemia.
- Check for eggs in the stools.
- Treat with niclosamide.

Ascariasis (Ascaridiosis)

Evaluate characteristics of *Ascaris lumbricoides:*
- It is one of the most common worms, transmitted by ingestion of contamined food or drink.
- It occurs mostly in areas of poor sanitation.

Evaluate clinical features of ascariasis:
- Pulmonary symptoms (infiltrates) occur during pulmonary migration.
- There are gastrointestinal symptoms; obstruction occurs in severe cases.
- Find eggs in the stools; rarely an adult worm will be vomited or passed in the stool.
- Treat with piperazine citrate; also may use pyrantel pamoate or thiabendazole.

Paragonimiasis

Evaluate clinical features of paragonimiasis:
- It is caused by *Paragonimus weastermani.*
- It is found in Asia, Africa, and South America.
- From snails the parasite passes into crabs and crayfish, which transmit the disease.
- There are no symptoms until eggs are being produced.
- There is fever, with cough; there may be hemoptysis.
- Pleuritic pain is felt.
- There is a slow progression of symptoms.
- Severe cases will present dyspnea, bronchitis and bronchiectasia, weakness, weight loss; and possibly gastrointestinal symptoms.
- If there is central nervous system involvement, there will be seizures, paralysis, etc.
- Find eggs in the stools.
- Treat with bithionol and chloroquine.

Ancylostoma and Necator Infestations

Evaluate characteristics of each hookworm:
- *Necator americanus* is the genus in America.
- *Ancylostoma duodenale* is the one in the Old World.
- Some 100 parasites are needed to cause symptomatology.
- Larvae remain in infected soil until coming into contact with the skin.

Evaluate clinical features of hookworm infestation:
- About 25% of the human population is infected.
- A maculopapular itchy rash (ground itch) develops at the site of infection.
- Pulmonary symptoms may appear during pulmonary migration.
- There are epigastralgia, iron-deficiency anemia, cardiac failure, and anasarca.
- There is growth retardation of affected children.
- Find eggs in the stools.
- Treat with pyrantel pamoate; also, tetrachloroethylene, bephenium hydroxynaphthoate, or thiabendazole.

Strongyloidiasis

Evaluate clinical features of this threadworm infection:
- It is caused by *Strongyloides stercoralis.*
- Larvae in the soil enter the skin.
- Autoinfection may also occur.
- The point of entry into the skin may present some rash and itch.
- Larger skin lesions may also occur.
- Pulmonary lesions occur when the worm passes the lungs.
- Gastrointestinal symptoms occur in severe infestations.
- Cases may be fatal.
- Larvae are found in the stools.
- Treat with thiabendazole.

Trichiniasis (Trichinosis)

Evaluate characteristics of *Trichinella spiralis:*
- Organisms are transmitted by ingestion of poorly cooked pork (bear, walrus).
- Only those reaching skeletal muscle will survive.
- These will encyst and remain alive for several years.
- Organism is more prevalent in temperate zones than in tropics (only 4% in United States in 1970).

Evaluate clinical symptoms and course of trichinosis:
- Initial gastrointestinal symptoms and fever will follow the ingestion of infected meat (1 or 2 days).
- One or two weeks later systemic symptoms will occur.
- Edema of the upper eyelids is almost a characteristic early symptom.
- It may be followed by photophobia, pain, and hemorrhages in the conjuctiva or retina.
- Fever, with chills, intense sweating, thirst, weakness, and prostration usually come after eye symptoms.
- Muscle soreness or actual myalgia is an important symptom.
- There are also subungual hemorrhage, dyspnea, dysphagia, difficult speech and mastication.

Other symptoms may occur, such as lymphadenitis, encephalitis or meningitis, nervous disorders, lung involvement, myocardial failure, and perhaps others.

Death may occur; recovery will begin about 1 month after the start of the disease.

Evaluate diagnostic procedures:

Initial eosinophilia.

Skin tests after the first week (delayed skin test) or after the third (immediate skin reaction).

Management of the disease:

Care is mainly supportive.

Use corticoids.

Thiabendazole may give results.

Malaria (Paludism)

Evaluate characteristics of malarial parasites:

Plasmodium vivax provokes paroxysms every 48 hours.

Plasmodium falciparum provokes paroxysms every 36 to 72 hours, but with some irregularity.

Plasmodium malariae provokes paroxysms every 72 hours.

Plasmodium ovale is rare (may substitute for *P. vivax* in some areas).

Parasite is transmitted by the bite of an anopheles mosquito.

It is also transmitted by transfusions or use of a common needle (addicts).

Evaluate clinical features of malaria:

Typical paroxysms occur in three stages.

First stage is the chill, usually severe, which lasts 15 to about 60 minutes; headache, nausea, and vomiting may occur.

The second, or hot, stage is characterized by spiking fever, even above 40°C (104°F).

Finally, there is the sweating stage with profuse sudoration and abatement of fever; usually it is followed by sleep.

At the beginning, paroxysms may not be regularly cycled.

The established disease will present regular periodicity; there will also be splenomegaly.

Evaluate the clinical course of each kind of malaria:

For all kinds there may be an incubation period of 10 to 35 days.

The opening symptomatology may be an influenzalike syndrome of 2 or 3 days' duration.

In vivax malaria paroxysms occur every 48 hours; fever lasts 8 hours.

In falciparum malaria temperature rises and falls at a slower pace, and fever lasts about 1 day (20 to 36 hours), paroxysms are not too regular (36 to 72 hours), and most patients never feel well.

In malariae malaria paroxysms occur every 72 hours.

The course of ovale malaria is similar to that of vivax malaria.

Falciparum malaria is the most serious disease; it may cause central nervous symptoms (cerebral malaria) and hemolysis with hemoglobinuria (blackwater fever).

Chronic malia may cause malaise, periodic headaches, mild fever, etc.; but also relatively typic attacks.

The diagnosis depends in all instances on the detection of the causative parasite in blood; it is better to take more than one smear.

Management of malaria:

Plasmodium vivax	Chloroquine, together with or followed by primaquine phosphate.
Falciparum malaria	Chloroquine; but for resistant parasites use quinine, pyrimethamine, and a sulfa, all at the same time.
Plasmodium malariae	As for *Plasmodium vivax.*
Plasmodium ovale	As for *Plasmodium vivax.*

Kala-Azar

Evaluate clinical features of this visceral leishmaniasis, caused by *Leishmania donovani:*

Children in Asia, Africa, or South America are mainly affected.

The main clues for diagnosis are fever, emaciation, and splenomegaly.

Fever is insidious, irregular, and chronic; there are two spikes a day.

Splenomegaly (usually together with hepatomegaly) may reach enormous proportions; doughy at the start, it becomes hard thereafter.

Emaciation is progressive, with darkening of the skin.

Death will occur in 90% of the untreated cases, but in only 10% of the treated cases.

Diagnosis is made by needle biopsy.

Treatment is with pentavalent antimonials; also aromatic diamidines may be used; in cases found in Sudan (resistant to antimony) use pentamidine.

American Leishmaniasis

Evaluate clinical features of this leishmaniasis, caused by *Leishmania mexicana* or *L. braziliensis:*

Lesions occur on exposed skin, mainly nose and mouth.

Ulcers will cause disfiguring erosions, including bone.

Lymph nodes are involved.

A positive Montenegro test is diagnostic; but test is meaningless if negative.

Diagnosis is with biopsy or material from the ulcer edge.

Treat with sodium antimony gluconate; in early stages by infiltration of the edge of the ulcer.

Oriental Sore

Evaluate clinical features of this leishmaniasis caused by *Leishmania tropica:*

- Found in the Old World (Asia and Africa).
- Transmitted by the bite of sandflies.
- Local swelling, ulceration, and discharge of pus; different local varieties of the parasite will cause wet (pus) or dry lesions.
- Spontaneous healing in months or years.
- Secondary infections frequent (mostly wet lesions).
- Parasites found in scraps from cleaned edges of the ulcer.
- Treat by infiltration of the edge of the ulcer with antimony sodium gluconate; may also give physical therapy; treat secondary infections.

Trypanosomiasis (African Sleeping Sickness)

Evaluate clinical features of the rapid *Rhodesian trypanosomiasis:*

- All forms of African trypanosomiasis are transmitted by the bite of a tse-tse fly (*Glossina palpalis, G. morsitans,* and others).
- It is caused by *Trypanosoma brucei* var. *rhodesiense.*
- There is irregular fever, with tachycardia.
- There are headache, and anorexia leading to malnutrition.
- There are personality changes, tremors, disturbances of speech and gait, delayed pain sensation with deep hyperesthesia.
- Transient skin rashes, circinate and edematous, are noted.
- Not rarely there is evidence of myocarditis, which may be lethal.
- Final apathy, convulsions, coma, and death may result.
- Find the parasite in lymph node aspirates.
- Treat early infections with suramin sodium; late, with melarsoprol.

Evaluate clinical features of the slower *Gambian trypanosomiasis:*

- It is caused by *Trypanosoma brucei* var. *gambiense.*
- There are irregular fever, tachycardia, headache, and anorexia.
- Personality changes, tremors, disturbance of speech and gait, and delayed pain sensation are found.
- Frequent and marked splenomegaly and large, rubbery, painless lymph glands in the back of the neck are noted.
- Final coma and death may occur.
- Find the parasite in lymph nodes aspirates.
- Treat with pentamidine; may also use melarsoprol or suramin.

Chagas' Disease (American Trypanosomiasis)

Evaluate clinical features of the disease caused by *Trypanosoma cruzi:*

- It is transmitted by the reduviid bugs (kissing bugs, "assassin," and other Triatomas).
- The chagoma may be the initial symptoms, as a hard, edematous, red, and painful cutaneous nodule.
- The Romaña's sign may also initiate the disease, as a unilateral conjuctivitis, with edema of the face and eyelid.
- Later, there will be intermittent fever, hepatomegaly, regional adenopathies at the site of the symptoms, tachycardia, etc.
- Involvement of the central nervous system or of the heart may also occur, mostly as a later manifestation.
- Efforts will be made to isolate the parasite; the Machado test will help.
- Try Bayer 2502.

Balantidiasis

Evaluate clinical features of balantidiasis:

- It is caused by *Balantidium coli.*
- Transmission occurs by ingestion of contaminated material.
- A large number of patients will remain asymptomatic.
- Diarrhea alternating with constipation is the most frequent symptom.
- There may be intermittent attacks or dysentery with colics, mucus, and blood.
- The *Balantidium* will be found in stools.
- Treat with a tetracycline, or with diiodohydroxyquin.

Toxoplasmosis

Evaluate characteristics of the causative *Toxoplasma gondii:*

- Transmission is by ingestion; most of the infected material comes from cats.
- Infection is widespread, some populations having only 7% infected, but others up to 94%.

Evaluate clinical symptoms and course of toxoplasmosis:

- Congenital toxoplasmosis may cause abortion (early infection) or the birth of a symptomatic child (mild or extremely severe).
- There may be chorioretinitis, thrombocytopenic purpura, intracerebral calcifications, convulsions, and psychomotor disturbances that may lead to blindness and mental retardation.
- An acquired lymphatic form may be the mildest manifestation of the disease, with enlarged nodes (cervical and axillary), myalgia, irregular febricula, anemia, hypotension, some liver impairment, etc.
- Chronic toxoplasmosis will present uveitis (posterior) usually of a severe type, weakness, diarrhea, weight loss, and headache.
- A fulminating infection is usually disseminated, with elevated fever, chills, a skin rash, and severe prostration, and occurs in patients with immunologic defects or patients using immunosuppressive drugs.

Evaluate diagnostic procedures:
- Isolation of the parasite.
- Biopsy or serology (the Sabin-Feldman test, or the indirect fluorescent antibody test).

Management of toxoplasmosis:
- Try sulfa drugs, particularly for the subacute and acute stages.
- Supplement sulfas with pyrimethamine.
- Corticoids may also help.

Echinococcosis (Hydatid Disease, Hydatid Cyst)

Characteristics of the causative tapeworm:
- The causative organism is *Echinococcus granulosus;* in multilocular or alveolar cysts the causative organism usually is *E. multilocularis* (Russia and eastern Europe).
- The definite host is the dog, and similar canines.
- Transmission starts in the fur of infected dogs.

Clinical features of the disease:
- It is usually asymptomatic, until noticeable because of its size.
- A suggestive triad is composed of biliary colic with jaundice and urticaria.
- Ruptured cysts also become symptomatic; the leaking of fluid and hydatid sand (scolices) will cause urticaria with pruritus, asthma, or other evidence of allergy.
- Sudden rupture may cause anaphylactic crisis, possibly very serious.
- Pulmonary cysts will cause obstruction when large enough; or may rupture into bronchi.
- Cysts in the brain will cause earlier symptoms, because of pressure seizures, or other evidence of intracranial pressure.
- Cysts in the liver are far more frequent (70%); there is hepatomegaly, with dull ache of the liver area, and abdominal distention.

Diagnostic procedures to be considered are:
- Casoni intracutaneous test, positive in 86% of the cases, even after resection of the cyst.
- Serologic tests, positive in 90% of the cases.
- X-ray films; scintillation scans; angiography.
- Examination of hydatid sand.
- Confirmation after surgical removal.

Management of hydatid disease:
- Surgical removal, whenever feasible.

Filariasis

Characteristics of the causal nematodes or roundworms:
- The important ones are *Wuchereria bancrofti* and *Brugia malayi.*
- *Aëdes, Culex,* and *Anopheles* mosquitoes transmit *Wuchereria.*
- *Anopheles* and *Masonia* mosquitoes transmit *Brugia.*
- *W. bancrofti* affects only humans; *B. malayi* is also found in animal hosts.
- The incubation period may last 2 months.

Clinical findings in filariasis:
- Earlier symptoms that are inflammatory in nature.
- Fever, with or without lymphangitis, chills, headache, malaise.
- Lymphadenopathy most frequent in *B. malayi* infections.
- Not rarely, funiculitis and orchitis; epididymitis.
- Later manifestations that are obstructive in nature.
- Chyluria, hydrocele, scrotal lymphedema, soft edematous swelling of the skin that precedes frank elephantiasis of parts, notably legs or scrotum.

Diagnostic procedures in filariasis:
- Check for microfilariae in smears prepared with wet films of anticoagulated blood.
- Eosinophilia, as in most similar diseases.

Management of filariasis:
- Diethylcarbamazine; antihistamines and corticoids for reactions.
- Surgical procedures, particularly for scrotal elephantiasis.

Onchocerciasis (River Blindness)

Clinical features of onchocerciasis are:
- It is caused by a nematode or roundworm, *Onchocerca volvulus.*
- It is transmitted by Simulium black flies.
- Incubation will last for months up to 1 year.
- About 40% of the patients will start with skin manifestations.
- Itching may cause skin excoriations.
- Lichenification, pigmentation, thickening, erythematous or papulovesicular lesions may occur.
- Later on, a few nodules (about three to six) will appear over bony prominences on trunk, head, shoulders, arms, etc.
- There is superficial punctate keratitis; later more serious iritis, cyclitis, pannus may also occur.
- Check for the microfilariae in skin or nodules.
- Use diethylcarbamazine; surgery for nodules.

Toxocariasis (Visceral Larva Migrans)

Clinical features of toxocariasis are:
- The causative factors are *Toxocara canis* and *T. cati,* which are normal parasites of dogs and cats.
- Transmission is by ingestion of contaminated soil.
- Very young children are usually affected.
- There are fever, cough, hepatomegaly; there may be wheezing.
- Nervous symptoms may also be a common occurrence.
- Skin rash, recurrent pneumonia, splenomegaly, and granulomas of the retina (which may be taken for retinoblastoma) may occur.

Check for the larva in granulomatous lesions.
Try thiabendazole; give symptomatologic treatment.

Cutaneous Larva Migrans (Creeping Eruption)

Clinical features of the cutaneous larva migrans:

- The causative organisms are the dog and cat hookworms *Ancylostoma braziliense* and *A. caninum.*
- It is transmitted by contaminated moist sandy soil.
- Lesions are mostly noted on feet, legs, buttocks, or back.
- Very small itchy papules develop at the site of entry.
- After 2 or 3 days, the characteristic serpiginous tract will start, with intense itching; scratch lesions are the consequence.
- The parasite may remain alive for a few months.
- It will advance continuously, but the total trail will be only a few inches; if not killed, it will succumb by itself.
- Topical application of thiabendazole (use the oral preparation) will afford relief and cure in a matter of hours.

Myasis

Evaluate clinical features of infestation with larvae of several species of flies, such as screw-worms, flesh-flies, etc.:

- Invasion of tissues of the nose, mouth, eyes, ears, by the larvae will provoke progressive inflammation.
- Great irritation of the affected cavity will follow.
- Gastrointestinal infestation will provoke vomiting and melena; larvae may be found in feces.
- Larvae may be seen in affected superficial sites.
- Ocular myasis will provoke extreme irritation and itching; the conjunctivae appear red and excoriated; in extreme cases necrosis with destruction of orbital contents may occur, even to reach the meninges.
- Diagnosis is made by finding the larvae.
- Remove the larva carefully after thorough cleansing of the area.
- Deep invasion may present a disastrous outcome.

Dermatophyte Infections of Head and Body

Evaluate causative agents:

Trichophyton (*tonsurans, violaceum*)	Tinea capitis (ringworm of the scalp), tinea unguium (of the nails), tinea corporis (of the body.
Trichophyton (*mentagrophytes, rubrum*)	Tinea pedis (athlete's foot),
Microsporum (*aoudouini, canis, gypseum*)	Tinea capitis.
Epidermophyton (*floccosum*)	Tinea pedis.

Clinical features of *tinea capitis* or ringworm of the scalp:

- Children are affected.
- There is spontaneous disappearance of the disease at puberty; some *Trichophyton* infections may persist thereafter.
- There are bald patches on the scalp, round, gray, scaly, and frequently itchy.
- There are broken hairs, rather than true baldness.
- Diagnosis is by fluorescence under Wood's light.
- Watch for the development of a nodular, exudative pustule that may cause scarring (Celsius' kerion).
- Treat with griseofluvin.

Clinical features of *tinea corporis* or body ringworm:

- Practically all dermatophytes can cause the disease.
- Lesions appear on exposed areas; there is a history of exposure to an infected cat.
- There is severe itch of lesions consisting of rings of vesicles with central clearing.
- Lesions are grouped in clusters; they are asymmetrical.
- Check for hyphae from the cap of a vesicle.
- Treat with griseofulvin; may use local treatment (salicylic acid, undecylenic acid, or other medications).

Clinical features of *tinea cruris* or jock itch:

- Most dermatophytes can cause the disease.
- It occurs in intertriginous areas, causing intense itch.
- Lesions appear as erythematous macules with sharp edges and clear center; vesicles may be noted on the borders.
- Preferred location is at the groins; it may cause pruritis ani.
- There is easy demonstration of hyphae from the lesions.
- Treat severe cases with griseofulvin; others, with local care and use of fungicidal preparations (iodine, carbolfuchsin, undecylenic acid, etc.).

Clinical features of *tinea pedis* or athlete's foot:

- Possibly all people carry the dermatophytes.
- Itching or other sensations may occur.
- Lesions appear as macerated and fissured toe webs.
- Infections with *T. mentagrophytes* start on the third and fourth interdigital spaces; may spread to the plantar surface of the arch.
- Infections with *T. rubrum* cause thickening and scaling of the soles.
- Similar lesions may also occur on the hands.
- Nails may also be affected in these cases, *tinea unguium,* then becoming thickened, destroyed, with debris accumulating under the free edge.
- Hyphae are easily demonstrated.
- Treatment in acute stage is with aluminum subacetate solution or permanganate if there is secondary infection; in the subacute stage, coal tar or miconazole; in the chronic stage, undecylenic acid compounds, or any other of the many available preparations.

Erythrasma

Evaluate clinical features of erythrasma:

It is caused by *Corynebacterium minutissimum.*

It may occur in the tropics, and affects adults preferentially.

Some maceration, with scales and fissures, will occur in third and fourth interdigital spaces between toes.

Irregular patches, first pink, later becoming brown, with fine scaling, will occur in the genitocrural area, where thighs and scrotum contact.

Patches will also appear on axillae, trunk, and perineum.

Obese middle-aged women or diabetic patients may present erythrasma.

Diagnosis becomes evident when it shows its characteristic coral-red fluorescence under Wood's light.

Treat with tetracycline or erythromycin.

Tinea Versicolor

Evaluate clinical features of tinea versicolor:

It is caused by *Pityrosporon orbiculares,* formerly called *Malassezia furfur.*

It is most frequent in young adults, particularly those who perspire greatly or who use heavy clothing.

Lesions will appear preferentially on the trunk, but also on upper arms, neck, abdomen, and at times the face.

Lesions are velvety, chamois-colored, tan or brown, coalescent macules.

Macules produce scales; but these are better noted after scraping the skin with a fingernail.

Areas presenting the lesions will not tan under the sun (may be mistaken for vitiligo).

Itching is rare and only slight, particularly after heavy sweating.

Diagnosis will be made by finding hyphae in scrapings; or by golden fluorescence under Wood's light.

Treat with sulfur and salicylic acid, 2% each, in a shampoo; or may use selenium sulfide, or other local measures; relapses may occur.

Loiasis (Calabar Swelling)

Evaluate features of Calabar swelling:

It is caused by a nematode, loa-loa, of the filarial type.

It is transmitted by a biting fly, possibly *Chrysops dimidiata.*

It takes about 12 months for the larva to get the adult size.

First symptoms are the Calabar swelling, several inches wide, of an edematous and painful reaction, erythematous and pruritic; or the migration of the parasite beneath the conjunctiva, with considerable irritation and sensation of a foreign body.

The Calabar swelling lasts only a few days; it may migrate a few inches before disappearance.

Calabar swellings may occur at different intervals.

Allergic symptoms may occur; generalized urticaria, edema, generalized itching, etc.

Other, more serious symptoms may occur, like meningoencephalitis.

Recover the parasite from sites of swelling, or from the blood.

Treat with diethylcarbamazine.

Dracunculiasis (Dracontiasis, Dracunculosis)

Evaluate clinical features of the "fiery serpent" or Guinea worm infection:

It is caused by another nematode, *Dracunculus medinensis.*

Transmission occurs by ingestion of infected crustacea (genre *Cyclops,* diminutive ones having only one eye).

Initial symptoms are local erythema, tenderness; also generalized pruritus, urticaria, nausea with or without vomiting, and dyspnea.

Several hours later a blister develops, then ruptures, and the former symptoms abate.

The ulcer (there may be one or several) stays indurated, tender, and red; about 90% of the cases present the lesions on legs, and work or walking is much impaired.

The head of the nematode is seen in the ulcer.

If the head is not seen, larvae can be detected by expression from the moistened ulcer.

Remove the worm slowly (perhaps taking a few days); use metronidazole, niridazole, or thiabendazole.

Pneumocystis Carinii Infection

For more information, please refer to the section on pneumonia in the chapter devoted to respiratory diseases. Some additional facts are given here.

The disease may last from 1 to 4 weeks, and will end fatally in half of the untreated patients.

Symptoms are those of pneumonia, but usually with mild intensity.

The causative *Pneumocystis carinii* probably is a protozoan.

Not only patients with leukemia or on immunosuppressive therapy may present the disease, but also premature infants, debilitated patients, those with altered immunologic responses, and those receiving relatively elevated doses of adrenocortical drugs.

For identification of the causative organsim several procedures are recommended, such as aspirates, biopsy, pulmonary lavage, etc.

Treat not only with trimethoprim plus sulfamethoxazole, but also may use pentamidine isethionate, or multiple therapy with sulfadiazine, pyrimethamine, and folinic acid.

Isosporosis (Coccidiosis)

Evaluate clinical features related to isosporosis:

- It is caused by a coccidia, either *Isosporo belli,* or *I. hominis.*
- Transmission is by ingestion.
- Symptoms are few, if any.
- There may be febricula, mild malaise, vague gastrointestinal symptoms, and diarrhea.
- Symptoms usually subside spontaneously in 2 weeks.
- More severe cases, even with death, may occur.
- Cysts can be found in stools.
- Just give a bland diet, and advise rest for a few days.

Scabies (The Itch)

Characteristics of the causative acarid:

- It is *Sarcoptes scabiei.*
- It is a common cause of disease because of its very easy and rapid transmission.
- It is spread by direct skin contact; usually not spread by using the same clothing or because of sleeping on the same bed.

Evaluate clinical features of scabies:

- There is marked itching, practically intolerable at night.
- Most lesions are found in the webs or sides of the fingers, the heels of the hands, the flexor side of wrists, elbows, axillae, areola of the female breast, the male genitals, buttocks; but very rarely on the face, except for infants.
- Lesions are pruritic vesicles and pustules at the end of "runs" or "galleries," these burrows appearing as fine wavy dark lines a few millimeters long.
- Burrows may be obscured and become difficult to find because scratching will darken them; also secondary infection may occur.
- Check for parasites by probing the fresh end of a burrow with a scalpel; the mite will cling to the tip of its blade; confirm by microscopic examination of specimens mounted on glycerin or mineral oil.

Management of scabies:

- Treat the whole household and contacts at the same time; otherwise, treatment will be wasted.
- Start with gamma benzene hexachloride, 1% cream, from neck down; repeat in 1 week.
- Possibly resistant forms will appear; then use crotamiton, 10% cream, the same way as the former.
- Application may be repeated the next morning, instead of the next week.
- Treat secondary infections.
- Carefully cleanse house and clothes.

Pediculosis

Evaluate the infective lice:

Pediculus humanus, var. *capitis*	Pediculosis of the head, or pediculosis capitis.
Pediculus humanus, var. *corporis*	Pediculosis of the body or pediculosis corporis.
Phthirus pubis, pubic louse or crab	Pediculosis of the pubis.

- Transmission occurs directly by contact in all instances; or indirectly with combs or hats, in case of pediculosis capitis; clothing, in case of pediculosis corporis; or also venereal contact, in pediculosis pubis.

Evaluate features of *pediculosis capitis:*

- It occurs not only on the scalp, but also other hairy portions on the face.
- There is severe itching.
- Discrete adenopathy may occur.
- Secondary infections may occur.
- Diagnosis is made by direct inspection; the nits adhere to the hair.
- Treat with 1% cream of gamma benzene hexachloride.

Evaluate features of *pediculosis corporis:*

- Nits are found on body hairs.
- Parasites and ova are seen in seams of the underclothing.
- Bites are noted as red points, usually associated with scratch markings, on shoulders, abdomen, and buttocks.
- Treat as above.

Evaluate features of *pediculosis pubis:*

- Parasites usually set on the anogenital area; but other hairs may also be infected (body, eyelashes, etc.).
- Ova are attached at the base of the hairs.
- Parasites are not easily detected; they may appear as small crusts of scratches.
- There may be sky-blue macules on inner thighs or lower abdomen, or dark brown specks on undergarments.
- Diagnosis is made by careful inspection for parasites or ova.
- Treatment is also as for pediculosis capitis, above.